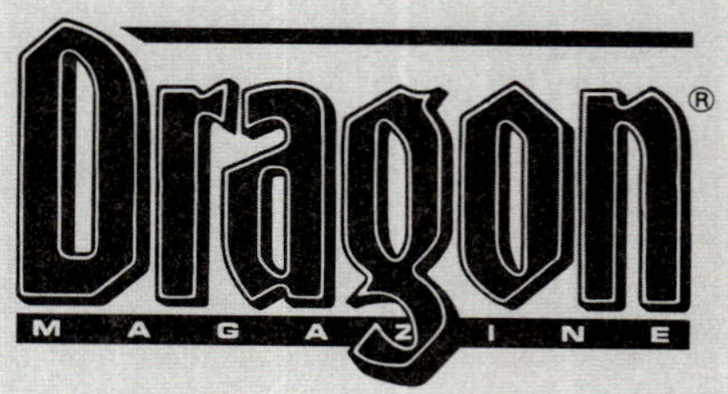

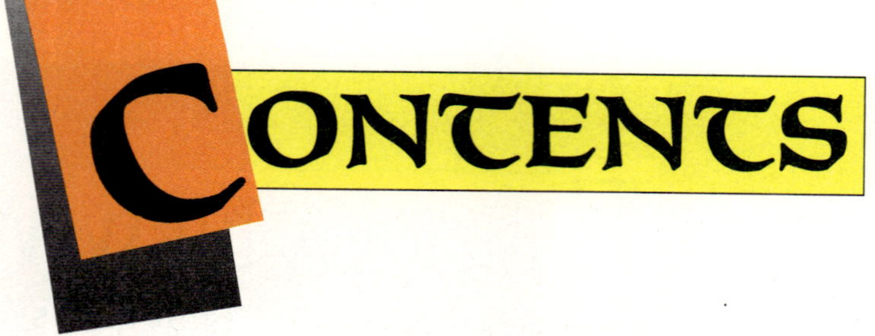

CONTENTS

Issue #194
Vol. XVIII, No. 1
June 1993

Publisher
James M. Ward

Editor
Roger E. Moore

Associate editor
Dale A. Donovan

Fiction editor
Barbara G. Young

Editorial assistant
Wolfgang H. Baur

Art director
Larry W. Smith

Production staff
Gaye O'Keefe   Tim Coumbe

Subscriptions
Janet L. Winters

U.S. advertising
Cindy Rick

*U.K. correspondent
and U.K. advertising*
Wendy Mottaz

SPECIAL ATTRACTIONS

FEATURES

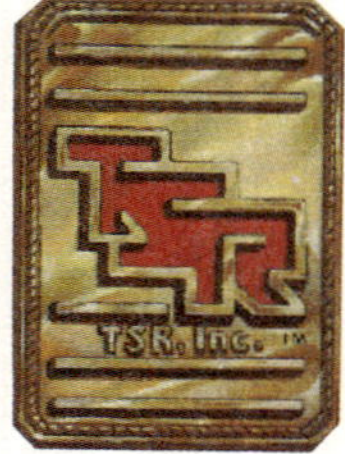

DRAGON® Magazine (ISSN 0279-6848) is published monthly by TSR, Inc., P.O. Box 756 (201 Sheridan Springs Road), Lake Geneva WI 53147, United States of America. The postal address for all materials from the United States of America and Canada except subscription orders is: DRAGON Magazine, P.O. Box 111, (201 Sheridan Springs Road), Lake Geneva WI 53147, U.S.A.; telephone: (414) 248-3625; fax (414) 248-0389. The postal address for all materials from Europe is: DRAGON Magazine, TSR Ltd., 120 Church End, Cherry Hinton, Cambridge CB1 3LB, United Kingdom; telephone: (0223) 212517 (U.K.), 44-223-212517 (international); telex: 818761; fax (0223) 248066 (U.K.), 44-223-248066 (international).

Distribution: DRAGON Magazine is available from game and hobby shops throughout the United States, Canada, the United Kingdom, and through a limited number of other overseas outlets. Distribution to the book trade in the United States is by Random House, Inc., and in Canada by Random House of Canada, Ltd. Distribution to the book trade in the United Kingdom is by TSR Ltd. Send orders to: Random House, Inc., Order Entry Department, Westminster MD 21157, U.S.A.; telephone: (800) 733-3000. Newsstand distrib-ution throughout the United Kingdom is by Comag Magazine Marketing, Tavistock Road, West Drayton, Middlesex UB7 7QE, United Kingdom; telephone: 0895-444055.

Subscriptions: Subscription rates via second-class mail are as follows: $30 in U.S. funds for 12 issues sent to an address in the U.S.; $36 in U.S. funds for 12 issues sent to an address in Canada; £21 for 12 issues sent to an address within the United Kingdom; £30 for 12 issues sent to an address in Europe; $50 in U.S. funds for 12 issues sent by surface mail to any other address, or $90 in U.S. funds for 12 issues sent air mail to any other address. Payment in full must accompany all subcription orders. Methods of payment include checks or money orders made payable to TSR, Inc., or charges to valid MasterCard or VISA credit cards; send subscription orders with payments to: TSR, Inc., P.O. Box 5695, Boston MA 02206, U.S.A. In the United Kingdom, methods of payment include cheques or money orders made payable to TSR Ltd., or charges to a valid ACCESS or VISA credit card; send subscription orders with payments to TSR Ltd., as per that address above. Prices are subject to change without prior notice. The issue of expiration of

Printed in the U.S.A.

REVIEWS

DEPARTMENTS

COVER

Nothing is so terrible that a huge red dragon can't make it just a hell of a lot worse. Eric Gooch catches a crimson wyrm reveling in dark triumph in this month's striking cover painting.

each subscription is printed on the mailing label of each subscriber's copy of the magazine. Changes of address for the delivery of subscription copies must be received at least six weeks prior to the effective date of the change in order to assure uninterrupted delivery.

Back issues: A limited quantity of back issues is available from either the TSR Mail Order Hobby Shop (P.O. Box 756, Lake Geneva WI 53147, U.S.A.) or from TSR Ltd. For a free copy of the current catalog that lists available back issues, write to either of the above addresses.

Submissions: All material published in DRAGON Magazine becomes the exclusive property of the publisher, unless special arrangements to the contrary are made prior to publication. DRAGON Magazine welcomes unsolicited submissions of written material and artwork; however, no responsibility for such submissions can be assumed by the publisher in any event. Any submission accompanied by a self-addressed, stamped envelope of sufficient size will be returned if it cannot be published. We strongly recommend that prospective authors write for our writers' guidelines before sending an article to us. In the United States and Canada, send a self-addressed, stamped envelope (9½" long preferred) to: Writers' Guidelines, c/o DRAGON Magazine, as per the above address; include sufficient American postage or International Reply Coupons with the return envelope. In Europe, write to: Writers' Guidelines, c/o DRAGON Magazine, TSR Ltd.; include sufficient return postage or IRCs with your SASE.

Advertising: For information on placing advertisements in DRAGON Magazine, ask for our rate card. All ads are subject to approval by TSR, Inc. TSR reserves the right to reject any ad for any reason. In the United States and Canada, contact: Advertising Coordinator, TSR, Inc., P.O. Box 756, 201 Sheridan Springs Road, Lake Geneva WI 53147, U.S.A. In Europe, contact: Advertising Coordinators, TSR Ltd.

Advertisers and/or agencies of advertisers agree to hold TSR, Inc. harmless from and against any loss or expense from any alleged wrongdoing that may arise out of the publication of such advertisements. TSR, Inc. has the right to reject or cancel any advertising contract for which the advertiser and/or agency of advertiser fails to comply with the business ethics set forth in such contract.

DRAGON is a registered trademark of TSR, Inc. Registration applied for in the United Kingdom. All rights to the contents of this publication are reserved, and nothing may be reproduced from it in whole or in part without first obtaining permission in writing from the publisher. Material published in DRAGON Magazine does not necessarily reflect the opinions of TSR, Inc. Therefore, TSR will not be held accountable for opinions or mis-information contained in such material.

® designates registered trademarks owned by TSR, Inc. ™ designates trademarks owned by TSR, Inc. Most other product names are trademarks owned by the companies publishing those products. Use of the name of any product without mention of trademark status should not be construed as a challenge to such status.

© 1993 TSR, Inc. All Rights Reserved. All TSR characters, character names, and distinctive likenesses thereof are trademarks owned by TSR, Inc.

Second-class postage paid at Lake Geneva, Wis. U.S.A., and additional mailing offices. Postmaster: Send address changes to DRAGON Magazine, TSR, Inc., P.O. Box 111, Lake Geneva WI 53147, U.S.A. USPS 318-790, ISSN 1062-2101.

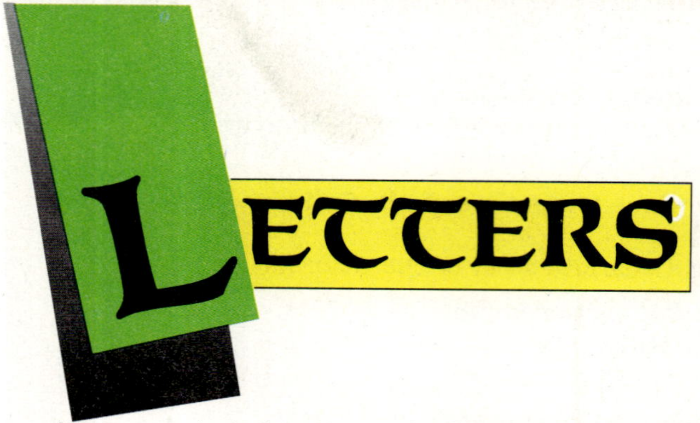

What did you think of this issue? Do you have a question about an article or have an idea for a new feature you'd like to see? In the United States and Canada, write to: Letters, DRAGON® Magazine, P.O. Box 111, Lake Geneva WI 53147, U.S.A. In Europe, write to: Letters, DRAGON Magazine, TSR Ltd., 120 Church End, Cherry Hinton, Cambridge CB1 3LB, United Kingdom.

African fan

Dear Dragon,
Finally, an African-like continent has been added to the AD&D® gaming world. I completely agree with David Howery when he says that it has been ignored. But I was wondering: Are there any books, games, or anything remotely relating to Africa or African heroes? Please print my address.

Bruce Jackson
17004 Belton, Apt. 249
Detroit MI 48228

We had a similar letter from a reader in issue #176, and our response listed a number of African-inspired game materials. (We may have articles in the future on this topic, too.) A number of books are now in print that describe African heroes, history, or myths and legends in detail; check any local bookstore or library. If no books are on the shelves about African tales, check a copy of Books in Print *(the subject index part) for titles, then order them. If anyone has other specific ideas on African materials, please write to Bruce Jackson and let him know.*

Uriah Heep & TSR

Dear Dragon,
Is it true that when the D&D® game was being developed in the early '70s, the name was taken from a Uriah Heep album that was popular at the time?
My friends and I have a bet going on this. Inquiring minds want to know.

Warren Mitchell
Woodinville WA

Uh . . . um . . . well, you've managed to catch the editors off guard with this one. We don't know anything about this, though we doubt Uriah Heep had anything to do with the naming of the D&D game. Your bet isn't going to be resolved anytime soon! (Which Uriah Heep album are you thinking of, by the way?)

Multiclassed gamers

Dear Roger E. Moore,
I'm actually from Istanbul, but three years ago I moved to Vienna in order to study elec-

tronics in the University of Vienna. I ended up studying aikido five times a week and running eight AD&D 2nd Edition campaigns on weekends (actually, six of them were in Istanbul during winter and summer breaks) in the FORGOTTEN REALMS®, DRAGONLANCE®, DARK SUN™, and SPELLJAMMER® campaigns.
My questions to you are: Are there more of our kind of multiclassed hobby gamer/aikidoists? If so, where are they? (I saw that you are practicing aikido in the forward to the *DRAGONLANCE Tales II Trilogy.*) And how do I get my AD&D game short stories (in English, of course) published?
Thank you for your attention.

Hasan Colakoglu
Vienna, AUSTRIA

You've been busy! Though I've regretfully had to leave off aikido practice to get my writing done, there are actually quite a number of multiclassed aikidoist/gamers running around. In my dojo in Milwaukee, there were one or two others who played role-playing games. Barbara Young, our fiction editor and also the editor of DUNGEON® Adventures, *is currently TSR's aikido expert, and she's met a number of gamers who also enjoy martial arts. Dale Donovan practiced aikido for a time, and Wolfgang Baur practiced tae kwon do. Several other TSR editors, designers, writers, and others are into different marital arts; Bruce Nesmith (a designer) and Gerald Brom (an artist) know tae kwon do, for example, and Bruce Nesmith and DARK SUN novel author Troy Denning enjoy kyuki-do. Now that I think of it, the only martial art I haven't heard of a gamer trying was sumo. (NOTE: Anyone who writes to us claiming to be a sumotori/gamer had better include a photo to prove it. Maybe we should have a contest . . . nah.)*
You can get our guidelines (which now include information on articles, fiction, artwork, and cartoon submissions, all in one) by sending a stamped, self-addressed envelope (long-type, please) to: Writers' Guidelines, DRAGON Magazine, P.O. Box 111, Lake Geneva WI 53147, U.S.A.

Tarding crads!

Dear Dragon,
I have several TSR trading cards with incongruent data on the backs. What is the rarity and value of such cards?

Steven T. Voigt
Pittsburg PA

That's hard to say, as you didn't mention which cards they were. I asked TSR's current "trading card tsar" (Thomas Reid) about this, since he pointed out a few flawed cards in his "Game Wizards" column in our last issue. He is extremely interested in hearing from readers who have "peculiar" cards—ones that are either misprinted or have information or pictures that

appear incorrect. If we get enough responses, we'll print some of the anomalies here. Write directly to: Thomas Reid—Trading Card Tsar, TSR, Inc., P.O. 756, Lake Geneva WI 53147, U.S.A., and tell him we sent you.

A review reviewed

Dear Dragon,
I would like to thank Rick Swan for his glowing review of the GURPS Old West* game (DRAGON issue #190). Liz Tornabene and I had a lot of fun writing this book, and we're glad some of our enthusiasm shows through. (Liz is especially proud of the transportation chapter, which Mr. Swan enjoyed reading as much as Liz enjoyed writing.) I was also pleased that Mr. Swan thought I handled Native American culture "with reasonable accuracy." That's exactly what I was aiming at when I wrote the Indians chapter.
However, I must take exception to Mr. Swan's statements that I was not "quite so reverent towards Indian religion," or that the section on Indian magic took a "patronizing" approach. And I certainly do not consider Native American beliefs—of either the 19th or 20th centuries—"quaint," as Mr. Swan implies.
In writing the rules for Indian magic, I decided to go on the assumption that magic in the GURPS Old West game would work *just as Native Americans, and especially medicine men, of the time period believed it would.* Of course, I was hampered by the fact that I had to base my information on sources local libraries could provide. (Although I have Native American blood in my ancestry, I have had little exposure to modern Native American culture.) I was also hampered by the lack of space; there simply weren't enough pages in the book to address Native American culture in any but the most superficial way—and that included religious beliefs.
I chose to base the Indian magic section on Plains Indians' beliefs for a number of reasons: There was more information available on Sioux religion than on any other Native American belief system (although Navajo chantways came in a close second); the Plains Indians are those most often thought of when gamers think of the Old West; and Sioux religion seemed to lend itself to easy translation into GURPS game mechanics. In adapting my knowledge of 19th-century Native American magic rituals to GURPS magic rules, I tried to maintain, at the very least, the "flavor" of Sioux religion. I also tried to maintain as much accuracy as possible, although game mechanics can never truly simulate real life.
Perhaps what Mr. Swan objects to is that I presented Native American beliefs in game terms at all. In most role-playing games with rule systems covering magic and spell-casting,

Continued on page 7

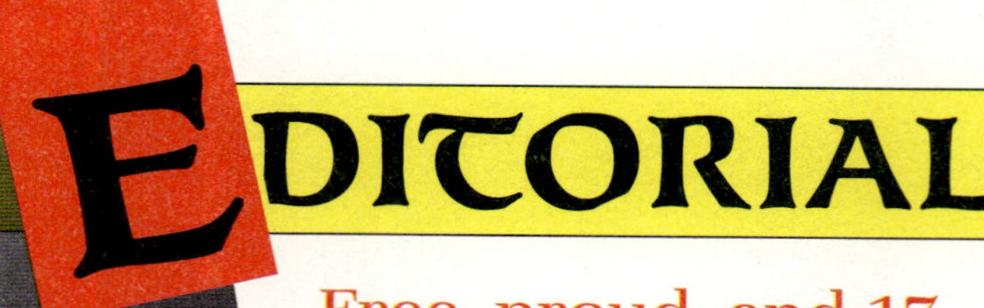

Free, proud, and 17

One of the less entertaining things about having a car radio with a "scan" feature is that you often listen, albeit briefly, to lots of radio stations you would never normally allow yourself to hear (country music, classical music, talk radio, etc.). About a month ago, on my way to work before the sun was even up, I punched "scan" and soon found myself listening to a warning being issued by a Christian fundamentalist radio station in Milwaukee. The warning was against a Walt Disney movie, *Beauty and the Beast*.

Before I go any further, I want to paraphrase a much more famous person and say that I will defend to my death the Constitutional right of that radio station to give air play to such views. I say this despite the fact that some of those views, such as the one I'm about to relate, might come across to some people as being a little on the lunatic side (as I am sure my editorial will come across to the people who have those lunatic views, but I can live with that).

The meat of the message to radio listeners was that parents should have nothing to do with *Beauty and the Beast*, despite its beauty and grandeur and warmth and moral lessons, because the movie contains, right at its very start, an episode of black magic—namely, the transformation of a heartless prince into a beast by a sorceress's spell. That's lycanthropy, the station said, and that's evil, so don't buy the video and expose your kids to it.

It's obvious that the people issuing the warning believe fully in the existence of black magic and lycanthropy, which does make me wonder if they also lock their closet doors every night to keep out the boogeyman. (I can already guess what they must think of fantasy role-playing games like ours.) Anyway, since these people believe in black magic, they want people to stay away from it, which is good advice for anyone under the age of three but might sound agonizingly ignorant to everyone else.

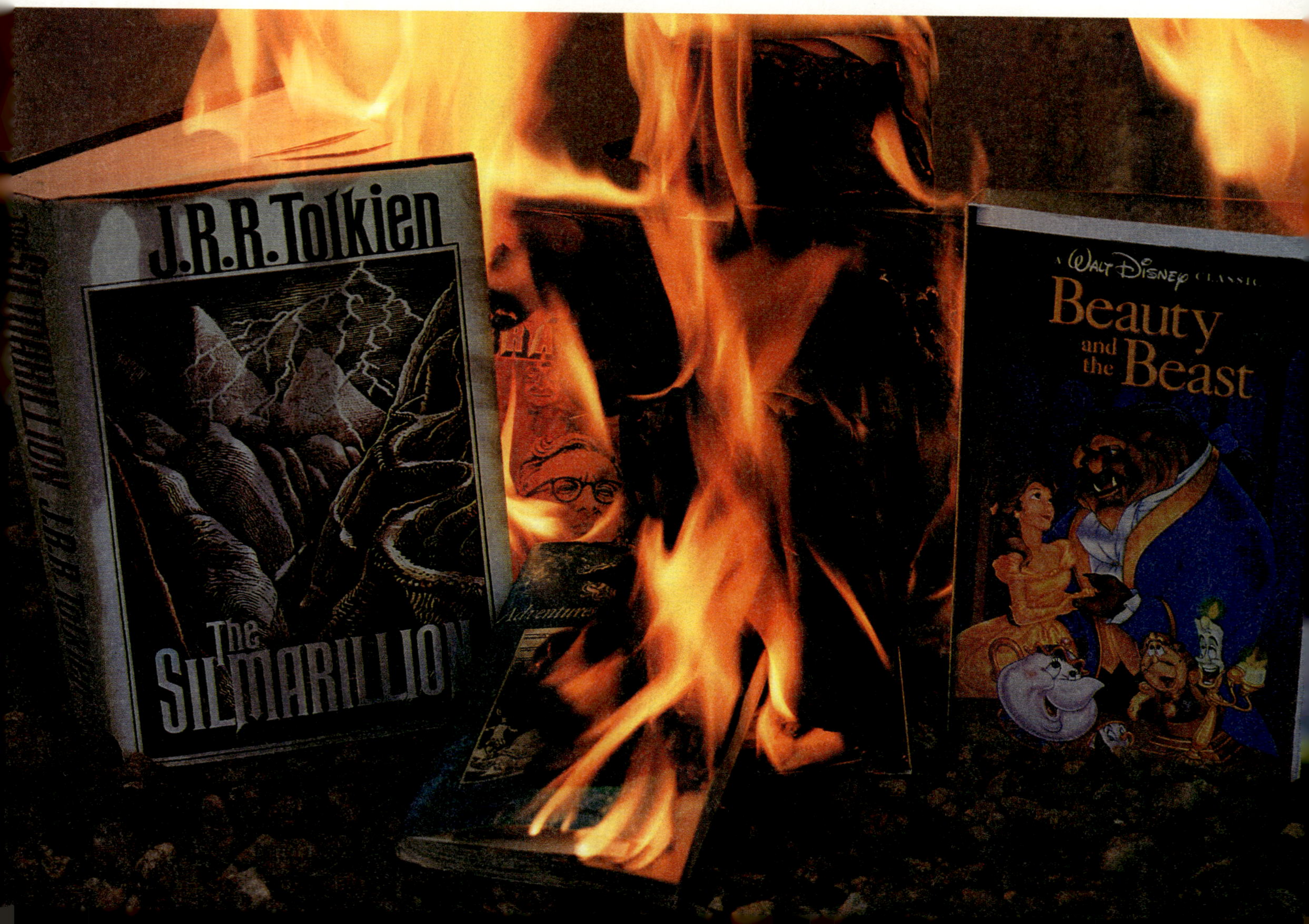

Obviously, some people in this country (and elsewhere) are very much afraid of fantasy, in whatever form it takes. Anti-fantasy attacks are not limited to arguments against *Beauty and the Beast*, of course. The same kind of reasoning that equates a Walt Disney film with black magic reappears in arguments against the DUNGEONS & DRAGONS® game, such as the one offered by a lawyer who tried to get nominated for the office of Virginia state attorney general in 1985: "The essence of D&D is violence. It teaches Satan-worship, spell-casting, witchcraft, murder, rape, suicide, and assassination along the way." (He lost the nomination.)*

Other fantasy materials have been under attack in this century, particularly fantasy and science-fiction novels and stories. *Alice's Adventures in Wonderland*, *A Clockwork Orange*, *The Martian Chronicles*, *The Lathe of Heaven*, Oscar Wilde's *The Happy Prince and Other Stories*, *1984*, *Slaughterhouse-Five*, *Tarzan of the Apes*, *Brave New World*, *Flowers for Algernon*, Stephen King's *The Shining*, John Gardner's *Grendel*, and *The Wizard of Oz*, among others, have run into trouble in this country because of their content. (Some people felt, incredibly, that *1984* promoted communism; bad language snarled a number of others, Tarzan and Jane were living in sin, and *The Happy Prince* was challenged because it was "distressing and morbid"— well, jeez!)

However, some fundamentalist groups have challenged fantasy books on the basis that they are supposed to be occult and connected with satanism or witchcraft—that's what snagged *The Wizard of Oz*, if you can believe that. The revolting but amusing "Dark Dungeons" pamphlet published by Chick Publications, which I described in the editorial for DRAGON® issue #182, urges the reader at one point to burn all "occult books" that he or she owns; a footnote clarifies this to include "C. S. Lewis and Tolkien, both of which can be found in occult bookstores." I even have a clipping from the February 27, 1992 issue of the *News Messenger*, a newspaper published in Marshall, Texas, in which one of TSR's old FANTASY FOREST™ multiple-plot paperbacks is accused of using "mind control" tactics on young readers. The argument put forth by those opposing the book is that reading this "pick-a-path" book will lead to satan worship and cult activities. There are parts of this article that I want very much to laugh at, but it's hard to laugh because you know these people are very, very serious about their accusations.

As annoying and stupid-sounding as anti-fantasy attacks can be, they are merely the tip of the Titanic's iceberg. The American Library Association's Office for Intellectual Freedom keeps tabs on attempts to ban or restrict public access to any books, and many public libraries have materials from the ALA on censorship and book-banning that you might find shocking. Among the other books that have come under attack in this country are some that you might even be reading right now. They include: *The American Heritage Dictionary*, *The Merriam-Webster Collegiate Dictionary*, *Catch-22*, *Lord of the Flies*, *Oliver Twist*, *Jaws*, *Gone With the Wind*, *The Adventures of Huckleberry Finn*, *A Farewell to Arms*, *The Merchant of Venice*, *Soul on Ice*, *Deenie*, *Native Son*, *Bury My Heart at Wounded Knee*, *To Kill a Mockingbird*, *Ulysses*, *Grapes of Wrath*, *All Quiet on the Western Front*, *Serpico*, *Elmer Gantry*, *The Bell Jar*, *The Sun Also Rises*, *Catcher in the Rye*, *Death of a Salesman*, *The Color Purple*, *Where the Sidewalk Ends*, and *The Lorax*—by Dr. Seuss!

The people who really burn me up, though, are the ones who have tried to ban *The Diary of Anne Frank*. It's been tried several times. People who think that *The Wizard of Oz* promotes witchcraft are laughably foolish; they merely wish to smack your hands with a ruler so you won't daydream. But I have difficulty imagining the bottomless abyss of moral and spiritual depravity to which someone has sunk who is trying to ban Anne Frank's story. These people would put out your eyes, blinding you to their bigotry, then lead you by the trusting hand into the inferno. You will hear the echoes of Gestapo jackboots in every word they utter, the most accursed of the cursed, the lowest of the low.

I've taken a break to calm down, so we can continue.

If the idea of boycotting *Beauty and the Beast* because it promotes lycanthropy sounds vaguely moronic to you (and I would be lying if I said it didn't to me), then I have some suggestions.

First, the next time you hear that a particular book has been banned from a local library or a new movie is being boycotted, think about exercising your First Amendment rights to read the book or see the movie. (Use your discretion, of course.) You can judge the content of those presentations for yourself, and you'll have a more informed opinion. Granted, after examining the material you may come away with the idea that it is perfectly awful, but at least now you know for sure. No one made up your mind for you. (I once watched a very controversial movie on home video and came away with the idea that it should have been banned because it was so *boooooring*.)

Second, if you think the reasons to ban the item are stupid at best, feel free to tell other people what you think and why. In this country—at least so far—free speech is your right. (People who want to ban controversial materials will already be speaking their minds, so you'll be in good company there.) Talk to friends, write to the local newspaper, make your thoughts known.

Third, even if you think a particular book, movie, or game is so bad that satanists would run screaming from it, feel free to criticize it to your heart's content— but **don't** push to ban it. We have the freedom to listen and read and make our own choices. Controversial books and movies often offer to teach us something, though the lesson may be very unpleasant. Even *Mein Kampf* is valuable in some sense, as it shows the highly disturbed mental workings of a major historical figure and throws light on the origins of World War II and the Holocaust. You can flip through it and get a feel for how something as horrific as the events in Anne Frank's diary could have possibly occurred—and why we should never allow that to happen to anyone else ever again.

Drop by your local library to ask about the ALA's materials on banned books and intellectual freedom. Check out the Banned Books Week displays at local libraries every September. Look up books like Dave Marsh's *50 Ways to Fight Censorship* (it's fairly radical but still rather entertaining). Keep an open mind and open eyes and ears.

And if you want something good to watch on TV, get a copy of *Beauty and the Beast* at the video store and watch it with a special friend or loved one. It's the best.

DRAGON Magazine celebrates its seventeenth birthday this month. In keeping with the rebellious spirit of that age, we present this editorial. We're free, proud, and 17. Enjoy.

Roger E. Moore

* Material quoted from the Christian Broadcasting Network pamphlet, *Dungeons & Dragons: Adventure or Abomination?*, page 4.

Letters
Continued from page 4

designers can concentrate on what works in the game (so far as playability and game balance are concerned) without worrying about offending anyone by getting it "wrong." After all, few people in the world today believe in magic as it's portrayed in most fantasy novels and games (e.g., powerful wizards casting *lightning bolts* and summoning fiends from the outer planes). But traditional Native American beliefs recognize the supernatural, and that human beings can gain some measure of influence over fate and the spirits through certain rituals. If I inadvertently offended some people by quantifying those beliefs in game terms, I apologize.

Ann Dupuis
Randolph MA

We contacted Rick Swan, who supplied us with this answer:

"Actually, it doesn't matter to me whether designers draw inspiration from Native American religion or the phone book. I merely point out that when you attempt to translate the real-life beliefs of real-life practitioners, you walk a fine line. And I still like Ann's book—a lot." Ω

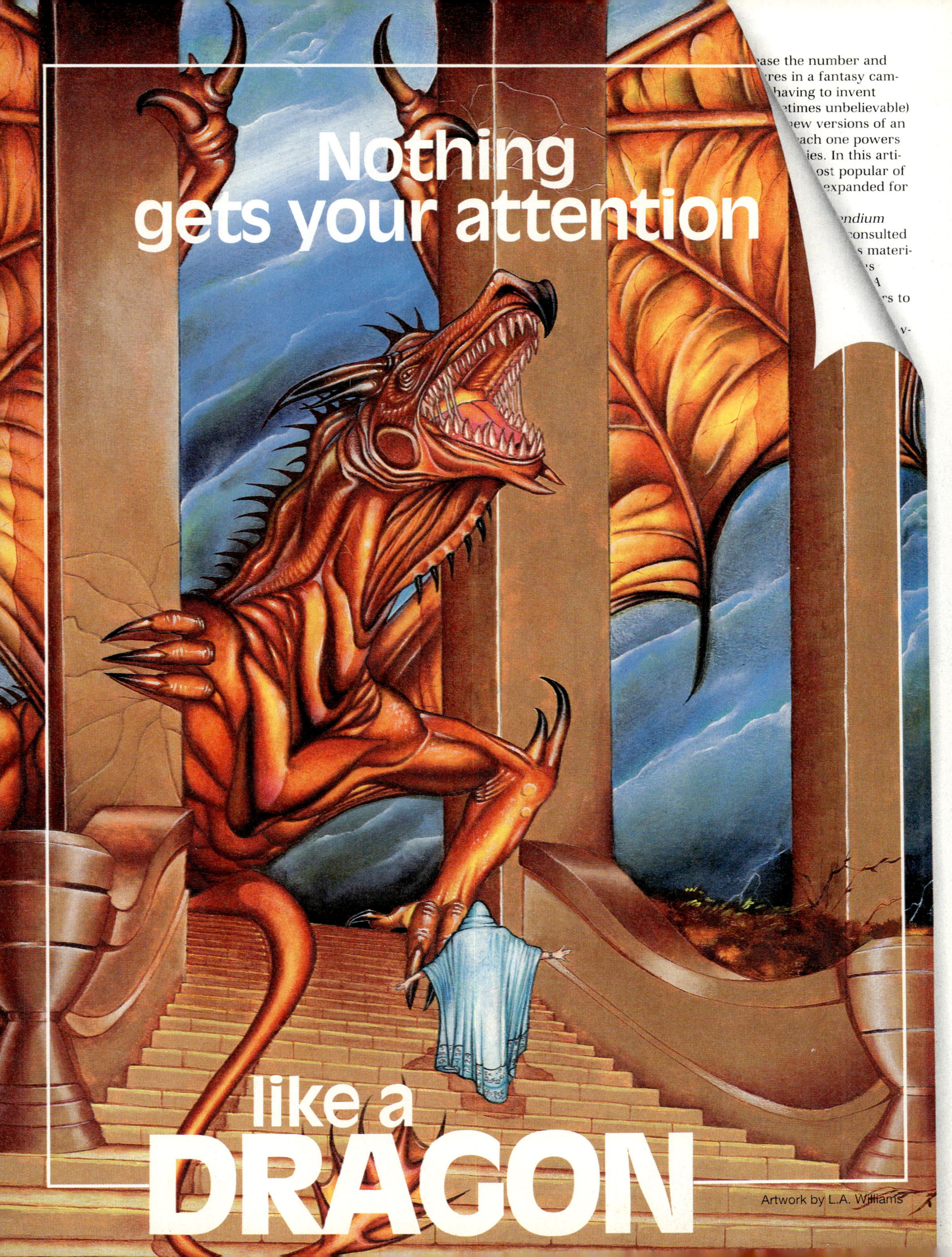

Nothing
gets your attention
like a
DRAGON
Artwork by L.A. Williams

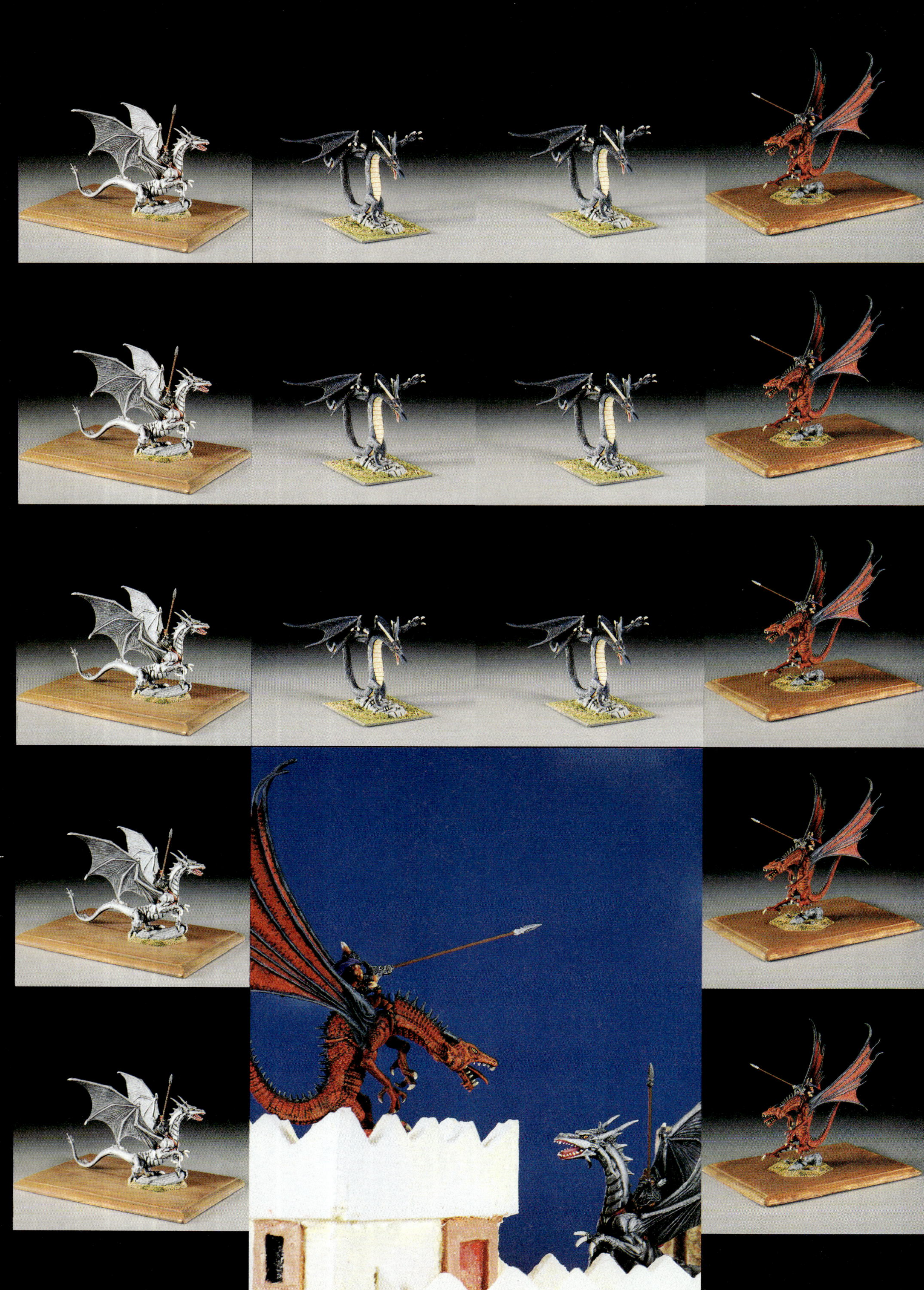

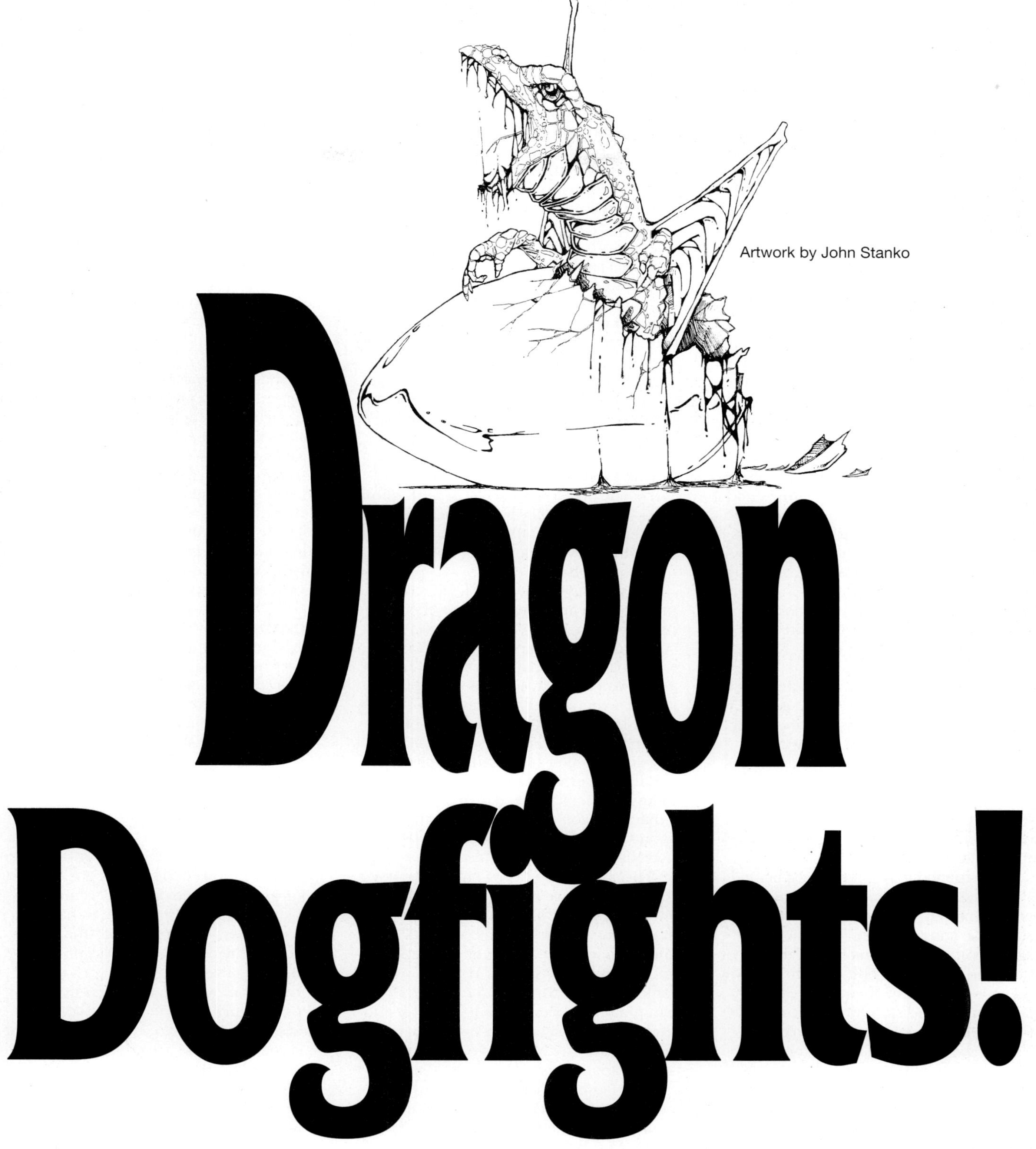

Dragon Dogfights!

Use your dragon miniatures for an aerial duel

by Anne Brown

There's a little event that takes place in Milwaukee, Wis., every August known as the GEN CON® Game Fair. It inspires a plethora of emotions—excitement, nervousness, financial anxiety, and anticipation of great fun and lack of sleep. But for us TSR folks, the primary emotion inspired by the mention of the GEN CON game fair (even in a whisper) is *panic.* Seminars? What seminars? Demos? I`m demonstrating *which* game this year?

Every year, around December, we are assigned to run demos for the various AD&D® game worlds. (A person learns quickly not to be out sick on the day that we sign up for game demos.) About July, we learn exactly what nifty visual aids will be provided for our demos. Then it's time to scramble and get a demo game put together.

Last year was no different. Demo sign-up day was indeed in December, and *sigh*—I was sick that day. (Had I known it was planning day, I'd have hobbled to work under almost any condition.) So my first taste of panic came the following Monday ("What? We signed up for demos last Friday? What's left? Oh, noooooo . . .").

It wasn't nearly as bad as I thought. The DRAGONLANCE® game demo was still available, and my buddy Rob King was still available as a demo partner. Since Rob had edited the *Tales of the Lance* boxed set and I had proofread large hunks of it, what could be more perfect? We scribbled our names onto the list, chattering away about bringing Lord Soth back for a visit.

We blissfully forgot about our demo until about July. I had stacks of pregenerated convention characters in my files, so all we needed was a quick adventure, right? Wrong.

The fateful day arrived when we learned what our demo table would look like. "You're getting a giant floating citadel and ten painted dragon miniatures, with a drop-cloth of an overhead view of farm fields and whatnot," we were cheerfully told. "Just run some aerial dragon battles. It'll be great!"

Rob and I moped our way back to our cubicles. No Lord Soth. No kender not knowing when to run in terror. No grouchy dwarves.

Reality set in. "There's no such thing as 3-D aerial combat in the AD&D game," we moaned. (At least nothing that we knew of—neither of us are big miniatures gamers!) We called upon my husband, Rick, a veteran miniatures gamer, and upon Jim Ward, an old war dog, for rules. "Nope," came the answers. "Not unless you want to play only one turn in an hour. Just make something up!"

Panic turned to desperation. I bribed Jim Ward with lunch one day (not a cheap proposition) to help me sketch out the rules. We roughed them out, then Rob and I took our red pens out. (If there's one thing we *can* do, it's edit.) We threw away the rules for facing, threw away breath immunities, and standardized the scores for all 10 dragons. In a real stroke of genius, we decided to tie a colored ribbon to each dragon to indicate its range of movement. Then we subjected a few co-workers to our game and made a few more modifications.

After scrounging for a thousand dice, dry-erase markers, and plastic covers for the character sheets, we were ready before the opening bell of the game fair.

Karen Boomgarden was scheduled to run the first few hours of the demos. After my early-morning seminars, I descended breathlessly on the TSR demo area. "How's it going?" I asked with trepidation. Karen pooh-poohed. "Great! After the first turn, they're running it themselves!" We exchanged gummi-bears as I watched in wonder. Ten gamers crowded around the table, rolling dice like crazy. All I could think was, "It works! Rob, you have to see this!"

We ended up with a hit on our hands. People even hung around to play more than one round. Karen was able to run the game even though she lost her voice on the second day of the convention. Even some of the most die-hard miniatures gamers (including my husband) thought it was pretty cool.

So that's what this article is about: running your own 3-D aerial dragon combats with our little game rules. Use it when you're bored with role-playing, or when you just feel like some hack 'n' slash combat. Two to 10 people can play, and the more the merrier. A game with ten people, each playing one dragon, takes just about an hour. You should know the rules after the first turn.

What you need

For our demo, we had 10 dragon miniatures—one gold, silver, bronze, brass, copper, red, green, blue, black, and white. Each dragon was mounted on a four-inch-square base.

Our playing surface was a felt cloth printed with an overhead view of farm fields, woods, rivers, and the like. Your surface can be as fancy or simple as you want—it doesn't matter to the play of the game. You can play it on the living room rug or a kitchen table if that's most convenient. Determine the boundaries of your playing surface—any size or shape is fine, but don't exceed six feet in any direction.

Each player will need one each of the following dice: d4, d8, d10, d20.

Each dragon figure needs a corresponding character sheet. Each player needs a method to keep track of hit points and breath-weapon uses on the sheet. For the game fair, we placed each character sheet in a plastic sleeve and used dry-erase pens to mark on the plastic. The sheets wiped off easily after each game. You can do it this way, or you may wish to make multiple copies of the sheets so you can mark on them, erase the marks, and throw them away as they wear out. Or simply track the hit-point damage on scrap paper.

For measuring devices, we bought colored ribbons corresponding to each color of dragon. A ribbon was tied to each dragon's right front foot and then cut to the dragon's movement rate in inches (18 inches, in this case). This eliminated messing around with rulers. It also simulated a dragon's maneuverability—since dragons in our game can fly wherever they want, it doesn't make sense to limit their movement to straight lines. But if you don't feel like messing with ribbons or string, by all means use rulers or tape measures.

If you wish to use ribbons (ordinary string will work just as well), buy one yard of ribbon for each dragon. First, tie one end to the dragon's foot, or attach it to the base. Next, measure out 9" of ribbon away from the dragon's foot. Tie a knot at the 9" mark. This represents the range of the dragon's breath weapon. Finally, measure out 18" from the dragon's foot and tie another knot. Cut off the excess. The knot at the end will keep the ribbon from fraying. A drop of white glue or super glue on the end knots will also improve their durability.

By the way, don't cut an 18" length of ribbon first, then tie the knots. You'll lose the length that's twisted up in the knots.

Set-up

Decide whether you want to play every-dragon-for-itself or in teams. For our game, the evil dragons defended their citadel, and each evil dragon began the game with its base touching the citadel. The good dragons started with their bases touching the edge of the gaming table and tried to defeat the citadel's guardian dragons.

Draw your battle lines and agree upon your starting positions. We didn't allow anyone to start off the board, but your group could decide to allow it.

Combat sheets

Included in this article is a dragon character sheet we used at the 1992 GEN CON game fair. To make this game as easy as possible, we gave all the dragons the same statistics. Essentially, everyone got the same character sheet—we just changed the dragon's color, name, and objective. If you'd like a more complicated game, see the advanced rules.

The basic game

Once you've chosen teams or individual play and established starting positions for all dragons, decide on victory conditions. For our demo, the first team to have all five members eliminated was the loser.

Follow the Sequence of Play on the character sheets, as follows:

Initiative: A d10 is rolled for every dragon figure (even if a player controls more than one dragon). The lowest number goes first. Ties are considered to be simultaneous actions. If your group prefers, ties can be resolved with another die roll.

Movement: Dragons always move first, then attack. A dragon can move a total of 18", curving or looping as desired. Movement in 3-D can be simulated ("I'm going to fly over this other dragon") without penalty. A dragon can face any direction at the end of its movement.

When a dragon is reduced to half its hit points, its movement is reduced by half.

Attack: At the end of a dragon's movement, the player declares its mode of attack: breath weapon, melee, or defend.

Breath weapon: A dragon's breath

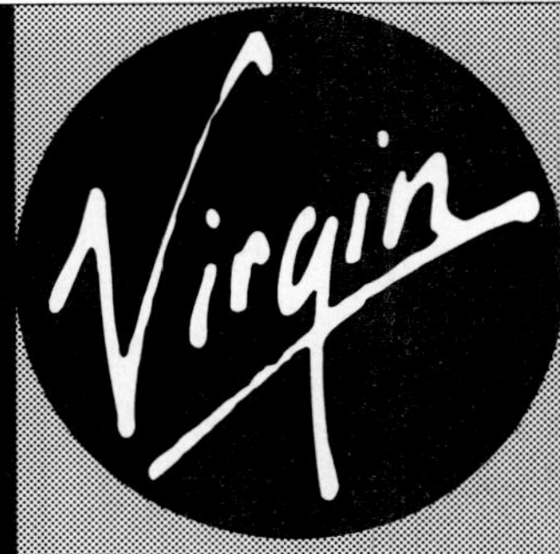

get giant games at elfin prices

middle earth box set £5.99

treasures of middle earth £5.99

lords of middle earth vol. 1 £4.99

nazguls citadel £4.99

creatures of middle earth £3.99

forest of tears £3.99

ghost warriors £2.50

warlords of the desert £2.50

more MERP available instore

now you're tolkien !

ADDITIONAL OFFERS AVAILABLE INSTORE • PRICES MAY VARY IN DUBLIN

Virgin

GAMES CENTRES

ahead of the game

Red Dragon

Objective

Defend Citadel by destroying the Metallic Dragons.

Age Category: Adult (156 years old)
Hit Points: 148
Attack Roll: 6   **Damage:** 1d4x10
Breath Weapon: Fire   *Range:* 9 inches
    Damage: 1d8x10   *Save:* half damage
Saving Throw: 6

Set Up

Chromatic dragons begin circling the Citadel.
Metallic dragons are placed with their bases
  touching the outer edge of the board.

Sequence of Play

1. Roll initiative (1d10).
2. Lowest number goes first. Dragon
   moves, then attacks.

Movement

Each dragon has a ribbon tied to its foot.
The dragon may move anywhere within the
  reach of the ribbon (18 inches).
The dragon may face in any direction.
A dragon at half its hit points moves half speed.

Attacks

Player declares *one* attack form: breath weapon,
  melee, or defend.
An attack ends a dragon's move.

**Breath Weapon (may be used 3 times during
the game—mark each use in the box provided)**
  A. Automatically hits one creature in range (9
     inches).
  B. Attacker rolls damage (1d8x10).
  C. Defender rolls saving throw (1d20). If
     defender rolls 6 or greater, defender suffers
     only half damage.

Melee
  A. Attacker rolls 1d20 once; a roll of 6 or
     greater is a successful hit.
  B. Attacker rolls damage (1d4x10).
  C. Dragons in melee must break off their
     attacks at the end of the round; in the next
     round, they must move at least 4 inches.

Defend
If a dragon is not in attack range when it
  finishes its move, it may defend. This allows
  the dragon to save its attack for use against
  an attacker. The defensive attack occurs
  after the enemy has rolled its attack.

Breath Weapon Roster

Hit Point Roster

A PUBLISHING EVENT!

The classic fantasy adventure serialized on Prodigy® is finally available in book form.

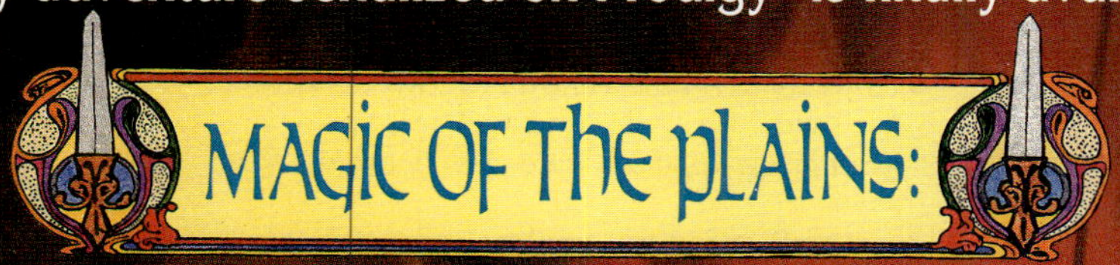

Volume I

By the Sword

GREG COSTIKYAN

THE FIRST NOVEL IN THE NEW SERIES
by the author of *Star Wars®: The Role Playing Game, Paranoia®,* and *MadMaze®* is one of the most popular features (game or otherwise) on Prodigy®...the largest commercial computer network in the world.

Prodigy® commissioned Greg Costikyan to write BY THE SWORD as a serial. For 26 weeks, tens of thousands followed the weekly adventure about Nijon, a barbarian from a small plains tribe, who is also the son of one of his world's gods.

Now you can own the complete story, filled with even more details than the Prodigy® version, in a deluxe hardbound edition of your own.

By the Sword
IS ONE BOOK YOU WON'T WANT TO MISS.

AVAILABLE WHEREVER BOOKS ARE SOLD

TOR BOOKS®

Publishers of the best science fiction and fantasy in the world weapon automatically hits one creature within 9". Even if several dragons are close together, only one is affected.

The attacking dragon rolls damage (1d8×10), with the victim is allowed a saving throw for half damage. A roll of 6 or greater on 1d20 indicates a successful save.

Breath weapons can be used three times during the game. Each use must be marked in the box provided.

Melee: A dragon can physically attack any one dragon in range (bases or figures touching). Although dragons typically attack with a claw/claw/bite routine, we used one attack roll (1d20—success on 6 or better) and one damage roll (1d4×10) to keep the game moving quickly.

Defend: This option is used most at the beginning of the game. Because of starting positions on the gaming table, a dragon may use its move but not be in range to attack any foes. Later in the turn, another dragon may move into range and attack that dragon. The *defend* option ensures that each dragon is allowed an attack in the round if any targets move into range during that turn. The defend can be either a breath weapon or melee attack and is rolled after an attacker's rolls.

That's it! You know everything you need to play the basic game. Now, for those of you who like lots of options and number-crunching, try the advanced rules that follow.

Advanced rules

Okay, you've mastered the basic rules for dragon dogfighting, and now you'd like more flavor, realism, and strategy. A list of optional, advanced rules is given here. Pick and choose among them for the degree of complexity your group desires.

Individualizing dragons: This option lets each player roll up some or all of a dragon's statistics. For this, you'll need the *Monstrous Compendium* entries for the appropriate dragons.

Age category: Decide whether all the dragons in the game will fall into the same age category. If so, choose a category randomly or by vote. If not, roll 1d10 for each dragon and assign age categories appropriately. However, since this could possibly pit a hatchling against a great wyrm, you may wish to choose a span of four age categories (for example, Very Old through Great Wyrm) and roll 1d4 to determine each dragon's age.

Hit points: Use the base hit dice listed for each type of dragon, modified by the hit-die modifier for age category. For example, an adult black dragon would have 14 hit dice (12+2). Roll hit points accordingly (14d8).

Attack roll (or THAC0): If you wish to calculate individual THAC0s, you also need to find the armor class for each dragon. Use the base THAC0 given for the dragon type plus the combat modifier for age to determine the dragon's THAC0. An adult black dragon has THAC0 3. To determine armor class, use the dragon's base AC modified by the hit die modifier for age category. Our black dragon's armor class is –1.

Damage: Use the damage listed in the *Monstrous Compendium* entry, modified by the combat modifier for age. Our black dragon's damage is 1d6+6/1d6+6/3d6+6.

Breath weapon: Use damage as listed in dragon entry. Range can be standardized for all the dragons in your game, or can be adjusted by dragon type. Saving throws for half damage are still allowed.

Saving throw: Determine a dragon's saving throw based on its hit dice for a warrior of the same level. Our black dragon has 14 hit dice, so her saving throw versus breath weapon is 5.

Movement: Allow dragons the choice of moving or attacking first, rather than requiring movement to happen first.

Melee options: Allow a dragon to split its claws and bite attacks between opponents as long as the attacker's base or figure is touching the base or figure of all its intended targets. The dragon then rolls its three attacks separately.

Immunities: Add appropriate immunities to the different dragon types. For example, our black dragon is immune to acid attacks.

Hit locations: Divide a dragon's hit points among its body, head, left wing, and right wing. For example, 40% of a dragon's hit points go to body, 30% to head, and 15% to each wing. In this manner, the dragon's flight may be crippled (halve the dragon's current flight speed) when a wing loses all its hit points; the dragon may be unable to make bite attacks when its head loses all its hit points; or the dragon may be unable to make its clawing attacks if its body loses all its hit points. Other options and penalties can be invented to increased variety and fun.

Spells: If you wish, allow dragons some or all of their spells or spell-like abilities as detailed in their *Monstrous Compendium* entries. Allow area-effect spells to affect more than one opponent (or teammate) engaged in melee combat. Track the dragons' spells on an extra sheet of paper or on the back of the dragon's character sheet.

Riders: Now it gets complicated! Roll up a character to serve as a dragon's rider. This is most likely a wizard, cleric, or even a lich, but almost any character is possible. You'll need to track the character's hit points, attacks, THAC0, and spell abilities, and rules for falling off a dragon are in order, too.

The sky's the limit (okay, bad pun) with this simple system for dragon dogfights, so dust off those dragon figurines and get started. May the best wyrm win!　Ω

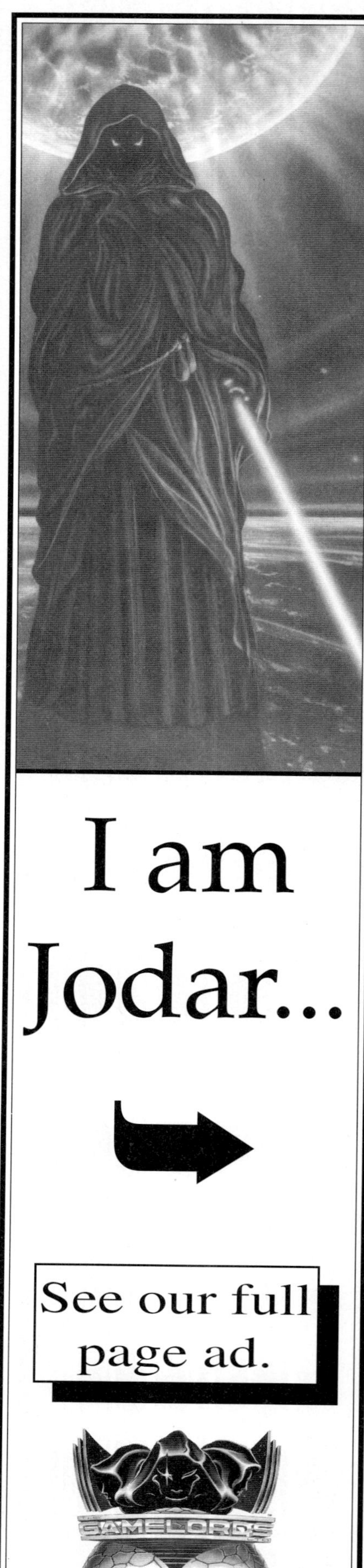

The DRAGON PROJECT

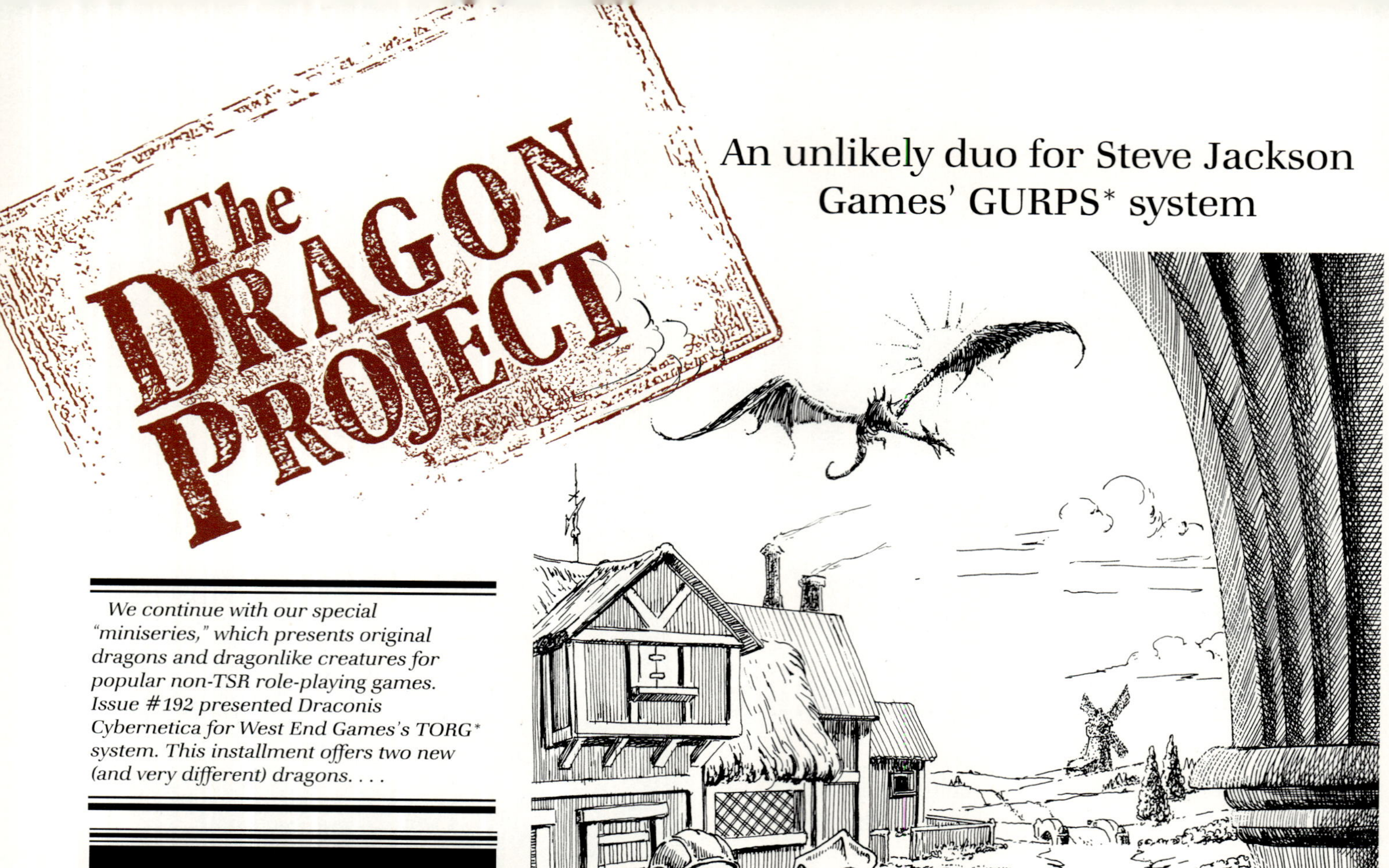

We continue with our special "miniseries," which presents original dragons and dragonlike creatures for popular non-TSR role-playing games. Issue #192 presented Draconis Cybernetica for West End Games's TORG system. This installment offers two new (and very different) dragons. . . .*

Dexter & Cornelius

©1993

by Loyd Blankenship

Artwork by Daniel R. Frazier

GURPS* stands for the Generic Universal RolePlaying System, an eight-year-old role-playing game from Steve Jackson Games, in Austin, Tex. The GURPS game is a point-based system: Each character is designed by spending points on attributes, advantages, and skills, and gaining points for disadvantages and quirks. The GURPS system covers almost every genre imaginable—fantasy, science fiction, super-hero, cyberpunk, and more—with one basic rule system. For more information, write to: Steve Jackson Games, at P.O. Box 18957, Austin TX 78760.

Dexter and Cornelius are an unlikely pair of con artists who roam the land extorting money and trade goods from small villages. Cornelius, a human, typically scouts out a town disguised as a wandering priest or beggar, ensuring that there aren't any warriors around who might be inclined to interfere with their blackmailing plans. Once convinced the coast is clear, he sends in Dexter, a dragon, to put on a show for the hapless village. After Dexter makes a few passes over the town square, with occasional flame bursts and a great deal of bellowing and roaring, the townspeople are convinced that they are doomed. During this time, Cornelius helps himself to the contents of any abandoned houses.

Then Cornelius arrives to "save the day." Typically, saving the day involves a payment of anywhere from $500 to $2,500 (or the same number of gold pieces), plus any small, valuable items that Cornelius might have discovered in his looting. Cornelius then warns the citizens that, should they be *too* helpful when their lord inquires into the affair, Dexter might be forced to return. In fact, the townspeople might be best served to just forget that this little incident ever happened.

Background

Cornelius was a rather unsuccessful sneak thief, pickpocket, and aspiring blackmailer when he stumbled into his fortuitous meeting with Dexter. He was attempting to trail a merchant caravan through a mountain pass when he became lost. After wandering for almost two days, he was attracted by the sounds of combat. Not one to run toward a fight, Cornelius cautiously approached. He arrived in time to see the untimely death of two great fighters—a heavily armed and armored human knight and a great reddish dragon. The dragon was slain by the two-handed sword thrust through her throat, but not before one last blast of flame parboiled the knight in her armor. Never one to miss an opportunity to make a quick and easy score, Cornelius waited to make sure that both were dead, then approached the dragon's cave. He had no sooner peered inside than he was bowled over by a horse-sized, newborn dragon with wild, frightened eyes. He felt a frantic touch at his mind as he locked eyes with the hatchling, and the clear sound of a voice (mentally translated into human speech) saying, "Mommy?"

Once he became convinced that the baby dragon was not going to eat him alive, Cornelius did his best to comfort the lizard. As the little beast began to trust Cornelius, the possibilities of the situation gradually dawned on the human and a scheme was born. Destroying villages was wasteful and dangerous—and was sure to attract every dragon-hunter in the realm. But it would be much harder for a knight to get worked up about a dragon that did nothing more than fly about, wouldn't it?

Cornelius spent the next two years living in the cave with the dragonling, making occasional forays into town for supplies he purchased with the dwindling stack of coinage Dexter's mother had accumulated. He played upon Dexter's instinctive lust for treasure to assure cooperation in the plan. Finally, slightly over six months ago, the pair embarked upon their current reign of terror.

Campaign role

So far, Dexter and Cornelius have been extremely successful in their operations. They must hit only one or two villages per month to live quite comfortably. Needless to say, this level of activity couldn't remain hushed forever. Even though no crops or towns have been destroyed, the sudden shortage of coinage in certain villages is sure to make tax collection more difficult than usual.

The GM could allow the adventurers to hear rumors of a great dragon that is laying waste to villages to the north. Perhaps the PCs would be contacted by the local nobility to investigate the mysterious partnership fleecing coinage from the baron's serfs, or the party might even be passing through a village when Dexter and Cornelius pay a visit.

Dexter

ST: 20   Move/Dodge: 6.5/6
DX: 11   PD/DR: 2/2
IQ: 11   Damage: 1d+1 cut claws/
                         1d breath
HT: 15/22   Reach: R,C,1
Size: 6 hexes   Weight: 730 lbs.

Dexter, although he looks terrifying to the average farmer or peasant, is actually a fairly small, young dragon. He is approximately the size of an elephant (not including his tail) and would not be a threat to most experienced parties in a straight battle. However, he has Cornelius to make sure no straight battles are necessary. Dexter completely trusts his deceitful mentor. He believes that Cornelius has his best interests at heart, and he won't listen to anyone claiming otherwise. While he doesn't particularly want to destroy villages or harm anyone, Dexter isn't against such activities, either. Dexter is very suspicious of anyone other than Cornelius. He usually attempts to flee a confrontation with more than one person. If forced to fight, however, he goes for the kill.

Continued on page 22

Attention, PARANOIA* Troubleshooters—
Meet D.R.A.G.O.N.-bot ver. 3.1!

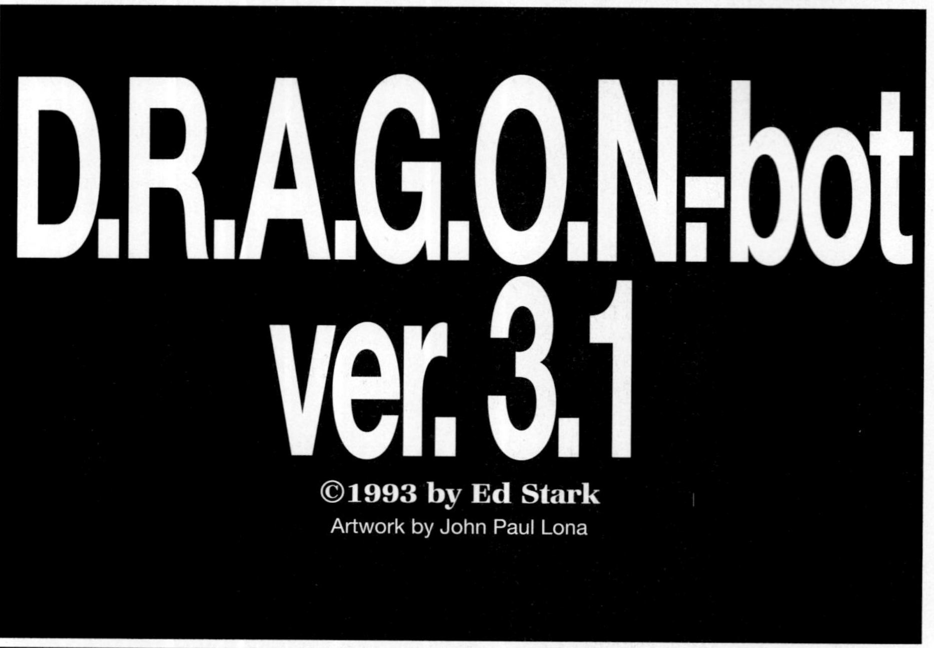

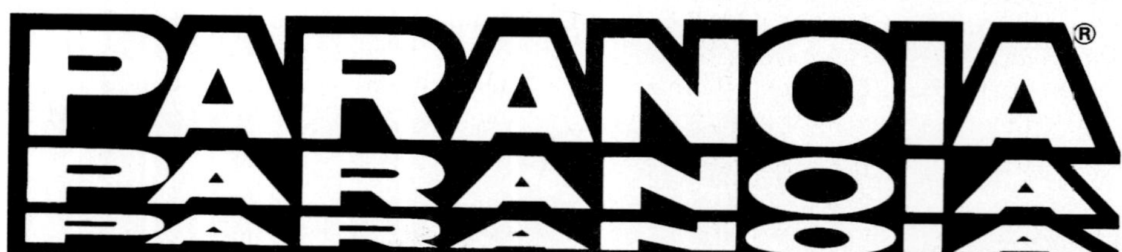

PARANOIA*, Second Edition: The Role-playing Game of a Darkly Humorous Future is West End Games's look at role-playing games in general, and the science-fiction genre in particular. The game is set in a future foreseen by Sartre, Orwell, and Huxley, but interpreted by Marx—*Groucho* Marx. Slapstick, cyanide, and laser weapons are all rolled into one extremely paranoid environment.

Everyone lives in a giant domed city called Alpha Complex, which is ruled by The (never "a") Computer. The Computer is Your Friend. The Computer wants you to be happy. You *will* be happy, Citizen—even if it kills you. To ensure your happiness, Your Friend The Computer has recruited you to eliminate any potential . . . *problems* that may arise in Alpha Complex. Doesn't this make you happy to help out Your Friend? It had better, or you might become one of those potential problems.

So, you are a Troubleshooter. You are given a laser pistol and all kinds of neat (and definitely dangerous) toys by The Computer to help you shoot trouble. What kind of trouble? Oh, standard stuff—Commies, Mutants, Traitors, that kind of thing.

Are *you* a Commie, Mutant, or Traitor? Probably—but we wouldn't want to annoy The Computer with that sort of bothersome knowledge, now would we? Of course not.

Instead, let's take a look at The Computer's newest Troubleshooting device:

The D.R.A.G.O.N.-bot ver. 3.1

The latest development from The Computer's most loyal Research and Design Service Group, the D.R.A.G.O.N.-bot ver. 3.1 has been added to the many and diverse military resources available to Troubleshooters all over Alpha Complex. The D.R.A.G.O.N.-bot ver. 3.1 is the greatest advance in technology produced for Troubleshooters in the war against unregistered mutation since the now-legendary MutaGenetic Handshake and Solicitous Greeting ("Hi! How are you? How's the clone-family? By the way, are you a mutant?" *RIIIP!* "Yow! Guess you are! Super-strong one, too!").

The D.R.A.G.O.N.-bot ver. 3.1[1] was originally designed as an infiltration device to be used by Troubleshooters in the mutant-dominated simplex known only as the Dungeon. No one knows when the

traitorous simplex came into being, but it has long been a temporary refuge for those terrible, ungrateful mutants who refuse to either register their mutations or submit to Summary Execution. Instead, they flee like cowards into the lower levels of Alpha Complex—even below the Food Vats—to hide in the dark, mutating still further and waiting for loyal Troubleshooters, whom the mutants tend to eat. It is not known whether these even more traitorous mutations (only one per customer, please) are caused by the eating of Troubleshooters or the consumption of Food Vat run-off, which leaks down through treasonously unplugged holes in the floor. (There are those that say the holes in the floor were caused by the run-off eating through the floor, but those who say that are promptly shown the error of their ways by being consigned to those very Food Vats. The run-off coats the walls, ceilings, and floor of the Dungeon with grayish ooze and greenish slime.) Extensive tests are currently being performed by R&D, under The Computer's direction, to determine the truth of these two hypotheses; volunteers are being accepted at any Production, Logistics, and Commissary cafeteria (for Food Vat Testing) or at the Armed Forces "Panicked Infrared" Target Range (for Clone Consumption Preparation).

Description

The ultimate melding of stealth and firepower, the D.R.A.G.O.N.-bot ver. 3.1 has been designed to carry its Troubleshooter Team deep into Dungeon territory, fight off mutant attacks, and get out again undamaged—either piloted by the original Team or, more likely, their clone brothers and sisters (Troubleshooters just aren't as durable as The Computer's prize creation). It is heavily armored, both above and below. There are no hollows, not even right over its left breast. Honest.

The D.R.A.G.O.N.-bot ver. 3.1 is exactly five meters long and three meters high at its extreme points. It is covered with armored plate and has been painted appropriately; appropriate colors not only correspond to the colors of the highest clearance level allowed inside each D.R.A.G.O.N.-bot ver. 3.1, but also to the appearance of the known mutant creatures inhabiting the area of the Dungeon simplex that the device is designed to emulate). A Red-clearance D.R.A.G.O.N.-bot ver. 3.1 is, naturally, the least well-armored and armed—since large, red, mutant creatures are obviously the lowest on the power end of the mutant scale. Then there is the ultrapowerful Violet clearance D.R.A.G.O.N.-bot ver. 3.1, designed to seek out and destroy violet mutant reptiles, should any ever show up in the Dungeon.

Regardless of coloration, each D.R.A.G.O.N.-bot ver. 3.1 has a common basic design. All are made to house a Troubleshooter Team of four. Usually, the four Troubleshooters assigned are chosen from the best and brightest clones the Armed Forces, R&D, Internal Security, and Power Services have to offer (it is well known that Technical Services, HPD&MC, Production, Logistics and Commissary, and Central Processing Unit have their own infiltration device currently on The Computer-board design table, but it isn't finished yet). The Armed Forces clone sits in the front of the D.R.A.G.O.N.-bot ver. 3.1 and operates both the steering and frontal weaponry of the device, usually a flamethrower. Next is the Power Services clone, who is in charge of motivating the D.R.A.G.O.N.-bot ver. 3.1 by using its unique "stealth drive." This drive is so quiet that no mutant would ever hear the camouflaged device approaching (hearing the device at all is, of course, treasonous, as The Computer has carefully pointed out).

The third clone is the R&D Troubleshooter, in charge of routine maintenance and secondary surveillance. The R&D clone is also in charge of communications—both with the Team's briefing officer (through Uplink—see later) and the outside world. To aid the Troubleshooter in her chore, PLC has graciously provided two megaphones (not just phones, *megaphones*), labelled respectively Uplink and Downlink. It is important that the Troubleshooter not mix up these two devices, as PLC has assured The Computer this would cause confusion and disaster. Finally, the IntSec agent is in charge of primary surveillance (of the Team, of course) and has the important job of Tail-Wagging, Demonstrating Lifelike Neurological Gratification, which has come to be known as "twiddling." The IntSec agent also has a small hole in the rear of the device that the clone can use for either viewing the outside area or waste disposal. Naturally, the Troubleshooter Team is equipped with Disposable And Munchable Savory Edible Lunches (D.A.M.S.E.L.s) for their long daycycle's journey into nightcycle (the Dungeon is notorious for being badly lit).

To the outside observer (who should be executed, obviously being a mutant from the treasonous simplex), the D.R.A.G.O.N.-bot ver. 3.1 looks like a long, reptilian creature with a large, mobile, nodding head; a scaled body that is brightly colored to show up against the dank interior of the Dungeon; and a long, wagging tail (which had better be wagging—that IntSec agent was bought and paid for, you know!). The head-nodding gives the unit a lifelike appearance, and the Armed Forces clone provides realistic sound effects; however, the nodding head gets in the way of the flamethrower occasionally (details will follow). The shape used for the D.R.A.G.O.N.-bot ver. 3.1 was gleaned from Old Reckoning pictures and texts by the

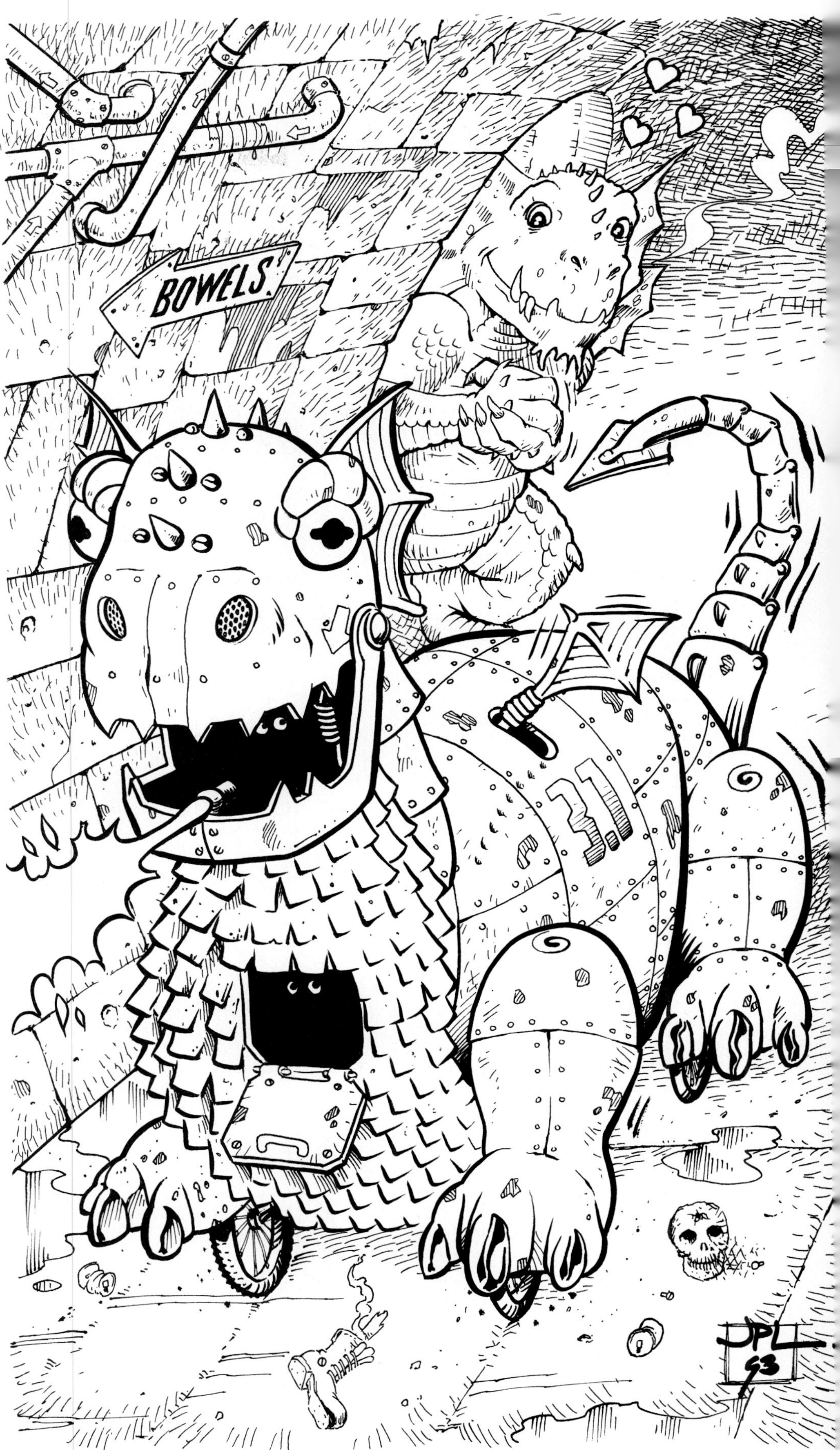

late, lamented, Infrared clone, Just Shoot Me-NOW-6.

The statistics for the basic, Red-clearance D.R.A.G.O.N.-bot ver. 3.1 are given here. They can be modified for higher clearance versions. (There is a treasonous rumor of one Ultraviolet D.R.A.G.O.N.-bot ver. 3.1 that leads the elite unit, though lower-level clones seem to confuse "Ultraviolet" with something called "Platinum.")

The D.R.A.G.O.N.-bot ver. 3.1

Mutant Powers by Internal Troubleshooters
No secret-society affiliations (at least, there'd better not be!)
S20 E18 A2 D11 M² C15 MA²
Armor: All (5)

Using the D.R.A.G.O.N.-bot ver. 3.1

The D.R.A.G.O.N.-bot ver. 3.1 is an infiltration and attack device designed by The Computer for use in the Dungeon simplex. It was not intended for use outside of the Dungeon, but it has already been employed in Transtube Clearance, Food Riot Stoppage, and Cutting Ahead in Line special operations. It is an impressive piece of equipment, even though it doesn't steer well (obviously the fault of the Armed Forces clone in charge of driving—is The Computer to blame because the useless clone can't see through a little smoke and flame?) or keep up a continuous rate of speed (thanks to those lazy Power Services clones). And there is absolutely *no* truth to the rumor that the head of the D.R.A.G.O.N.-bot ver. 3.1 bobs randomly, sometimes (5% chance per shot) causing the flamethrower's automatic blast to shoot back into the interior. The flamethrower can be fired by the Armed Services clone on command, but it fires once every 10 minutes anyway, no matter what anyone else does.

So, go out and explore the Dungeon in perfect safety—at least until D.R.A.G.O.N.-bot ver. 4.0 comes out!

[1] In case you haven't noticed, it is treasonous to call the D.R.A.G.O.N.-bot ver. 3.1 by anything other than its full name. Rumors—which are treasonous—state that this is because versions prior to 3.1 were less than successful. While no one believes this reflects badly on R&D or The Computer—just as no one thinks Cone Rifle Penetration and Blast Radius Survey Research is something they'd really, really like to do—these past failures are still something of a sore diode in The Digital Dictator's side.

[2] These two attributes, as well as the skills of the D.R.A.G.O.N.-bot ver. 3.1, are dependent on the clones inside. Chutzpah is derived from the impressive appearance of the device, but can be higher if the R&D clone (the one doing the communicating) has a higher rating.

Keep in mind that the Agility statistic is for the overall movement of the device, and the Dexterity stat is the maximum allowable inside the D.R.A.G.O.N.-bot ver. 3.1; it should also be used as the maximum stat for firing the front-mounted flamethrower (Damage column: 15; Type: F; Range: three meters—with mouth open and head up; see following for more details).   Ω

* indicates a treasonous product produced by a company other than TSR, Inc. Most treasonous product names are trademarks owned by the companies publishing those treasonous products. The use of the name of any treasonous product without mention of its trademark status should not be construed as a challenge to such status. Carry on, Citizen.

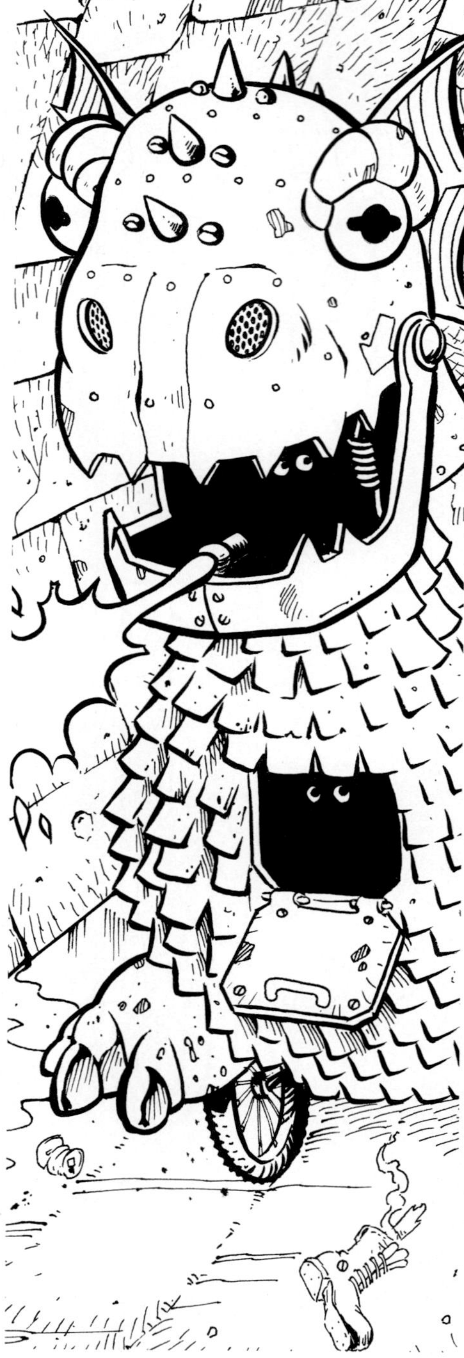

GURPS Dragon
Continued from page 19

Cornelius

ST: 9   **IQ:** 13
DX: 12   **HT:** 10
Dodge: 7   **Thrust:** 1d-2
Parry: 8 (w/knife), 7 (w/sword)
Block: n/a   **Swing:** 1d-1
Speed: 5.5   **Move:** 5

Advantages: Voice
Disadvantages: Wealth (Struggling), −1 Reputation (Thief and Blackmailer), Cowardice, Greed
Quirks: Any five of the GM's choice
Skills: Broadsword-11; Carousing-12; Climbing-12; Disguise-13; Fast-Talk-16; First Aid-13; Knife Throwing-13; Knife-12; Lockpicking-13 Performance-14; Pickpocket-12; Riding (Horse)-10; Shadowing-12; Stealth-13; Streetwise-14; Swimming-11
Equipment: Broadsword (1d cut, 1d-1 cr.), large knife (1d-3 cut, 1d-2 imp.), three throwing knives (1d-2 imp.), light leather armor (PD 2/DR 2), waterskin, simple first aid kit (+1 to skill), personal basics, one-person tent, blanket, large pouch, large backpack, light riding horse, one week's food, lantern, $1,500 (in bags on horse), $150 (in pouch)
Total Points: 50

Cornelius is completely ruthless concerning Dexter. He uses the young dragon to further his own fortune and has full intention of abandoning his charge once he has accumulated a suitable fortune. After a drink or two, he doesn't hesitate to describe his plans to anyone who seems to offer a sympathetic—or impressed—ear. If Dexter ever overhears Cornelius talking while he's in his cups, it will probably engender a radical change in their relationship.   Ω

* indicates a product produced by a company other than TSR, Inc. Most product names are trademarks owned by the companies publishing those products. The use of the name of any product without mention of its trademark status should not be construed as a challenge to such status.

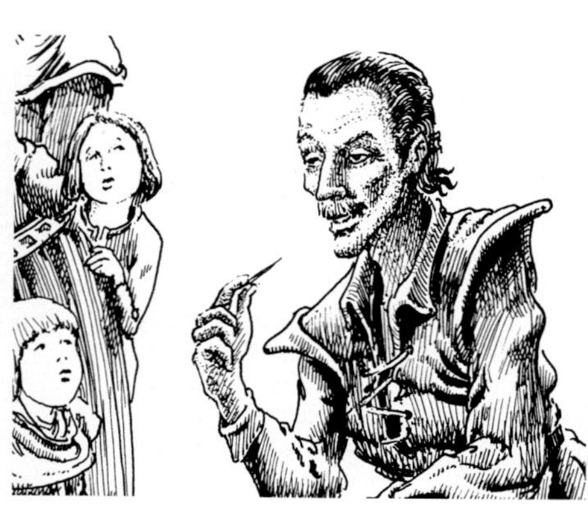

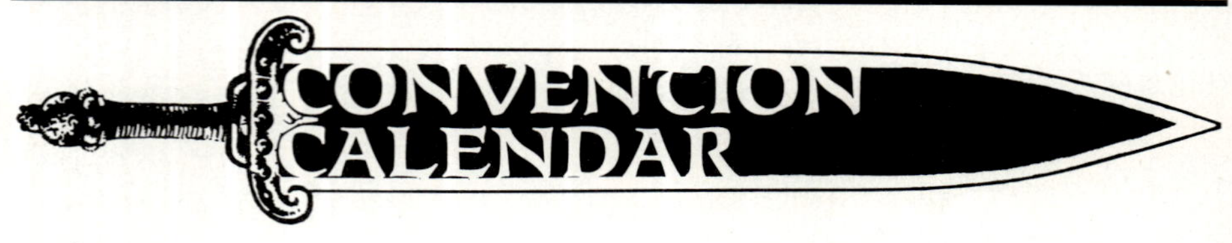

CONVENTION CALENDAR

* indicates a product produced by a company other than TSR, Inc. Most product names are trademarks owned by the companies publishing those products. The use of the name of any product without mention of its trademark status should not be construed as a challenge to such status.

CONQUEST I, June 11-13　　　　　MD

This convention will be held at the Ramada Inn in Hagerstown, Md. Guests include Jonathan Frid, Eric Menyuk, John Anthony Blake, and Sandy Petersen. Activities include an art room, dealers, workshops, a charity auction, and a video room. Send an SASE to: CONQUEST I, P.O. Box 1007, Hagerstown MD 21741-1007; or call: (301) 733-4649.

HEROES '93, June 11-13　　　　　NC

This convention will be held at the Charlotte International Trade Center in Charlotte, N.C. Guests include Mark Bagley, Dick Giordano, George Perez, and Dave Sim. Activities include contests, art seminars, workshops, and exhibits. Registration: $25/weekend or $10/day. Write to: HEROES '93, P.O. Box 9181, Charlotte NC 28299; or call: (704) 394-8404.

SAN DIEGO GAME CON IX, June 11-12　　　CA

This convention will be held at the Howard Johnson-Harborview hotel in San Diego, Calif. Events include strategic, board, role-playing, and card games. Write to: SDGC, 4409 Mission Ave., #J208, Oceanside CA 92057; or call: (619) 599-9619.

BOGGLECON '93, June 12　　　　　PA

This convention, originally scheduled for March 13 but postponed due to heavy snow, will be held at the Wind Gap Fire Hall in Wind Gap, Penn. Events include RPGA™ Network events and other role-playing games plus war games. Other activities include a painted miniatures contest, a games raffle, and a dealers' area. Registration: $10 at the door. Game fees are usually $1. Send an SASE to: Michael Griffith, 118 S. Broadway, Wind Gap PA 18091; or call: (215) 863-5178.

CAPITALCON IX, June 12-13　　　　IL

This convention will be held at the Prairie Capital Convention Center in Springfield, Ill. Events include role-playing, miniatures, war, and board games. Other activities include an auction, a flea market, and a figure-painting contest. Registration: $10 at the door. Write to: John Holtz, 400 E. Jefferson St. #508, Springfield IL 62701; or call: (217) 753-2656.

RECONN '93, June 12-13　　　　　CT

This convention will be held at the Holiday Inn in Norwalk, Conn. Events include role-playing, miniatures, war, and board games. Other activities include a movie room and a dealers' area. Write to: Jim Wiley, Gaming Guild, 100 Hoyt St. #2C, Stamford CT 06905; or call: (203) 969-2396.

SARASOTA-MANATEE FANTASY FAIR
June 13　　　　　　　　　　　　FL

This convention will be held at the Sarasota, Fla., Holiday Inn. Guests include Michael White. Activities include gaming, dealers, trading cards, anime, and door prizes. Registration: $3 at the door. Write to: The Time Machine, 5748 14th St. W., Bradenton FL 34207; or call: (813) 758-3684.

ATLANTICON '93, June 18-20　　　MD

This convention will be held at the Baltimore Convention Center in Baltimore, Md. Guests include numerous gaming personalities. Activities include role-playing, miniatures, and board games, plus a dealers' area. Registration: $20 preregistered; $30 at the door. Write to: ADF Inc., P.O. Box 91, Beltsville MD 20704; or call: (301) 345-1858.

CONTINUUM '93, June 18-20　　　MO

This convention will be held at the Holiday Inn Convention Center in Cape Girardeau, Mo. Guests include Mark Lenard and Robin Curtis. Activities include gaming, a dealers' room, an art show and auction, a masquerade, a costume contest, a video room, and a charity auction. Registration: $40/weekend. Single-day rates are available. Send an SASE to: CONTINUUM '93, 1617 Lyndhurst, Cape Girardeau MO 63701; or call: (314) 334-4386.

G.A.M.CON '93, June 18-20　　　　IL

This convention will be held at the Day's Inn in Quincy, Ill. Events include role-playing, board, and miniatures games. Other activities include a dealers' area. Write to: Andy Bowen, 7 Whispering Oaks, Quincy IL 62301; or call: (217) 228-2556.

GLATHRICON '93, June 18-20　　　IN

This convention will be held at the Executive Inn in Evansville, Ind. Events include AD&D®, MARVEL SUPER HEROES™, SHADOWRUN*, and CHILL* games. Other activities include an art show and auction a masquerade, panels, dealers, and a charity event for the American Cancer Society. Registration: $20. Write to: GLATHRICON, c/o Evansville Gaming Guild, P.O. Box 15414, Evansville IN 47716; or call: (812) 477-9508.

HEXACON III, June 18-20　　　　　AZ

This convention will be held at the Camelview Resort in Scottsdale, Ariz. Events include role-playing, board, and miniatures gaming. Other activities include a miniatures-painting contest, a game auction, dealers, anime, panels, guests, and computer gaming. Registration: $10 preregistered; $15 at the door. Write to: HEXACON, P.O. Box 62613, Phoenix AZ 85082; or call: (602) 497-9554.

MICHICON '93, June 18-20　　　　MI

This convention will be held at the Southfield Civic Center in Southfield, Mich. Events include board, role-playing, and miniatures games. Other activities include a dealers' room. Registration: $16/weekend or $9/day preregistered; $18/weekend or $10/day at the door. Write to: Metro Detroit Gamers, M-93 Pre-reg., P.O. Box 656, Wyandotte MI 48192.

NEW ORLEANS SF & FANTASY FESTIVAL
June 18-20　　　　　　　　　　　LA

This convention will be held at the Clarion hotel in New Orleans, La. Guests include Robert Silverberg, Walter Jon Williams, George Alec Effinger, and Aaron Allston. Activities include 24-hour open gaming. Write to: NOSF3 1993, P.O. Box 791089, New Orleans LA 70179-1089; or call: (504) 837-0125.

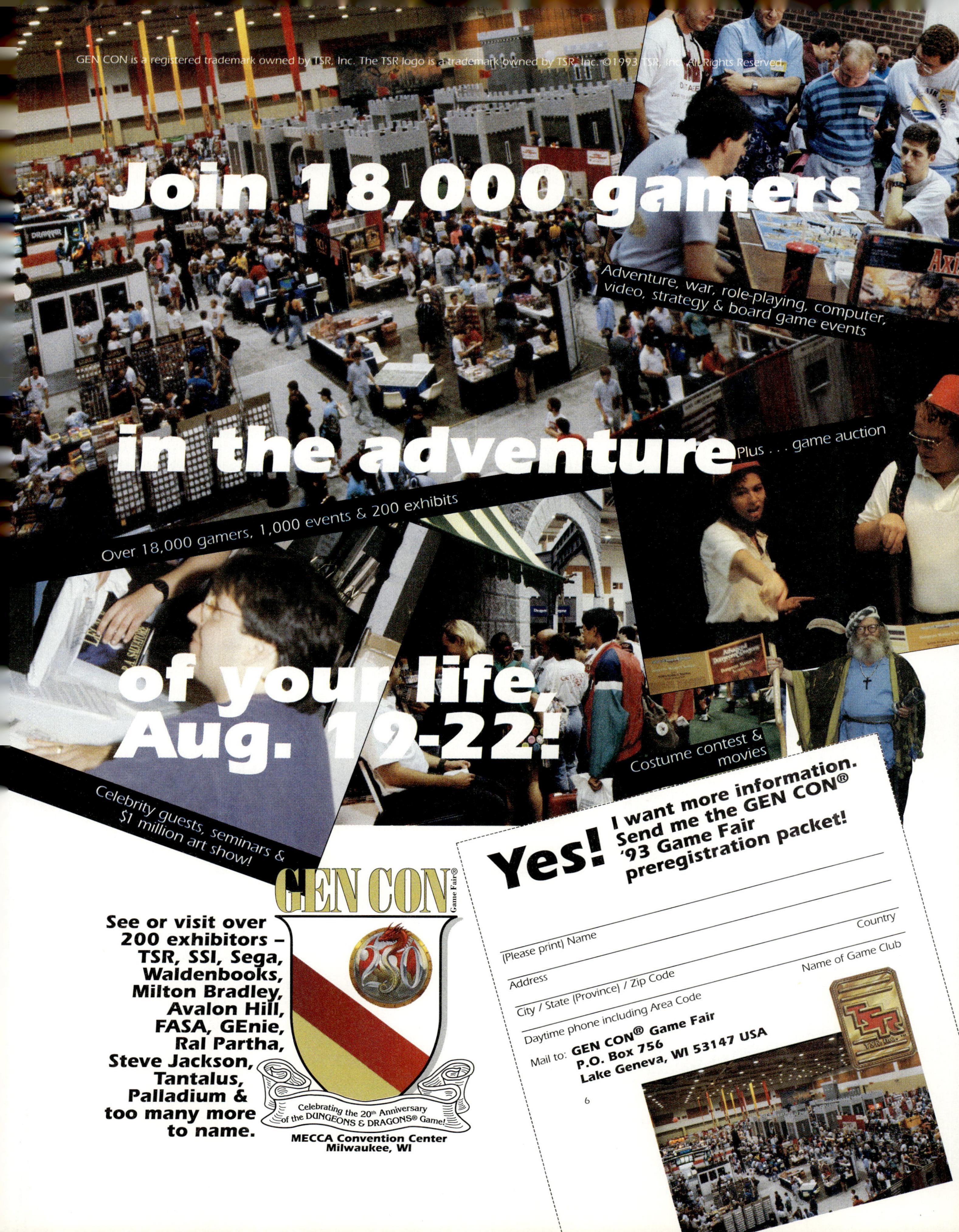

GEN CON is a registered trademark owned by TSR, Inc. The TSR logo is a trademark owned by TSR, Inc. ©1993 TSR, Inc. All Rights Reserved.

Join 18,000 gamers

Adventure, war, role-playing, computer, video, strategy & board game events

in the adventure

Plus . . . game auction

Over 18,000 gamers, 1,000 events & 200 exhibits

of your life, Aug. 19-22!

Costume contest & movies

Celebrity guests, seminars & $1 million art show!

GEN CON
Game Faire®

Celebrating the 20th Anniversary of the DUNGEONS & DRAGONS® Game!

MECCA Convention Center
Milwaukee, WI

See or visit over 200 exhibitors –
TSR, SSI, Sega, Waldenbooks, Milton Bradley, Avalon Hill, FASA, GEnie, Ral Partha, Steve Jackson, Tantalus, Palladium & too many more to name.

Yes! I want more information. Send me the GEN CON® '93 Game Fair preregistration packet!

(Please print) Name   Country

Address   Name of Game Club

City / State (Province) / Zip Code

Daytime phone including Area Code

Mail to: GEN CON® Game Fair
P.O. Box 756
Lake Geneva, WI 53147 USA

6

RIVERCON '93, June 18-20 — OH

This convention will be held at the campus of the University of Cincinnati, College of Applied Science in Cincinnati, Ohio. Events include role-playing, miniatures, computer, and board games. Other activities include a dealers' area, open gaming, and door prizes. Registration: $15. Write to: RPS RIVERCON, Univ. of Cincinnati, College of Applied Science, 2220 Victory Pkwy., Cincinnati OH 45206; or call: (513) 232-6213.

ST. JOSEPH VALLEY GAMERS' CON '93 June 18-19 — IN

This convention will be held at the IUSB campus in South Bend, Ind. Events include role-playing, board, and historical and fantasy miniatures games. Other activities include dealers, demos, a flea market, raffles, contests, and door prizes. Send an SASE to: St. Joseph Valley Gamers, 121 W. Colfax, South Bend IN 46601.

WYVERCON '93, June 18-20 — WA

This convention will be held at the Skagit Valley Fairgrounds in Mount Vernon, Wash. Events include a wide variety of role-playing and board games. Other activities include a miniatures-painting contest, videos, door prizes and a dealers' room. Registration: $20. Daily rates are available. Write to: WYVERCON, P.O. Box 2325, Mount Vernon WA 98273; or call Larianne or Todd: (206) 428-5900.

VEGASCON III, June 26-27 — NV

This gaming/SF/comics convention will be held at the Sahara hotel in Las Vegas, Nev. Activities include RPG tournaments, videos, panels, auctions, dealers, and 24-hour open gaming. Registration: $20. Write to: VEGASCON, 1149 E. Desert Inn Rd. #9039, Las Vegas NV 89109; or call: (702) 658-0667.

ORIGINS '93, July 1-4 — TX

This convention will be held at the Tarrant County Convention Center in Ft. Worth, Texas. Events include hundreds of gaming events, numerous seminars by industry notables, a huge game auction, and over 200 exhibitor booths. Write to: GEMCO, P.O. Box 609, Randallstown MD 21133.

ALOHA CON '93, July 3-4 — HI

This convention will be held at the AIEA High School on Oahu. Events include historical demonstration, an "artist alley," costume and miniatures-painting contests, a charity raffle, an auction, and miniatures, board, and role-playing games including RPGA™ Network events. Registration: $3/day or $5/weekend. Write to: Just For Fun, 4510 Salt Lake Blvd., Ste. B8, Honolulu HI 96819.

NAMELESS CON '93, July 3 — ✪

This convention will be held at the Victoria Hall, Sheepcote Rd., Harrow, Middlesex, England. Events include many role-playing games including RPGA™ Network events. Registration: £4. Write to: Darrell Impey, c/o 104 Dorchester Waye, Hayes, Middlesex, UB4 0HY, UNITED KINGDOM.

ARCANACON XI, July 8-11 — ★

This convention will be held at Collingwood College in Melbourne. Activities include a wide variety of role-playing game events. Write to: ARCANACON, P.O. Box 125, Parkville 3052, AUSTRALIA; or call Fraser at: (03) 380 5016.

IV-KHAN, July 9-10 — CO

This convention will be held at the Holiday Inn North in Colorado Springs, Colo. Guest of honor is John Stith. Activities include gaming, movies, a dealers' room, a miniatures-painting contest, an art show, and an author's banquet. Registration: $15 until July 4; $20 thereafter. There are $1 game fees. Write to: Miniatures Wargaming Guild, 695 S. 8th St. #55, Colorado Springs CO 80905; or call Perry at: (719) 630-8332.

DOVERCON IX, July 10-11 — NH

This convention will be held at the University of New Hampshire's Memorial Union Building in Durham, N.H. Guests include Barbara Young, editor of DUNGEON® Adventures. Activities include RPGA™ Network events and other role-playing, board, and war games, plus seminars, art, costume, and miniatures-painting contests, and a dealers' room. Registration: $15 preregistered; $20 at the door. Single-day rates will be available at the door. Write to: DOVERCON, P.O. Box 753, Dover NH 03820.

FARCON '93, July 16-18 — AR

This convention will be held at the Fayetteville, Ark., Hilton hotel. Activities include tournament and open gaming, an art show and auction, a costume contest, a 24-hour video room, dealers, and door prizes. Registration: $10/weekend preregistered; $15/weekend at the door (single-day passes are also available). Write to: FARCON, P.O. Box 2022 Station One, U. of A., Fayetteville AR 72701; or call Jesse at: (501) 521-1000, ext. 482.

KINGCON '93, July 16-18 — ✳

This SF/fantasy/gaming convention will be held at the Delta Brunswick hotel in Saint John, N.B. Events include gaming, a costume contest, an art show and auction, and seminars on writing, virtual reality, computer gaming, and haunted houses. Registration: $20 (Canadian) until July 1; $25 (Canadian) thereafter. Write to: KINGCON, MPO Box 1212, Saint John, N.B., CANADA E2L 4G7; or call: (902) 542-1798.

GRAND GAME CON '93, July 17 — MI

This convention will be held at American Legion Post #179 in Grand Rapids, Mich. Events include board, war, and role-playing games. Registration: $5 preregistered; $7 at the door. Write to: Will Holden, 1023 California N.W., Grand Rapids MI 49504; or call: (616) 454-0112.

STAFFCON '93, July 18 — ✪

This convention will be held on the Staffordshire University campus-Stafford. Guests include Terry Pratchett. Activities include role-playing and on-line games, plus merchants. Prizes will be awarded to competition winners. Registration: £25 including meals, £2 admission fee at the door. Write to: Chris Grice, c/o S.U. Office, Staffordshire Univ., Beaconside, Stafford, ST18 0AD, ENGLAND; or call: (0785) 211738.

IMPACT 3, July 23-25 — NE

This convention will be held at the Holiday Inn Old Mill in Omaha, Neb. Guests include Larry Niven, Marion Zimmer Bradley, and Lucy Synk. Activities include RPGA™ Network events, role-playing, miniatures, and board games, an art show and auction, videos, seminars, a masquerade, and dealers. Registration: $25. Write to: IMPACT 3, P.O. Box 4486, Omaha NE 68104-9998; or call Rahlyns at: (402) 345-9362.

You Wanted it —

You Got it!....!

Now running for FOUR DAYS!

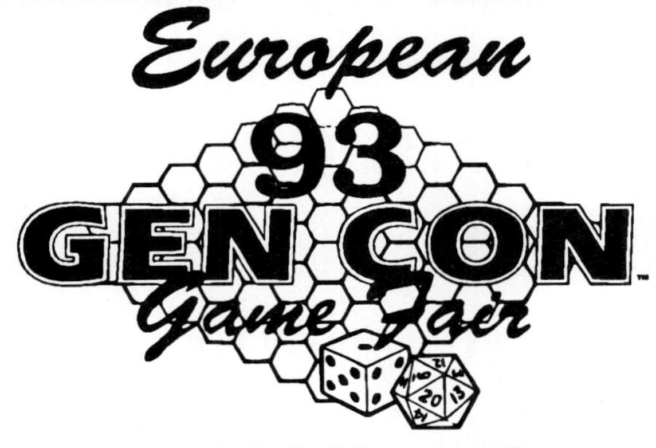

Everything you could want to play, learn and see about gaming under one roof! Come along for the weekend or .. for all four days! - How much can _you_ handle?

Contact TSR Limited now for your European GEN CON™ 1993 information pack on (International 44) 0223 212517 or write to 120 Church End, Cherry Hinton, Cambridge CB1 3LB, England to find out more!

OPERATION: GREEN FLAG '93
July 24-25   **PA**

This BATTLETECH*-only convention will be held at the Embers in Carlisle, Pa. Events include single and lance competitions, a miniatures-painting contest, gaming, and dealers. Registration costs vary. Write to: M. Foner's Games Only Emporium, 200 3rd St., New Cumberland PA 17070; or call: (717) 774-6676.

GAMEFEST '93 II, July 30-Aug. 1   **IL**

This convention will be held at Friends' Hobby Shop in Waukegan, Ill. Events include miniatures, role-playing, and board games. Write to: Friends' Hobby, 1411 Washington, Waukegan IL 60085; or call: (708) 336-0790.

WINDSOR GAMEFEST XI, July 30-Aug. 1   ✱

This convention will be held at the University of Windsor in Windsor, Ontario. Guests include Richard Tucholka. Activities include board and role-playing games, prizes, special events, contests and movies. Registration: $7/day or $12/weekend preregistered; $8/day or $15/weekend at the door. Write to: Sandwich Postal Station, P.O. Box 7463 Windsor, Ontario, CANADA.

CANGAMES '93, July 30-Aug. 2   ✱

This convention will be held at the Citadel Inn in Ottawa, Ontario. Events include role-playing, miniatures, and board games. Other activities include an auction, dealers, movies, and 24-hour gaming. Write to: CANGAMES, P.O. Box 3358, Station D, Ottawa, Ontario, CANADA K1P 6H8.

GAMEFEST XIV, Aug. 4-8   **CA**

This convention will be held in Old Towne in San Diego, Calif. Events include role-playing, board, and miniatures games. Other activities include figure-painting contests and trivia. Registration: $20 before July 31; $30 at the door. Write to: GAMEFEST XIV, 3954 Harney St., San Diego CA 92110.

AVALONCON '93, Aug. 5-8   **MD**

This convention will be held at the Hunt Valley Inn in Baltimore, Md. All activities are Avalon Hill and Victory Games board games, with single and team events, demos, and special events for junior players. Write to: Don Greenwood, c/o The Avalon Hill Game Co., 4517 Hartford Rd., Baltimore MD 21214; or call: (301) 254-9200.

CUBICON '93, Aug. 6-8   **MI**

This convention will be held at the Recreations and Organizations Center on the University of Michigan-Dearborn campus. Events include role-playing and board games. Registration: $4/day or $7/weekend. GMs are welcome. Write to: CUBICON '93, c/o SF3, Room 210 ROC, 4901 Evergreen, Dearborn MI 48128; or call: (313) 593-5390.

KINGCON '93, Aug. 6-8   **OH**

This convention will be held on the University of Dayton campus. Events include role-playing, board, and miniatures games. Registration: $10 preregistered; $15 at the door. Write to: KINGCON, P.O. Box 71, Dayton OH 45401; or call: (513) 223-8973.

SUMMER GAMES '93, Aug. 7   **PA**

This convention will be held at the Fire Hall in Kenhorst, Pa. Events include many role-playing game events. Registration: $7. Write to: SUMMER GAMES, c/o Nathaniel Lee Fischer, 516 March St., Shillington PA 19607; or call Nathaniel at: (215) 775-1548.

CAMELOT V, Aug. 13-15   **AL**

This convention will be held at the Tom Bevill Center on the University of Alabama-Huntsville campus. Guests include David "Zeb" Cook and Troy Denning. Activities include RPG events, dealers, videos, and open gaming. Registration: $20 preregistered; $25 at the door. Write to: SAGA, P.O Box 14242, Huntsville AL 35815-0242; or call: (205) 461-8827.

GOLD CON II, Aug. 14   **NJ**

This convention will be held at the American Legion Post in Clark, N.J. Events include role-playing, miniatures, board, and RPGA™ Network events. Other activities include a miniatures-painting contest. Registration: $8 before July 31; $10 at the door. There are no event fees. Write to: AU Gamers, P.O. Box 81, Whippany NJ 07981; or call: (201) 402-9239.

1993 GEN CON® Game Fair
Aug. 19-22   **WI**

For more information on the world's greatest game fair, turn to page 48!

BUBONICON 25, Aug. 20-22   **NM**

This convention will be held at the Howard Johnson Lodge in Albuquerque, N.M. Guests include Kevin J. Anderson and Robert C. Cornett. Activities include gaming, panels, signings, movies, a masquerade, an art show, an auction, hucksters, and filking. Registration: $21 before July 31; $24 at the door. Write to: NMSF Conference, P.O. Box 37257, Albuquerque NM 87176; or call: (505) 266-8905. No collect calls, please.

Important: To ensure that your convention listing makes it into our files, enclose a self-addressed stamped postcard with your first convention notice; we will return the card to show that your notice was received. You might also send a second notice one week after mailing the first. Mail your listing as early as possible, and always keep us informed of any changes. Please avoid sending convention notices by fax, as this method has not proved to be reliable.

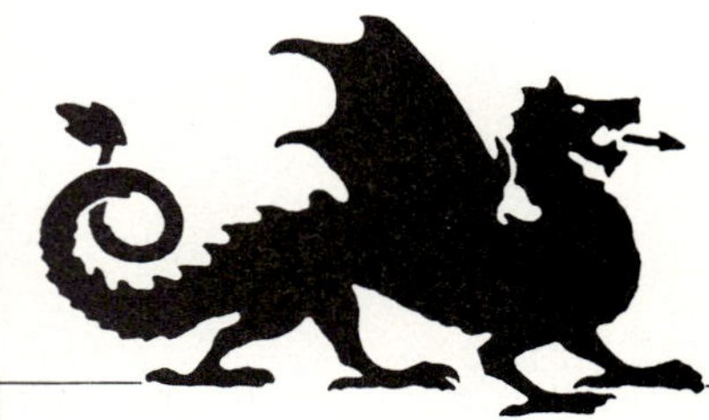

Give us the word!

What do you think of this magazine? What do you like best or want to see changed most? What do you want to see next? Turn to "Letters" and see what others think, then write to us, too!

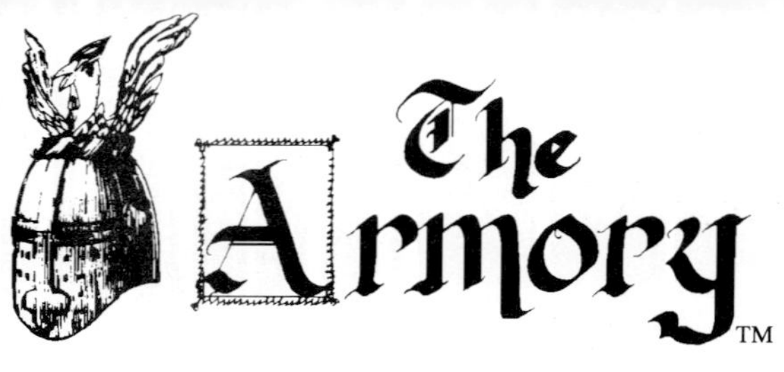

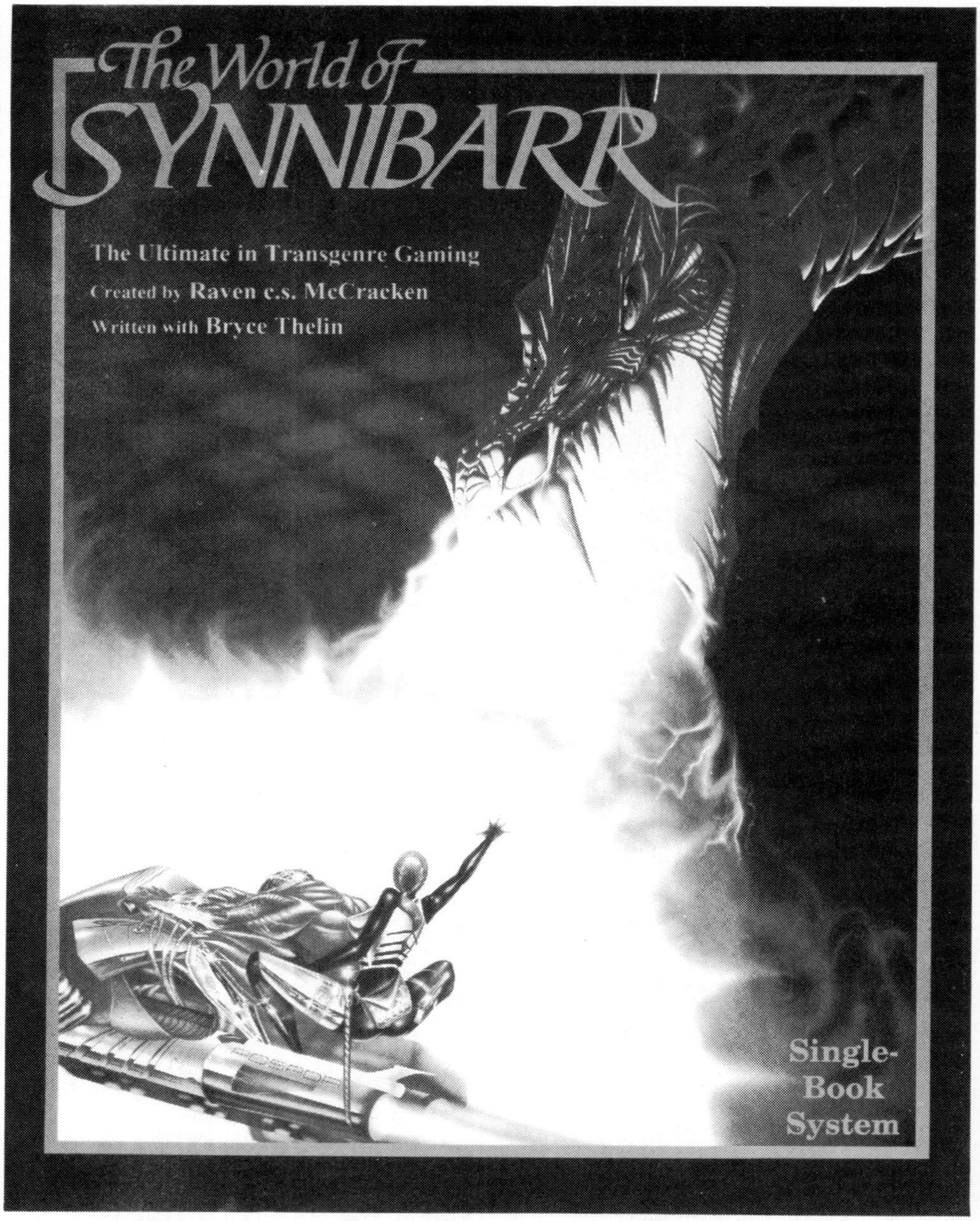

Tired of being forced to buy book after book to play a game? Equally frustrated with gaming systems that limit not only your imagination but your character's abilities as well?

If the answer to any of these questions is yes, then welcome to *The World of Synnibarr*, the ultimate in transgenre gaming, which contains all the necessary rules to play the game within one single comprehensive book.

The planet Synnibarr is in reality a starship created by the god Aridius from the planet Mars. It was transformed into an ark to carry the descendants of Earth to a new home star system to save them from a galactic holocaust.

The World of Synnibarr was created to put life back into gaming. The system covers the specifics for all types of play, from fantasy to science fiction and combinations of both, even warfare within dreams. The game is a complete system that maintains a balance of rules while allowing you the versatility of exploring your own horizons. Within this book's pages is an entire universe at your fingertips, waiting to be explored.

AVAILABLE NOW! $29.95

(800) NOW-GAME • (410) 764-8100

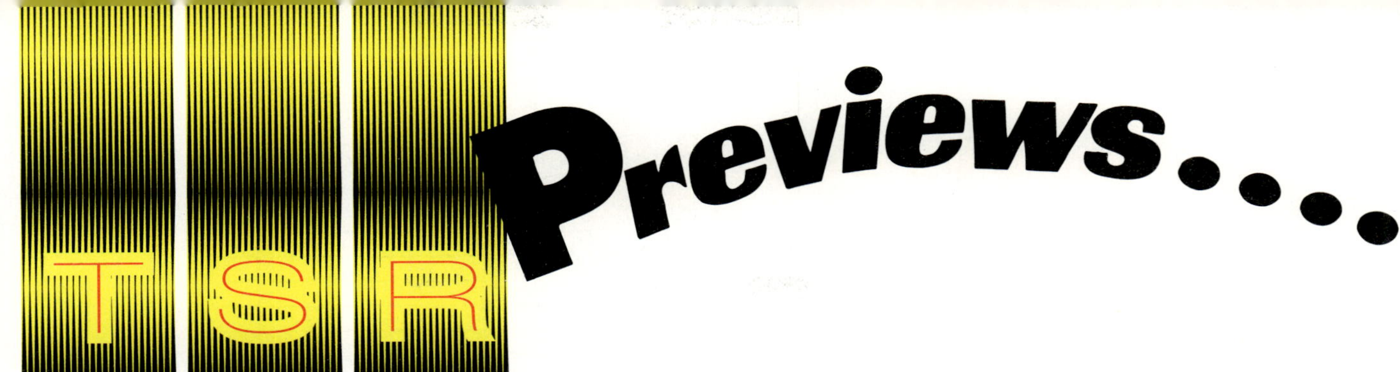

NEW PRODUCTS FOR JUNE

For Faerie, Queen, and Country game
The AMAZING ENGINE™ system
by David "Zeb" Cook

The first in a brand-new game line, this package contains the 32-page core rulebook and the 128-page campaign book of the *For Faerie, Queen, and Country* world. The rulebook gives all the game system's basic rules, and the campaign book details the Victorian England where pixies, boggarts, red caps, and hobs lurk in the streets of London, not in the depths of superstition. Plus, the concept of a *player core* allows players to apply earned experience points to any of their characters, no matter which world they were created for.
$24.95 U.S./$29.95 CAN./£14.99 U.K.
TSR Product No.: 2705

BUGHUNTERS™ game
The AMAZING ENGINE™ system
by Lester Smith

The second world for the AMAZING ENGINE™ system, this 128-page SF setting of the BUGHUNTERS™ adventure world also comes packaged with a copy of the 32-page core rulebook. In the BUGHUNTERS™ setting, the player characters are Interstellar Marines who protect the frontiers of space from all varieties of unbelievable alien menaces. The *player core* concept allows the players to transfer experience earned in the *For Faerie, Queen, and Country* setting to better their BUGHUNTERS™ game characters, or vice-versa. Get in on the ground floor of this exciting, innovative new facet of role-playing games with the AMAZING ENGINE™ game system.
$24.95 U.S./$29.95 CAN./£14.99 U.K.
TSR Product No.: 2706

The Created
AD&D® game RAVENLOFT® module
by TSR staff

A bizarre puppet master pulls the strings in this introductory adventure for low-level player characters. A mad puppeteer has moved to a small village. By day, he runs a toyshop where he sells his creations. By night, however, he creates horrific, living puppets to spread his evil.
$6.95 U.S./$8.50 CAN./£4.50 U.K.
TSR Product No.: 9414

The Jungles of Chult
AD&D® game FORGOTTEN REALMS®
accessory
by James Lowder and Jean Rabe

This 64-page book leaves your campaign's PCs shipwrecked and washed ashore on the coast of Chult. The characters must travel through a land forgotten by time, learn the secrets to surviving there, and return home. Will the PCs reach their destination when tribes of natives and ferocious dinosaurs stand in their way?
$9.95 U.S./$11.95 CAN./£5.99 U.K.
TSR Product No.: 9389

NEW PRODUCTS FOR JULY

MCC1 Monstrous Manual
AD&D® game accessory
by TSR staff

This 384-page hardbound tome collects all the most popular AD&D® game monsters and creatures in one place. Included are virtually all the monsters from MC1 and MC2, plus many creatures from the FORGOTTEN REALMS®, DRAGONLANCE®, and WORLD OF GREYHAWK® *Monstrous Compendium* appendices. Some of the creatures have been revised to eliminate errors and typos, and each creature's entry also includes all-new, full-color art.
$24.95 U.S./$29.95 CAN./£14.99 U.K.
TSR Product No.: 2140

FORGOTTEN REALMS® Campaign Setting
AD&D® game revised boxed set
by Jeff Grubb and Ed Greenwood

Since the debut of the FORGOTTEN REALMS® setting in 1987, godly interventions, a Mongol invasion, and the discovery of new continents and cultures have changed the face of Toril. This new edition of the FORGOTTEN REALMS® boxed set pulls together everything that has happened and will act as the "hub" for all future Realms material. This boxed set includes three 96-page books, four poster maps, and 16 MC pages.
$29.95 U.S./$38.50 CAN./£17.99 U.K.
TSR Product No.: 1085

City of Delights
AD&D® game AL-QADIM™ game accessory
by Tim Beach

The mightiest city in the Land of Fate comes to life in this full-sized boxed set. Medina Al-Huzuz, the City of Delights, is the "Baghdad" of the Land of Fate. Detailed here are all the wonders of the city, from the daily lives of the common merchants to the exalted intrigues of the Grand Caliph and his court, harem, and viziers. This set includes two 96-page books, eight MC pages, and two poster maps—including the Grand Caliph's sprawling palace.
$20.00 U.S./$24.00 CAN./£11.99 U.K.
TSR Product No.: 1091

CGR2 The Complete Gladiator's Handbook
AD&D® game DARK SUN® accessory
by Colin McComb

Everything players want to know about gladiators—their lives, techniques, and weapons—is revealed in this 128-page book. This volume contains new kits, equipment, and never-before-published details on gladiators, the greatest warriors on the face of Athas.
$15.00 U.S./$18.00 CAN./£9.99 U.K.
TSR Product No.: 2419

RM2 Web of Illusions
AD&D® game RAVENLOFT® module
by Eric Haddock

Come to the land of Sri Raji, where the ancient rakshasa, the evil masters of illusion and shapeshifting, await you. This 64-page adventure features a perilous journey through the deadly domain inspired by East India, where savage tigers and lost temples abound in the steamy jungles.
$9.95 U.S./$11.95 CAN./£5.99 U.K.
TSR Product No.: 9415

Cardmaster Adventure Design Deck
AD&D® game boxed accessory
by Rich Borg

This attractively designed set makes setting up challenging adventures for group or solo play as easy as shuffling cards. These cards break down the often complex task of designing an adventure into simple techniques. This set includes over 200 full-color and black-and-white cards.
$18.00 U.S./$21.50 CAN./£12.99 U.K.
incl. VAT
TSR Product No.: 1090

In the Phantom's Wake
D&D® game module
by Dale "Slade" Henson

In this 16-page adventure, four to six player characters have found a strange, magical astrolabe rumored to have come from a haunted place. They accidentally trigger its power and find themselves transported aboard a magical, haunted skyship.
$6.95 U.S./$8.50 CAN./£4.50 U.K.
TSR Product No.: 9436

Carnival of Fear
RAVENLOFT™ novel
by J. Robert King

A murder has occurred along the sideshow boardwalk of the Carnival l'Morai. Three of the carnival performers decide to track down the killer. Their investigation leads to more murders and the discovery of an evil conspiracy. Soon, they too are marked for death.
$4.95 U.S./$5.95 CAN./£3.99 U.K.
TSR Product No.: 8061

Hammer and Axe
Dwarven Nations trilogy, Volume Two
by Dan Parkinson

The humans of Ergoth threaten Thorbardin, but the intense differences between the dwarven clans result in warring cultures. The hill dwarves leave their homeland and become a renegade clan, dwelling aboveground. They soon become the most energetic and forward-looking of the clans, but they still cannot avoid the political intrigue that threatens to tear them apart.
$4.95 U.S./$5.95 CAN./£3.99 U.K.
TSR Product No.: 8350

Role-playing Reviews

©1993 by Rick Swan

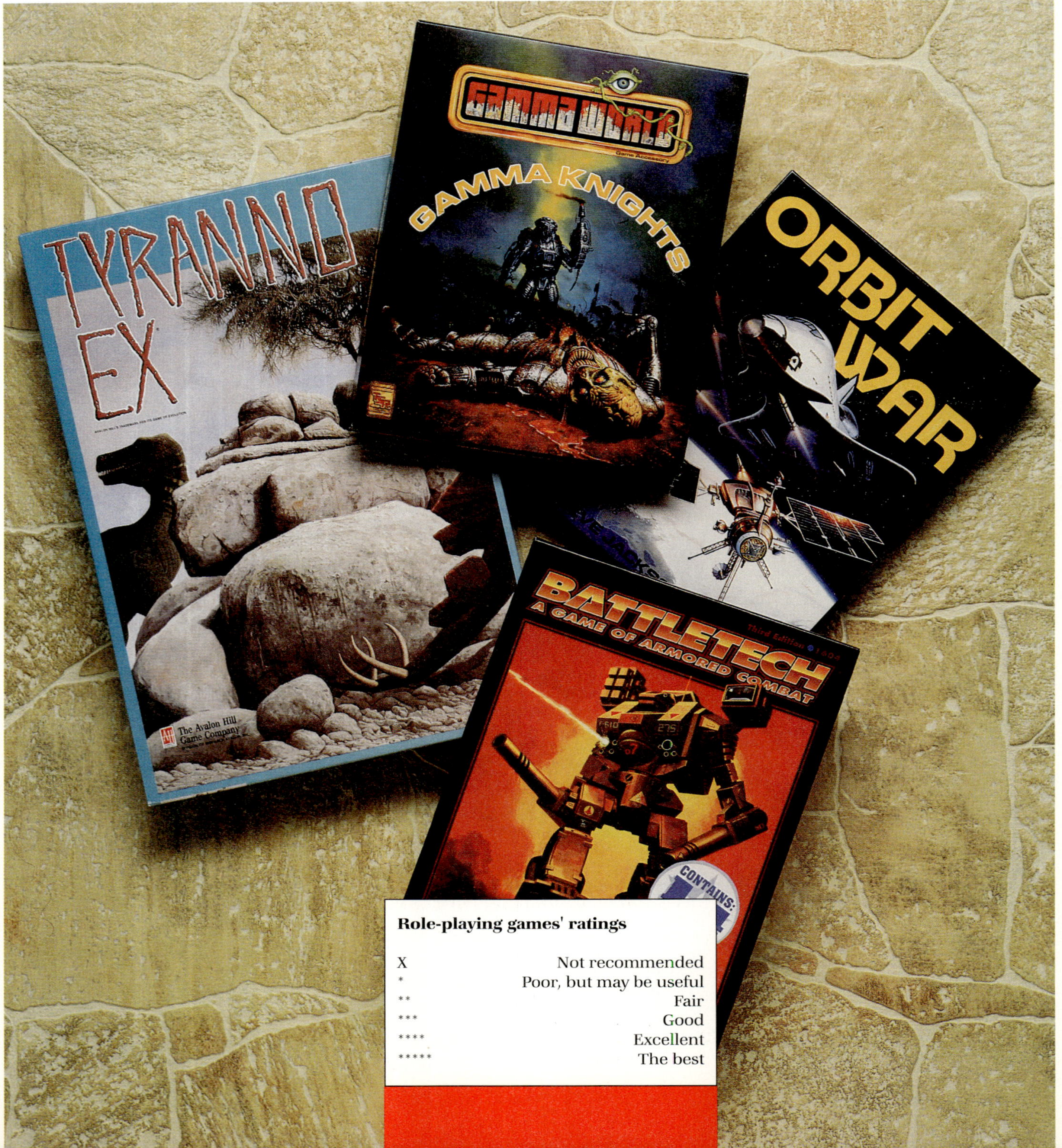

Role-playing games' ratings

X	Not recommended
*	Poor, but may be useful
**	Fair
***	Good
****	Excellent
*****	The best

Feeling powerless?
Recharge yourself with these science-fiction games

Friday was a miserable day. My cat threw up all over the carpet in my office, my accountant called to tell me I owed $700 in extra taxes, and my computer ate the first draft of this column. To top it all off, I discovered my wife had taped over the first four episodes of *Deep Space Nine* that I'd been waiting two months to see.

For relief, I turned to the stack of science-fiction games I'd been saving for just such an occasion. I spent the weekend stomping pip-squeaks with giant robots, blowing away mutants with torc grenades, and scorching the Earth with nuclear missiles. By Sunday night, I was manipulating the environment to engineer the extinction of entire species.

By Monday morning, I felt *much* better.

BATTLETECH* third-edition game *****

Boxed game with one 56-page rulebook, one 16-page record sheet booklet, two 22"×17" map sheets, 14 plastic miniatures, two six-sided dice
FASA Corporation $25
Design: Jordan K. Weisman, L. Ross Babcock, and Sam Lewis
Development: Michael Nystul
Editing: Donna Ippolito and Sharon Turner Mulvihill
Art director: Jeff Laubenstein
Cover: Alan Guitierrez and Jim Nelson

Perhaps the most durable science-fiction game of the last decade, FASA's BATTLETECH* game is one of those why-didn't-I-think-of-that concepts that keeps game designers awake at night, gnashing their teeth and slapping their foreheads. And no wonder. The basic idea—gargantuan robots, operated by human pilots, meet on bleak terrain to bash each others' mechanical brains out—could've been dreamed up by an imaginative 10-year-old. But what might have been just another clever premise became a gaming milestone, thanks to brilliant mechanics, flawless execution, and nearly a decade of refinement. Appallingly addictive, this game is no mere diversion but a hobby unto itself.

While the previous version was a class act (reviewed in DRAGON® issue #131), the third edition (here called "BATTLETECH Three") stands as the definitive treatment, a handsome upgrade worth the purchase price even for owners of the old editions. The package includes a pair of attractive color maps, a pack of record sheets (clutter-free and a joy to use), and—best of all—2" plastic miniatures of Thunderbolt, Battlemaster, and a dozen other BattleMech war machines. Meticulously detailed right down to Rifle-man's detachable autocannons and Locust's pincer feet, I half-expected them to march off the table and take over the house.

I've heard skeptics grumble that the BATTLETECH system is less than user-friendly, what with its emphasis on war-gaming concepts and endless expansion sets. BATTLETECH Three clears the decks and starts from scratch, presenting the fundamentals in clear, simple language. The lavishly illustrated rulebook leads newcomers through a series of four "Training Exercise" scenarios that introduce the rules in bite-size chunks. Players choose their BattleMechs, locate the corresponding record sheets, then deploy the plastic figures on the map sheet as directed by the scenario. A turn begins with the players determining Initiative by rolling 2d6. The player who loses the Initiative roll moves first. The record sheets indicate movement allowances for each 'Mech type; the Locust can spend 8 points to walk or 12 points to run, while the Griffin can spend 5 points to walk, 8 points to run, or 5 points to leap like a kangaroo. Extra points may be spent to navigate hostile terrain or change facing.

Following movement, the 'Mechs attack, utilizing a devastating battery of weapons attached to various parts of their exoskeletons. The relatively benign Locust comes equipped with a chest-mounted laser beam and two machine guns where its arms ought to be. The Crusader, which looks like a cross between an offensive lineman and a jackhammer, sports missile launchers in its legs, plus a half-dozen additional weapons sprouting all over its armored shell. Each weapon has distance limits and to-hit numbers for short, medium, and long ranges. A machine gun, for instance, has a short range of one hex and a long range of three hexes. To make a successful machine-gun assault at short range, the attacker must roll a 4 or better; at long range, he must roll at least an 8. The to-hit number may be modified by movement (+2 if either the attacker or defender was running) and terrain (+1 if light woodland conceals the target).

If an attack hits, the attacker rolls on the Hit Location Table to determine which part of the defender was damaged. The defender notes damage by filling in the appropriate number of dots on the armor diagram of his record sheet. If a successful machine gun attack inflicted two points of damage on the left arm of a Locust, the defending player fills in two of the four dots on the left arm. If all the dots of a particular area have been filled, excess damage may be transferred to other areas of the 'Mech, as indicated by the Damage Transfer Diagram (excess damage to the left arm is transferred to the left torso). When no more damage can be transferred, the affected location is disabled; all weapons in that area become inert. If a leg was eliminated, the 'Mech is immobilized. 'Mechs continue moving and attacking until one 'Mech bites the dust or a fixed number turns have passed. Whoever does the most damage wins.

By the third training scenario, a MechWarrior (the BattleMech pilot) has learned to twist his 'Mech's torso to improve its aim and maneuver a fallen 'Mech back to its feet. MechWarriors must also contend with heat build-up, which can cause a 'Mech to shut down if not closely monitored. Virtually every action creates heat; walking generates one heat point per turn, while firing an autocannon can generate as many as seven. Though a 'Mech's heat sinks absorb some of these points, the excess must be noted on the record sheet's Heat Scale by marking off the appropriate number of boxes. As the Heat Scale rises, the 'Mech suffers a variety of adverse affects. At 5 on the scale, the 'Mech loses a movement point. At 14, it shuts down unless the player rolls a 4 or better. At 23, the 'Mech suffers an ammunition explosion—which zaps the pilot with two points of electrical feedback damage—unless the player rolls at least a 6.

In the final scenario, the player must roll for a critical hit whenever his 'Mech suffers internal damage. A roll of 8 or more refers the player to the Critical Hit Table on his record sheet, with subsequent rolls indicating the specific types of damage. Critical hits range from a disabled leg actuator to a blown-off head, which instantly kills the MechWarrior inside. The advanced rules encourage Mechs to supplement their weapon attacks with physical assaults, such as punches, pushes, and kicks. My favorite tactic is to beat an enemy 'Mech over the head with its own detached arm.

Most combat games tend to bog down in a morass of modifiers and tables long before the players make their way through the advanced rules—but not this one. Because of the bare-bone mechanics and logical presentation, BATTLETECH game players can concentrate on studying the game map instead of the rulebook. Most attacks boil down to pair of dice throws, and attentive players should have the relevant tables memorized after one trip through the training scenarios.

Any quibbles? Just a few. If an attack has an equal chance of hitting two different sides of a 'Mech, the defender gets to pick which side take the damage. Wouldn't it make more sense to resolve

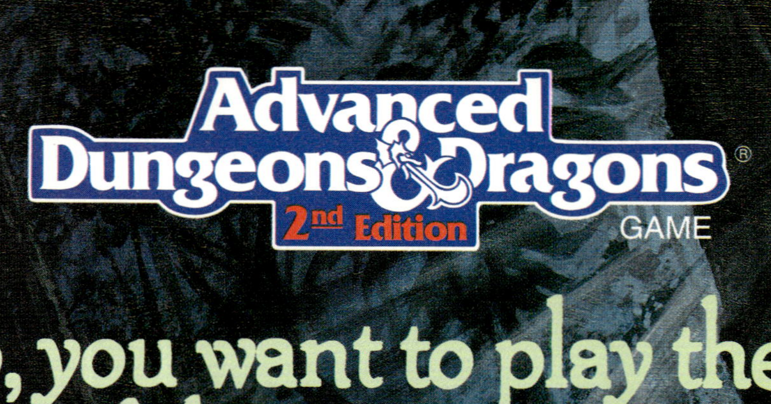

So, you want to play the role of the monsters...

Go right ahead! PHBR10 *The Complete Book of Humanoids* describes in detail over 20 humanoid races that can be run as player characters — from mischievous pixies to stubborn minotaurs, lizard-like saurials to the savage half-ogre — and many more in-between! New proficiencies, humanoid kits, unusual equipment, and a few surprises that open realms of adventure within any ongoing AD&D® game campaign also are featured. Don't miss *The Complete Book of Humanoids*, available now at book, game, and hobby stores everywhere!

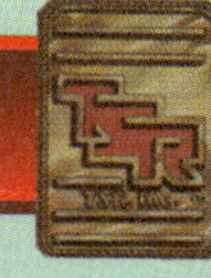

this randomly? I find it hard to swallow that machines this sophisticated can't target specific areas for their attacks; why can't a skilled pilot aim for the head or arm rather than leaving it up to a Hit Location Table? And the maps may be functional, but they're dull. How come the backs of the maps have blank hexes instead of terrain?

Evaluation: As if terrific rules, an evocative concept, and a stunning package weren't enough, the BATTLETECH game boasts one of the hobby's richest settings. Hundreds of years in the future, a once-united Star League has splintered into five Successor States engaged in a violent struggle for control of the cosmos. A group of elite warriors handles much of the front-line combat, waging war in their BattleMechs throughout the Inner Sphere. FASA has explored the ramifications of the Succession Wars in a staggering number of supplements, novels, and expansion sets, with no end in sight.

Where do you go next? After you've mastered the BATTLETECH game, I recommend moving on to the MECHWAR-RIOR second-edition game (reviewed in DRAGON issue #183) for its extensive role-playing rules. Then take a look at the *Technical Readout* series, which features descriptions and statistics for dozens of 'Mech variants; *Technical Readout: 3055* (FASA, $15) has some especially nasty ones. The deluxe *Solaris VII* box (reviewed in DRAGON issue #185) contains a tantalizing assortment of new maps, combat rules, and personalities. I also suggest you make plenty of copies of the BATTLETECH record sheets. You'll be playing this a long time.

GAMMA KNIGHTS game   ***½

Boxed game with one 16-page rulebook, one 32-page sourcebook, one double-sided 32"×21" map sheet, one sheet of reference tables, 24 die-cut playing pieces, 24 plastic stands, 208 cardboard counters, four 10-sided dice
TSR, Inc. $20
Design: Steve Winter and Slade Henson
Editing: Steve Winter
Illustrations: Mark Nelson
Cover: Fred Fields

With the possible exception of the BULLWINKLE AND ROCKY™ game (reviewed in DRAGON issue #144), the GAMMA WORLD® game remains TSR's most eccentric design. Apocalyptic role-playing for the deranged, the GAMMA WORLD game takes place in a war-ravaged future populated by giant rabbits, friendly robots, and talking plants. Players assume the roles of mutant grasshoppers and sentient fungi, with a few ordinary humans tossed in for good measure. Though great fun for the open-minded, this game may be a bit too weird for those demanding at least the pretense of science in their science fiction.

Hard-liners, then, should welcome the GAMMA KNIGHTS supplement, a more or less straightforward tactical military game that nudges the GAMMA WORLD game back in the direction of reality. Gamma Knights—no relation to the hateful Knights of Genetic Purity from the GAMMA WORLD rulebook—comprise an order of free-lance warriors outfitted in elaborate power suits left over from the wars of centuries past. Nobody seems to get along, so even casual encounters tend to erupt into violence. Hence the game's simple premise: Opponents duel to the death on barren landscapes in sort of a pint-size version of a BATTLETECH campaign.

The GAMMA KNIGHTS game, however, opts for more sophisticated and complicated game mechanics than in the BATTLETECH game. As in the latter game, players begin by locating the playing pieces (cardboard counters with plastic bases) representing their units, then gather their record sheets and deploy the pieces on the map as indicated by the scenario. But the resemblance to BATTLETECH games pretty much ends there. Before starting play, players have the option of drawing up to four systems markers from a cup, which grant random bonuses and penalties to the Knights' equipment. The Heavy Armor marker, for instance, allows the Knight to ignore the first hit made against his power suit, while the Fragile Weapon marker increases the first hit made against a weapon by 1. The system markers set the tone of the game, which emphasizes unexpected complications and a parade of variables.

Players move and attack by expending Action Points (APs). Each Knight has a fixed number of APs depending on his armor type—e.g., Assault Armor provides 8 APs, while Powered Plate Armor supplies only 4. The first player, determined by the scenario instead of an initiative roll, decides whether his Knights operate in Attack Mode or Movement Mode during the current turn. Attack Mode Knights begin the turn with an Initial Fire Phase, making as many attacks as their AP totals allow (each weapon attack costs 2 APs, a sensor attack costs 1). Units that don't make an initial attack are considered to be in the Movement Mode.

In the Movement Phase, which follows the Initial Attack Phase, Movement Mode Knights can expend as many APs as they like to move; it costs 1 AP to enter an open hex, 2 APs to enter a building. Some Knights also can fly, expending 1 AP per hex when airborne. Attack Mode Knights may move only a single hex during the Movement Phase. During the Terminal Fire Phase, Movement Mode Knights can make a single attack; Attack Mode Knights sit tight. The turn ends with the Recovery Phase, where the first player repairs damaged equipment, revives stunned units, and regenerates force fields. The second player then repeats all four steps, and the turn ends. A player wins by meeting the scenario's victory conditions, which usually require him to eliminate the other side.

Unsurprisingly, most of the rulebook is devoted to combat. The basics are simple enough—you merely compare the combatants' strength ratings and cross-index the result on the Attack Table—but finding those strength ratings in the first place requires some serious calculator time. The attacker's strength, for instance, equals the sum of the primary sensor value, secondary sensor value, weapon strength, and a 2d10 roll (1d10, if attacking in the Terminal Fire Phase). Totalling the defender's force field rating, armor number, and terrain value gives the defensive strength. Other factors include range, line of sight, and attack type (saturation, pinpoint, or close). Special cases require additional rules: A unit subjected to pinpoint or saturation fire has his attack strength reduced by two, rolling doubles gives the attacker an extra attack die, sensor locks can be lost four different ways . . . you get the idea. Players draw markers from a cup to determine if successful attacks hit weapons, systems, or armor sections, and whether they suffer light or heavy damage.

Though there are a lot of numbers to juggle, the sheer variety of variables keeps combat encounters unpredictable and fresh. Weapons range from high-tech gadgetry (such as the black ray pistol, which can vaporize an enemy in a single shot) to a delightfully anachronistic arsenal straight out of the Middle Ages—picture a robotic desperado with a heavy crossbow in one hand and a whip in the other. Over a dozen armor options are available, along with 16 pages of instructions for designing original models. The six scenarios, including a challenging solitaire showdown with the Iron Society, are imaginatively staged and well balanced.

The GAMMA KNIGHTS game suffers from a few lapses in logic, none of them game-breakers but puzzling all the same. A Knight spends 1 AP to enter an open hex, regardless of whether he's on the ground or airborne; he must be running like an antelope or flying in slow motion. Air and ground movement can't be combined in the same turn, even though there's ample time to do both (one turn represents a full minute). For no apparent reason other than dramatic effect, opponents instantly regain their allotment of APs when they begin close combat, regardless of how many points were spent moving into the contested hex. And the rules encourage lengthy, sometimes interminable, combat encounters; I'd suggest speeding things up by suspending the rule that allows force fields to regenerate automatically.

Evaluation: Familiarity with the GAMMA WORLD game isn't required for playing a GAMMA KNIGHTS session. In fact, the latter works better as a stand-alone game than as a role-playing supplement. (How often do Knights pop up in a typical campaign, anyway? And what are the other characters supposed to do while the Knights spend an hour or so whacking each other?) On its own terms, the GAMMA KNIGHTS set succeeds as a new approach to tactical combat, combining traditional mechanics with some appealing quirks. While I miss the whimsical touches that make the GAMMA WORLD game so much fun, there's plenty of room for expansion. Fightin' fungi, anyone?

ORBIT WAR* game   **½

Boxed game with one 12-page rulebook, one "Quick Start" rules sheet, one 22"×17" mounted map, 390 counters, ziplock bag, two six-sided dice
Steve Jackson Games $25
Design: Wallace Wang
Development: Steve Jackson
Counter graphics: J. David George
Cover: Alan Gutierrez

Steve Jackson first launched the ORBIT WARS game back in 1983, including it as a bonus in issue #66 of *Space Gamer* magazine. That version featured components you could store in a business envelope, including a cheesy paper map and dinky little cardboard counters that—if memory serves—had to be cut apart from the subscription card. Now it's back, this time as a classy boxed set with upscale production values and a price to match.

While the package has improved, the game itself hasn't changed much. Set in the year 2020, two players representing the United States and the Asian-Polish Union vie for control of Earth's skyways by engaging in satellite warfare, vaguely similar to what Ronald Reagan had in mind with his Strategic Defense Initiative (he *was* kidding, wasn't he?). Each side spends a fixed number of points on orbital rockets, space stations, and other self-powered hardware, then loads them up with mines and nuclear warheads. Once in orbit, they proceed to blast each other to oblivion. Satellites may also spew nukes at Mother Earth, leveling cities and incinerating an unsuspecting populace. Whoever does the most damage earns the most Victory Points and wins the game.

The action takes place on a hex map of outer space, designed as a series of 10 concentric "orbit lines" encircling a single-hex Earth. Orbiting units may move twice in a turn, once automatically and once voluntarily. Automatic movement represents the inherent motion of orbiting objects, requiring all units to move a fixed number of hexes along their orbit lines. The closer the orbit line is to Earth,

the more the satellite moves; satellites on the outermost line move one hex per three turns, while those on the innermost line move four hexes *every* turn. Voluntary movement represents a satellite's ability to move under its own power, indicated by the movement allowance on its counter. Satellites may move in any direction and may position themselves on different orbit lines to bring them closer to enemy units.

After both sides finish moving, opposing units attempt to blow each other up. Normal combat occurs between enemy satellites occupying the same hex. Units are also subject to attacks from space mines (orbiting booby-traps affecting multiple targets) and nuclear missiles (fired at targets two hexes away). To resolve combat, the attacker subtracts his unit's strength from that of the defender, then cross-indexes the result with a die-roll on the Combat Results Table. If the roll is high enough, the enemy unit disintegrates. Successful attacks against the Earth result in Victory Points rather than disintegration. (For visual appeal, we piled little cotton balls on the Earth hex to indicate the mounting carnage.)

The ORBIT WAR game would've been just another fly-'em-and-fry-'em board game if not for its inventive options. With 17 different units to choose from, players can experiment with an endless variety of fleets. Space Marines can spill from an ELR (Earth-Launched Rocket) to assault enemy satellites, supported by mine-laying shuttlecraft and orbital weapon platforms. Suicide satellites, detonated at the owner's discretion, can blow enemy space stations into the next galaxy. The advanced game includes rules for targeting nuclear attacks on industrial sites, inflicting damage on satellites instead of destroying them outright, and repairing inoperative equipment.

However, while the rules are clever, they're often a pain to execute. Adjusting the positions of all the orbiting satellites gets awfully tedious awfully fast, especially in the advanced scenarios where dozens of counters may be on the board at the same time. Bland counter graphics makes it hard to distinguish one unit from another. There's far too much bookkeeping for a premise this humble, as players must keep track of their missile launchings, mine deployment, and reinforcement allocations on paper. Common sense also takes a few lumps. If an exploding mine can pick and choose which units in its hex are affected, why can't an exploding suicide satellite? How come you have to pay for satellites, but rockets and nuclear warheads are free? And how come all of this takes place in two-dimensional space?

Evaluation: I enjoyed the challenge of this game, but I had a hard time working up much enthusiasm after the first couple of plays. Despite the interesting premise,

the ORBIT WAR game lacks personality. It's intellectually engaging but not particularly memorable, like something Mr. Spock might use to amuse the kids on a slow day on the U.S.S. *Enterprise*. Whatever this game's pleasures, they don't come cheap. The ORBIT WARS game was a steal at $3.00 (the 1983 price, complete with a magazine), but at $25.00 you might want to stick to crossword puzzles.

TYRANNO EX* game   ****

Boxed game with one six-page rulebook, one 22"×16" mounted map, 32 playing cards, four cardboard screens, 160 counters, six six-sided dice
The Avalon Hill Game Company $35
Design: Karl-Heinz Schmiel
Development: Don Greenwood
Card and marker art: Dave Dobyski
Cover and map: Charlie Jarboe

We here at the testing center usually arrive at a consensus without too much dissent. Not so with the TYRANNO EX game, Avalon Hill's oddball board game about evolution and environmental survival. After one play, I was jumping up and down, screaming, "Five stars! A masterpiece!" Everyone else thought I was nuts. "Good, not great," they said. "Two stars, maybe three." Subsequent plays didn't affect their opinion, despite my reminding them that I'm always right.

We all agreed that the TYRANNO EX game was one of the most original designs we'd seen in a long time. Each player receives a stack of Animal Cards (representing the Stegosaurus, Iguanadon, or one of 26 other prehistoric creatures, with a colorful illustration on one side and a historical description on the other), a dozen Element Disks (depicting Fish, Water, Trees, and other environmental factors), and a Primeval World Track (a row of boxes on the game board symbolizing evolutionary advancement). A turn begins with the players selecting Animals from their respective decks and placing them in the first box of their Primeval World Tracks (PWTs). Players then attempt to manipulate the environment by placing Element Disks face-down in the Evolution Boxes adjacent to the PWTs. Using an ingenious system driven by bluffs, strategic positioning, and blind luck, players displace old Elements with new ones, competing to create environments favorable to their own Animals. After three to five rounds of Element displacement, the phase ends, with a particular Element dominating in each Track.

Every Animal has three Elements required for survival, indicated on its card; the Stegosaurus, for example, requires Brush, Sun, and Water. During the Element Displacement phase, if a player instigates a change that results in all three of an Animal's Elements domi-

nating in the Evolution Boxes, the Animal's strength increases by one. For the Stegosaurus, this means that Brush must dominate in one of the Evolution Boxes, Sun in another, and Water in a third. The owning player indicates the increased strength by placing a marker on the Stegosaurus's card. At the end of the Element displacement phase, any Animal that doesn't have at least *one* of its Elements dominating a PWT immediately becomes extinct and vanishes from the board.

Surviving Animals are subject to predator attacks in the Battle phase. The aggressor attacks with a number of dice equal to the number of disks in the Evolution Boxes corresponding to the Element symbols on its card (e.g., if there are three Suns and two Waters in the boxes, the Stegosaurus attacks with five dice). The defender's dice are determined the same way. Every die roll less than or equal to the Animal's strength counts as a hit. Whichever Animal scores the most hits wins the round. If an Animal wins two consecutive rounds, the opponent becomes extinct. If an Animal wins two out of three rounds, the loser receives a Suppressed marker. A Suppressed Animal remains alive but has its strength reduced.

At the end of the Battle phase, Animals advance one box on their PWTs. Players then tally victory points; the further along the PWT, the more points an Animal earns. The game continues until all of the Animal Cards have been depleted. Whoever has the most victory points wins.

I loved it, despite a few awkward rules. Combat involves an endless amount of die-rolling; even the example in the rulebook requires 48(!) dice to resolve. A victorious Animal receives a strength bonus only if it begins combat with fewer strength points than its opponent, a clumsy restriction to keep powerful Animals from taking over. Though it's possible to mount a game with two or three players, you need four to get the full effect. And forget about solitaire.

My playtesters, on the other hand, objected to the approach as a whole. The TYRANNO EX game, they said, addressed evolution only obliquely, treating it as a superficial abstraction—and a dull one at that. While the PWTs portray a dense jungle, a volcanic wasteland, and two other distinct landscapes, the different terrains have no effect whatsoever on play. The Animals are so colorless they might as well have been called X, Y, and Z. All Animals begin with the same strength and appear at random, without any consideration given to the era in which they actually belonged. Any Animal can attack another without regard to its terrain, appetite, or disposition. Animals don't evolve in any meaningful sense; they just get a little stronger as they march off the side of the board. Though the playtesters gave the

TYRANNO EX game a reluctant thumbs up, it impressed them mainly as a collection of missed opportunities. They've got a point, but . . .

Evaluation: . . . I still think they're wrong. Truly original board games are so few and far between that the debut of a good one is cause for celebration. The TYRANNO EX game is a virtuoso performance, an ingenious take on an underused topic, rendered with insight and elegance. Easy to learn but impossible to master, it may not be everyone's idea of an acceptable simulation or even a good time. However, from where I'm sitting, it looks to be an early contender for the best new board game of the year.

Short and sweet

Minion Nation, by Lester Smith. GDW, Inc., $4.50. The trouble with using cards and tables to generate random encounters is that sooner or later you run out of surprises. The *Minion Nation* expansion kit rejuvenates the MINION HUNTER* board game (reviewed in DRAGON issue #188) with a bonanza of variants. Two pages of tables, replacing the original game's Encounter Chart, generate hostile minions from the Interstices, Plaguelands, and Mechaniaca. Sixteen additional equipment cards supply hunters with horses, vampiric swords, and chameleon suits. A Random Plot Table, featuring 100 different entries, replaces the Plot Deck, which anyone who's played the game more than twice should be ready to retire. Despite the quality of the package, it's no bargain. The booklet is a skimpy eight pages—one of them a title page, another a useless glossary—and you've got to cut the cards apart yourself (it must be the work of a minion in the marketing department).

RIFTS Sourcebook Two: The Mechanoids*, by Kevin Siembieda. Palladium Books, $12. Meet the bad guys who won't stay dead. This race of alien killers originally reared their steely heads in the now-defunct MECHANOID INVASION* game, Palladiums' first and worst RPG. They rose again in 1985's MECHANOIDS* game, which designer Siembieda dismisses as "a so-so rework" (he's too modest—I'd rank it among the most inventive science-fiction RPGs of the decade). Now the Mechanoids have clawed their way out of the cosmic junkyard, as nasty as ever, in this stylish supplement for the RIFTS* game. How nasty are they? Not only do they hate you and me, they hate anything that even *looks* like us. Siembieda opens with a compelling overview of Mechanoid history, then packs the rest of book with statistics and playing notes for the Multi-Brain Combat Vehicle, the Tunnel Crawler, and the rest of the Mechanoid armada. Siembieda misfires, though, when he suggests that Mechanoids can be used as player charac-

ters; these things were born to be bad. As good as it is, *RIFTS Mechanoids* merely scratches the surface of the vast Mechanoid universe, which Siembieda promises will be explored in the forthcoming MECHANOID SPACE* game. I can't wait—my containment chamber's twitching already.

Rick Swan has worked as a rock musician, suicide-intervention counselor, and newspaper publisher. He now writes full-time. You can contact him at: 2620 30th Street, Des Moines IA 50310. A self-addressed stamped envelope increases the chance of a response. Ω

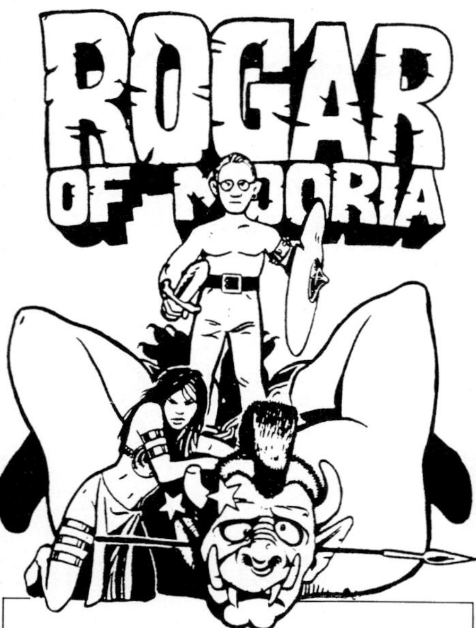

Were we great or what?

What do you think of this magazine? What do you like best or want to see changed most? What do you want to see next? Turn to "Letters" and see what others think, then write to us too!

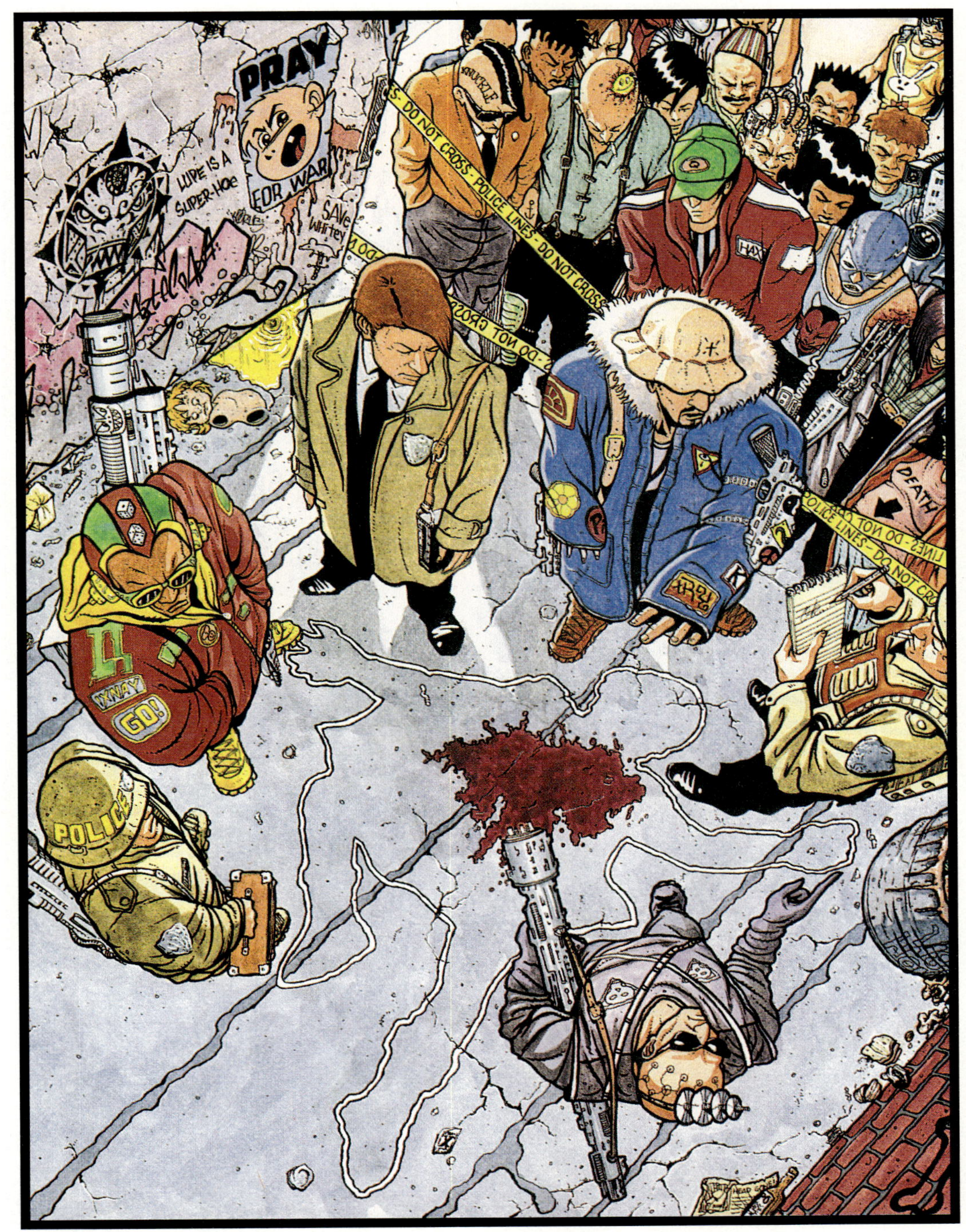

Coming this summer.

MG

MAYFAIR GAMES INC

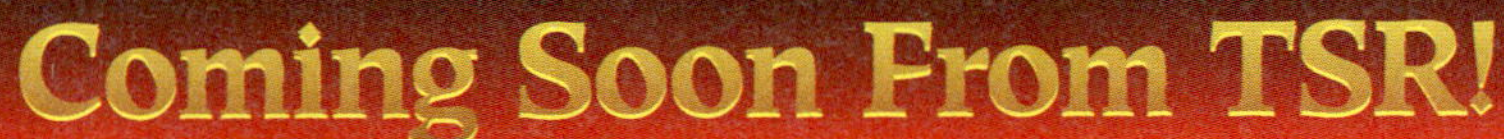
AL-QADIM™
CAMPAIGN

Discover
the mystery
and intrigue
beneath the
glitter of
Golden
Huzuz

AL-QADIM
CITY OF DELIGHTS
Advanced Dungeons & Dragons

Coming Soon From TSR!

TSR

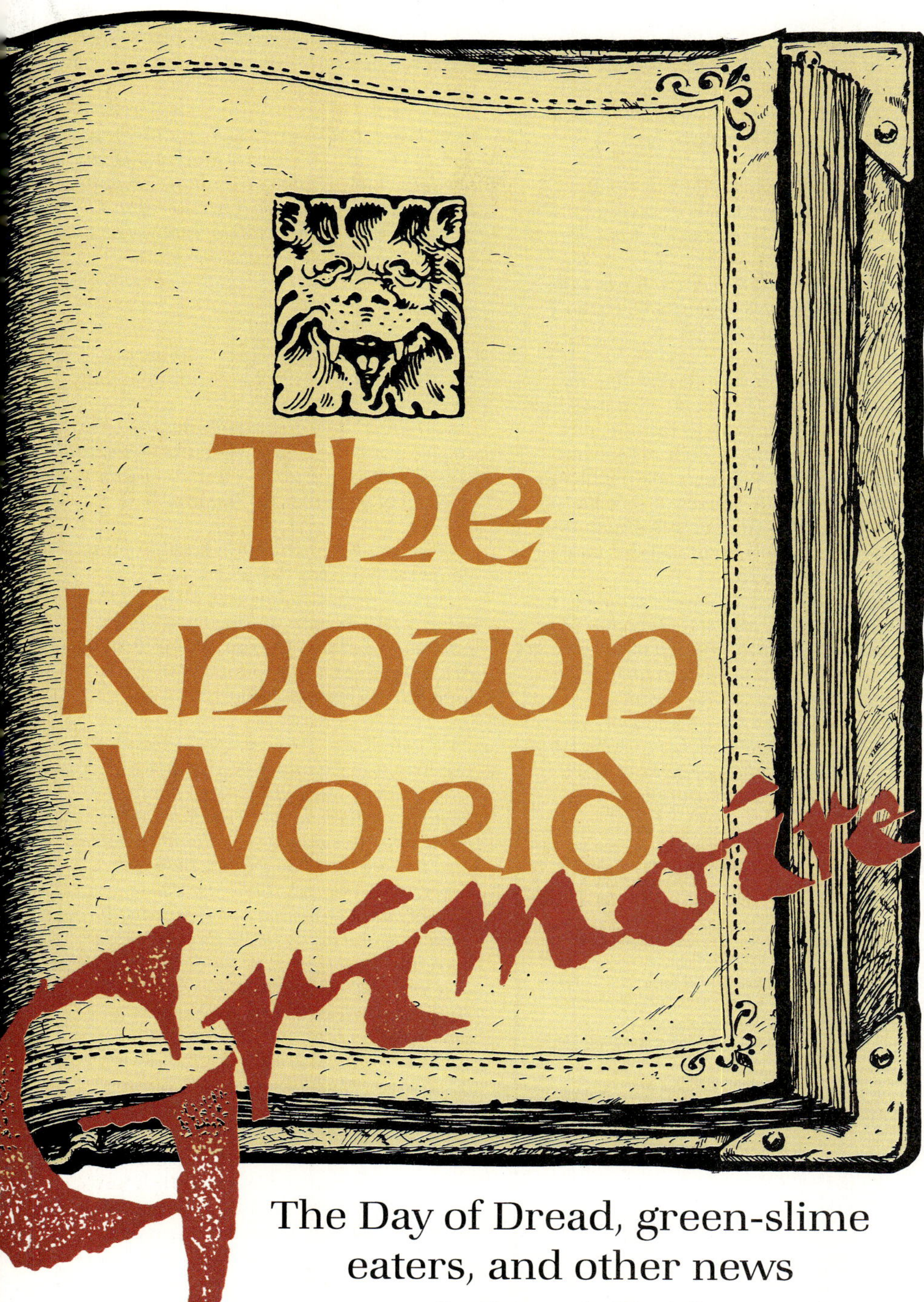

The Known World Grimoire

The Day of Dread, green-slime eaters, and other news

by Bruce A. Heard

This regular feature offers answers to letters on the D&D® game, its worlds and products, occasional articles, or "first glance" reviews of D&D game products. The reader is welcome to send questions, suggestions, or criticism on the game or on the material published here. We can't promise all letters will be answered in this column, but they all will get our attention.

Letters

The adventure presented in *Wrath of the Immortals* calls for a day without any magic at all. Although it seemed like a great idea, it causes a number of problems in my campaign (magically rejuvenated characters dying of sudden old age, the Flying City of Serraine or the Floating Islands of Ar crashing, etc). Did you really mean "no magic at all"?

As far as drama was concerned, the idea worked well, but for a long-lasting campaign, the effects should be limited to prevent campaign-busting problems. A full explanation of the Day of Dread appears in *AC1011* Poor Wizard's Almanac, with suggestions on how to manage its repercussions. Here is a summary of what's already written in *AC1011's* present draft:

Essentially, all mortal-level spells and spell-like effects fail. This includes spells cast from magical items (rings, scrolls, wands, etc.) and natural spell effects inherent to certain monsters (see below). The Day of Dread does not affect artifacts, Immortals, or anti-magic at all. The magical blackout is limited to the prime plane and the Mystara planetary system only.

Other permanent magical items may retain their effects during the Day of Dread (magical swords and armor and rings of protection, for example). Roll 1d4 for each magical item, and compare the score with the guidelines for damaged items on page 145 of the Rules Cyclopedia. "Damaged" items cease to function during the Day of Dread, from midnight at the site of Glantri City to the following midnight (watch for time differences east and west of that position; Thyatis runs a little under one hour later than Glantri).

Here's an example: The owner of a sword of flying +3 should roll to see if the item retains its +3 magic. Regardless of the score, this sword will not allow its owner to fly during the Day of Dread.

The Day of Dread's effect on potions is rather nasty. Their contents automatically become inert during that day, and if the die roll calls for a "damaged" result, the potion is permanently spoiled. Poison is not affected.

Here's a rule of thumb for determining which innate magical abilities monsters can retain. The ability still works if it is a permanent effect affecting only the monster itself (e.g., immunities to nonmagical weapons, a beholder's ability to levitate). The ability does not work if the monster can use that ability only a certain number of times a day (e.g., lycanthropic or metamorphic transformations, breath weapons), or if its ability normally affects something or someone else than the monster (e.g., a beholder's eye-stalk rays, a harpy's charm-song, an undead's level-draining). Shape-changers would remain stuck in whatever form they adopted prior to the Day of Dread.

Magically aged people come in two sorts, and each is affected differently. There are those who were permanently rejuvenated (and thus are unaffected by the day without magic) and those whose apparent ages depend on continuous magical effects (and thus would succumb to a total magical blackout). The former is the most common sort of magical aging. Likewise, major enchantments affecting the campaign world should remain mostly unaffected. For example, Floating Ar or Serraine might only lose altitude or become immobilized. Major magical objects that do not threaten a campaign's balance (like skyships, gargantoids, and other magical "sponges") could almost automatically be neutralized, considering the vast number of different enchantments they required during their creation.

Remember, this event was created more for campaign drama than rules-lawyering.

No rules will replace a DM's best judgment, so feel free to adjust the severity or the game mechanics of the Day of Dread in your campaign.

There was an Alphatian-controlled land called Minaea in the *Dawn of the Emperors* boxed set. Does any information exist about Minaea?

Very little. Minaeans were referred to as pirates many years ago in module M2 Vengeance of Alphaks. Minaea never fell under Alphatian domination. It marks the far-eastern limit of Alphatia's power and influence, prior to the latter's disappearance from the surface world (see the Wrath of the Immortals *boxed set). It is virtually unknown to typical Known World people because it is so remote. The only "civilized" people who would really know about the Minaeans are Bellissarians, especially those at the heavily fortified town of Spearpoint. The latter view Minaeans as bloodthirsty pirates. Based upon the location of the races in Mystara described in the* HOLLOW WORLD® *boxed set, Minaeans would have to be descendants of the fierce Jennites (horse-riders derived from real-world ancient Scythians). The present Minaeans could also be derived from Conan's mysterious Pictish warriors, given some additional seafaring experience.*

Within a few years following the disappearance of mainland Alphatia from the Known World (AC 1012 or later), Minaean raids into southeastern Bellissaria, if not major invasions, would be likely.

Is there a complete chart of weapon mastery for the weapons described in the HOLLOW WORLD accessory, *Kingdom of Nithia*?

Yes, as well as some errata. It was published in DRAGON® *issue #182, in the "Princess Ark" column.*

This is a question about *Wrath of the Immortals*. Page 71 of Book Two says that characters on the path to Immortality receive a +5 bonus to their arrival and petition modifiers if they seek Benekander's sponsorship. However, it costs 100 PP for an immortal to create a manifestation (which 1st-level Benekander cannot afford). Is there a fix?

Benekander, as a 1st-level Immortal, has 300 PP. The rules also state on page 72 of Book One that newly created immortals get their very first manifestation form for free, directly from their sponsor. Since Benekander didn't have a sponsor, assume that he automatically got his manifestation form (as described on page 17 of Book One) when he attained Immortality.

Shouldn't green slimes rule places like forests, since only fire or extreme cold can harm them?

Ever heard of green-slime-guzzlers? Neither have I, but sure enough, mother nature certainly has some kind of obscure predator for anything swimming, creeping, or crawling on Mystara. Care to submit a grimoire of low-life predators, anyone? (And no, you can't use a green-slime-guzzler as a wizard's familiar—it loves ear wax).

If a monster with a *charm* ability dies, are the victims of its *charm* automatically freed from its effects?

Nothing in the rules states that the effect ceases when the caster dies. The victim still gets to roll saving throws as described on page 45 of the Rules Cyclopedia.

What is a Night Dragon? Are there any game statistics for them?

They were first published in DRAGON *issue #163, in my column. They will be published again in the upcoming "Princess Ark" boxed set, Champions of Mystara (due out in October 1993).*

Will all of the "*Princess Ark*" episodes be published in *Champions of Mystara*?

Because of space limitation, the first 15 episodes will be summarized. All of the other episodes appear in full, up to part 35. Also included will be a more detailed description of Sind, the Great Waste, and the Serpent Peninsula; two maps displaying these regions in the usual hex format; a complete description of the Princess Ark *and its crew, along with two maps of the ship's main decks (in 25-mm scale); and new rules on building skyships, along with cards providing various skyship examples (Heldannic Warbirds, gnomish blimps, etc.).*

After reading issue #190, I just had to write. The complaint by the individual regarding the D&D game boxes was definitely unjustified. I've been involved with D&D and AD&D® games since the late '70s, and I found these products to be perfect for teaching new players.

This past Christmas, I bought the DRAGON QUEST™ game for my family, hoping they would like it and join one of my hobbies. Needless to say, they did, and we bought all four of the D&D boxed games. The cardboard stand-ups and game tiles add the realism I missed when all the monsters looked like dice.

Thanks for the vote of confidence! Ω

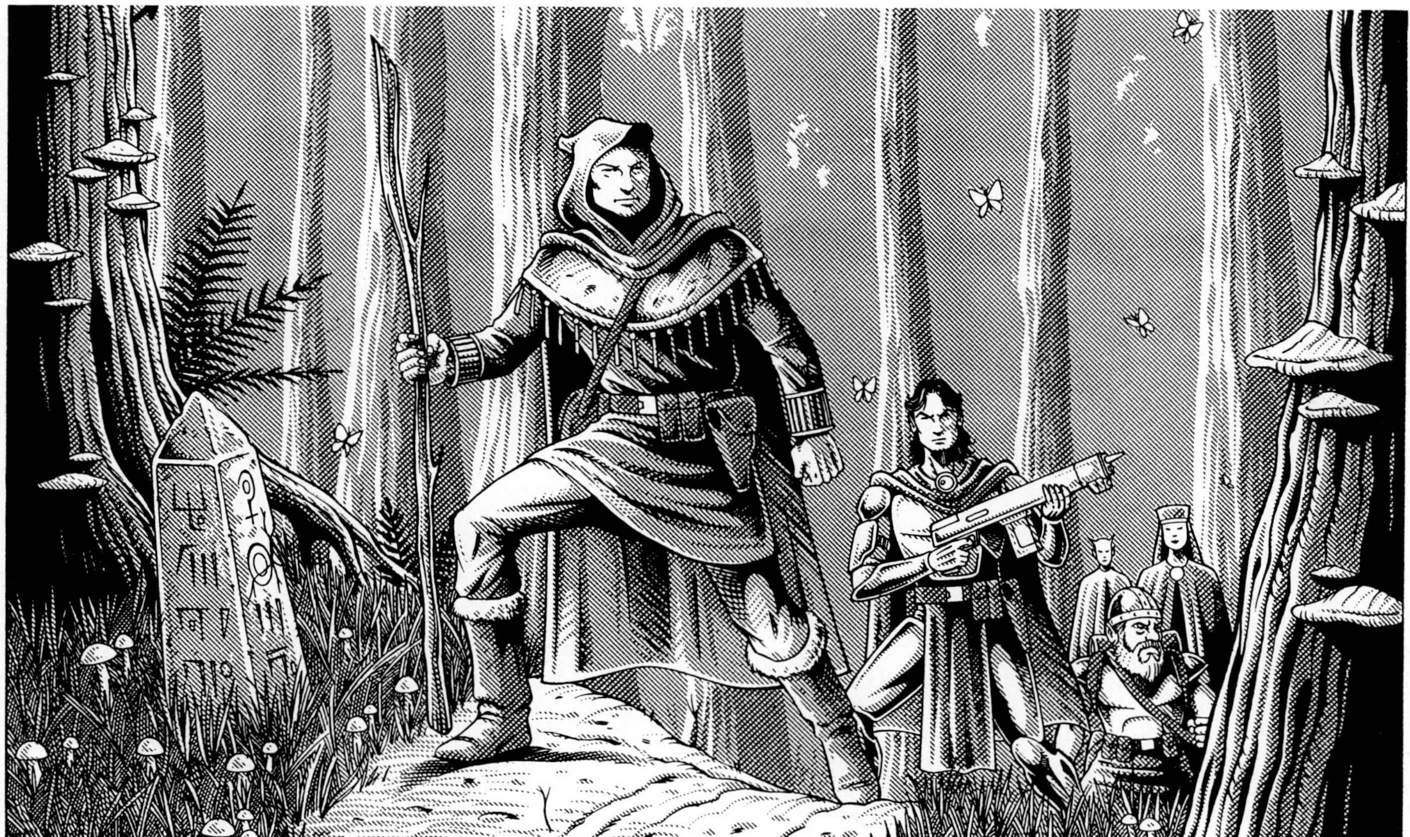

The Palladium® Fantasy World

Copyright © 1993 Kevin Siembieda

Island at the End of the World™

Is it the end of the Palladium World as foretold in the Tristine Chronicles?

The ocean is disappearing. Strange storms and ill winds smother the coasts. The cause of it all? Nobody knows with certainty, but the answers seem to rest at a legendary island at the end of the world.

Epic adventures carry our heroes through the Old Kingdom, ancient tombs, crystal palaces, and the south seas. Crystal magic, death traps, strange encounters, insanity, and dark secrets are all part of the adventures. Travel beyond the known world to a mysterious island locked in a deadly confrontation that threatens the entire world.

Highlights Include:
- **Crystal magic, swords, wands and weapons.**
- **Five powerful rulers, their fortresses, their insanities and their subjects.**
- **The mysterious lord of the Crystal Fortress.**
- **The Ghost Kings of the haunted tombs, filled with death traps and the dead.**
- **The maniacal Lord Axel and his evil minions. His goal, to reshape the world to his own twisted vision.**
- **More data about Changelings, their powers, history and future.**
- **Many adventures, adventure ideas and more.**
- **Written by Thomas Bartold and Kevin Siembieda**
- **160+ pages — $15.95 plus $1.50**
- **Available May or June, 1993**

The Palladium Role-Playing Game®

The Palladium fantasy RPG creates an exciting world of epic fantasy. Players can be any number of unique creatures such as the werewolf-like wolfen, the bearmen of the north, or the loathsome changeling who can assume the form of any humanoid creature. Additional player creatures include ogre, troll, goblin, orc, dwarf, elf, human, and dozens of optional races.

Magic is unparalleled, with the inclusion of the spell casting wizard, elemental aligned warlock, ward wielding diabolist, circle using summoner, psionically empowered mind mage, the metamorph druid and others.

Combat is realistic and fast playing. The world intriguing. If you play any of our other games then you're already familiar with the game mechanics. This is the original RPG system that all the other Palladium role-playing games grew out of.

274 pages. Compatible with *Rifts* and other Palladium RPGs. **$19.95 plus $2.00 for postage and handling.**

Fantasy Source Books

Book II: Old Ones™ is a giant book of cities, mapping and exploring 34 major communities in and around the *Timiro Kingdom*. Plus adventure in the mysterious dwarven ruins known as the *Place of Magic*. The dreaded Old Ones and six adventures. 208 pages. **$14.95 plus $1.50 for postage and handling.**

Book III: Adventures on the High Seas™. A super source book that maps and explores the islands around the Palladium Continent, including the *Isle of the cyclops*. Source material offers the gladiator and seven other new character classes, new skills, over 30 new magic items, faerie food, magic curses, herbs and gems, ship to ship combat, six adventures and ideas for a dozen more. 208 pages. **$14.95 plus $1.50 for postage and handling.**

Monsters & Animals™ presents nearly a hundred new monsters. Many, like the Bearmen, Coyles, Rahu-men, Ratlings, and Lizard Mages are optional races available as player characters. Most are quite new and original, not your usual repeat of monsters from myth. This source book also contains 200 different, real life animals all with complete stats and maps indicating their location in the Palladium Fantasy World. *Compatible with RIFTS and the entire megaverse.* **$14.95 plus $1.50 for postage and handling.**

Adventures in the Northern Wilderness™ is a 96 page, action packed adventure and source book that provides new data on the *Great Northern Wilderness* and the *Wolfen*. Six adventures pit characters against elemental forces, an insane dragon, ancient rune magic, the demonic Omicron, and, of course, the wolfen. Keith Parkinson cover. Interior art by Talbot and Long. **$9.95 plus $1.00 for postage and handling.**

Palladium Books®   12455 Universal Drive
Dept. D   Taylor, MI 48180

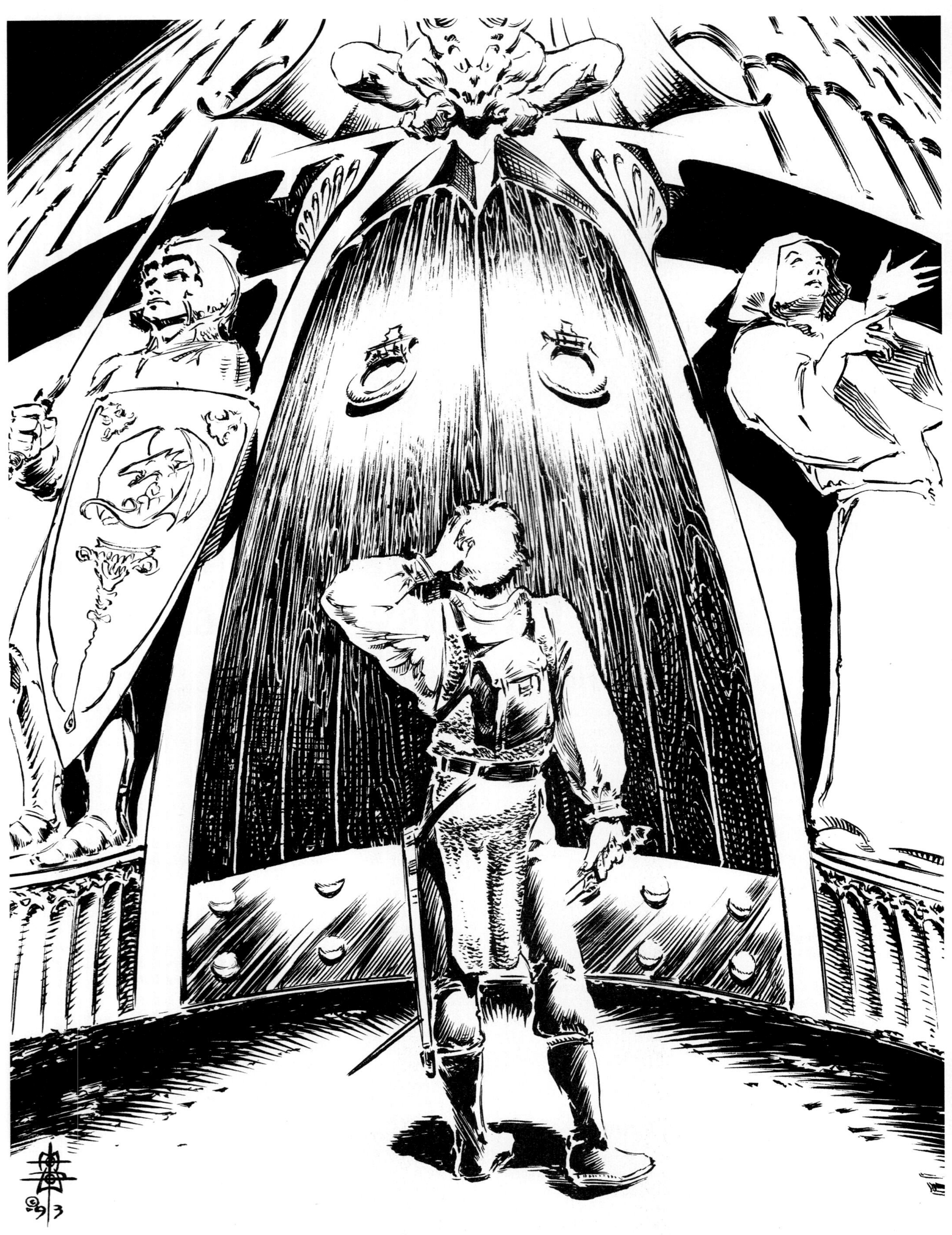

Breaking Them In

Incorporating novice players into your campaign

by Neil McGarry

Artwork by Tom Dow

Novice role-playing game players can be a trial to the most knowledgeable and experienced gaming groups. There is so much for them to learn, and the older players often do not want to wait for them to learn it. How do you, as the DM, bridge the gap?

The key lies in making the training of the new RPG player the job of the *entire group*, not just the DM. This spreads out the responsibility and speeds up the awkward period of adjustment the group goes through when taking on a new member. Here are a few tips to help you, the DM, help your new players get adjusted.

1. Set aside some time to work with the new player alone. Start the new player off by having her roll up her character's statistics, then let her choose a class. This will be one of the biggest decisions early on, so be prepared to give good advice. Try to remain impartial, however, or else she may wind up choosing the class she thinks you want her to use, rather than relying on her own preferences.

Once that is out of the way, you can get her familiar with armor class, hit points, saving throws, and the other mechanics of role-playing, so she will at least know what you mean when you say, "Make a saving throw versus poison." Ironically, I

find that most new players have more of a problem in identifying the type of dice they need to roll than in why they need to roll them (where else do you ever use 12-sided dice?). Keep this in mind as you and your veteran players are throwing around terms like "d20" or "d12."

When the player begins to choose the specifics of her character (spells for wizards, weapon proficiencies for fighters, etc.), try to maintain a "hands-off" approach. Answer her questions, but don't create the character for her. When complicated rules arise, such as the fighting styles in PHBR1 *The Complete Fighter's Handbook*, don't try to explain everything at once. Unless your new player is a whiz, this will confuse and aggravate her. Go slowly and give her time to understand the more complex rules. In extreme cases where a difficult choice must be made, recommend specifics that you know she will be happy with, and be willing to let her change these retroactively as she gains experience. The other players may howl when you let her change one proficiency to another, but they should be willing to compromise to accommodate the new player (and if not, then a few good DM growls should suffice to convince them). Finally, be prepared to stop game-play when the new player runs into a

problem; this slows down play at first but should happen less often as time goes by and the novice gains confidence.

Beware of the novice who nods too much, because it probably means that she doesn't understand what's going on but is afraid to slow down the game to ask for an explanation. Take the time to explain anything she doesn't understand, and make certain she knows that you are willing to answer *any* questions.

Most importantly, be sure that the novice turns first to you, the DM, for advice on specific rules. The other players may be well-intentioned in their efforts to advise her, but as we all know, many players have their own versions of the rules ("Oh, sure, you can bring a war elephant into a dungeon!"). This requires the DM have a working knowledge of the rules herself, a necessary prerequisite for any good referee.

2. Emphasize preparedness. The new player must be willing to spend the time and effort to learn the rules, or else your best efforts will be wasted. Of course, he cannot be expected to become a rules expert after just a few sessions, but he should have a willingness to read the rulebooks on his own. Again, if you let him lean on you too much at first, you'll wind up playing his character for him. To help him out, write or type out a summary of the most important rules needed during play, such as calculating THAC0, initiative, etc., that he can keep within easy reach and refer to as needed. This will save countless minutes of frantic flipping through the *Player's Handbook* for a table or chart. One idea that works particularly well is drawing up an attack matrix (see the AD&D® 1st Edition game's *Dungeon Master's Guide*, pages 74-75), according to his character's chance to hit. THAC0 can be a difficult concept to master, and this will ease him into calculating his chance of success for himself. Another useful addition to the summary is on page 93 of the AD&D 2nd Edition game's *PH*, entitled "What You Can Do in One Round." I find that one of the most frequently asked questions of new players is "Well, what can I do?" so this information should give them a head-start on the answer.

If the player is using a spell-caster (something that is not recommended for most novice players), photocopy or type out the spell listings on pages 126-128 of the *PH* and highlight those his character has access to. This comes in especially handy for priest characters, whose major and minor access to various spheres is certain to confuse a new player. Allow the player to use these aids freely, while stressing that they exist to supplement the rules, not substitute for them. Getting familiar with the rules themselves requires a little time away from the gaming table, but as all experienced players know, it's worth the effort. If the player is lagging on his "homework," a word to the wise should be sufficient to motivate him. The best advice a DM can give a new player is "Know your character." Learn what he can do, and what he can't.

3. Assign another player to be a guide for the novice. Ask for volunteers or assign someone you trust to lend responsible guidance. Your players may not be inclined to do this, so simply remind them that breaking in the new player is everyone's job, not just the DM's. If that doesn't work, try a small bribe to sweeten the pot (extra experience points, for example, depending on the guide's performance). If all else fails, the threat of a vampire or two can be a marvelous incentive to perform such a service.

Once the "guide" has been chosen, tell the novice that she would do well to follow the example of her new guide during play. Emphasize, however, the importance of innovation; in other words, see that the novice isn't blindly parroting the experi-enced player. Warn the other players that while outside suggestions to the novice are welcome, you will not allow her to be verbally bombarded ("Cast a spell!" "No, throw a flask of oil!" "Don't do that! Help my character!"), a tactic virtually guaranteed to discourage new players from ever returning to the gaming table. Ideally, the novice should rely more heavily on her guide at first, then less so as she gains knowledge and confidence. This expedites play, keeps your players happy, and makes your job as DM a little easier.

These suggestions may not fit all gaming groups; some DMs may prefer a "hands-on" approach to training, while others may leave it entirely to the novice to sink or swim. However it is done, the addition of a new player should not be a trial for the DM, but an experience shared by the whole group. If it's done properly, it can result in a sharp new player, a tougher party of PCs, and a more enjoyable game for all involved. Ω

Rolemaster

ORIENTAL COMPANION

Oriental Companion is your guide for using *Rolemaster* in the land of the Orient; an adventurous world with Samurai and Ninja, *Rolemaster's* Orient is a hybridization of many Far Eastern cultures injected with a mix of fantasy and wonder.

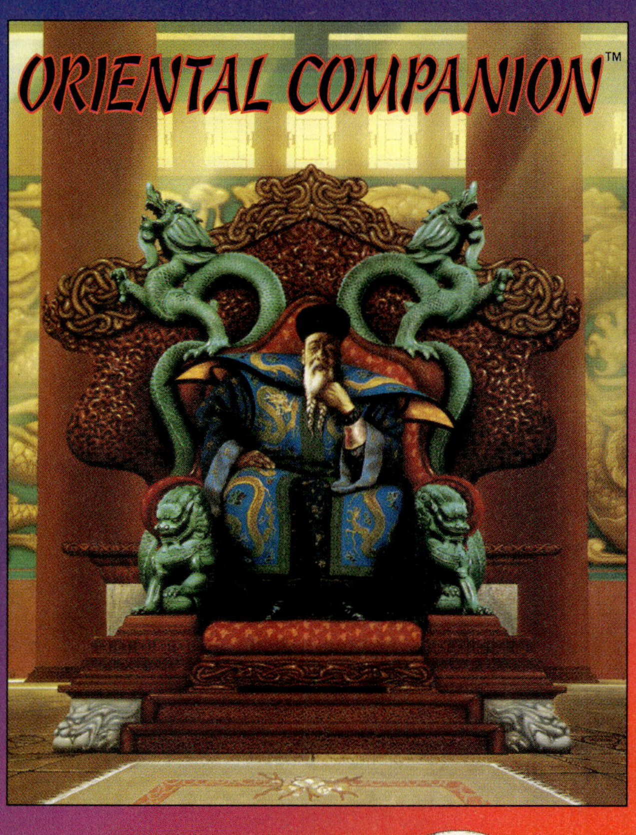

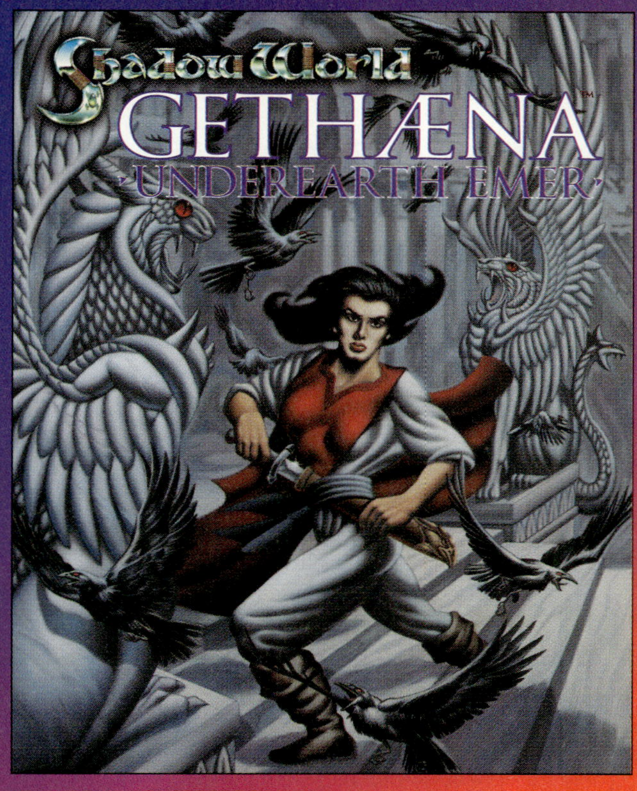

GETHÆNA
UNDEREARTH EMER

Vast caverns thread the earth beneath the *Shadow World;* one of these natural vaults contains Gethæna, lit by a magical sky-roof of brass. Six immortal, evil lords overlook the deserts and the steppe, vying among themselves for supremacy, unaware that their holdings may all be destroyed by events set in motion millenia in the past.

Treachery, rebellion, and the chances of war challenge adventurers in Gethæna!

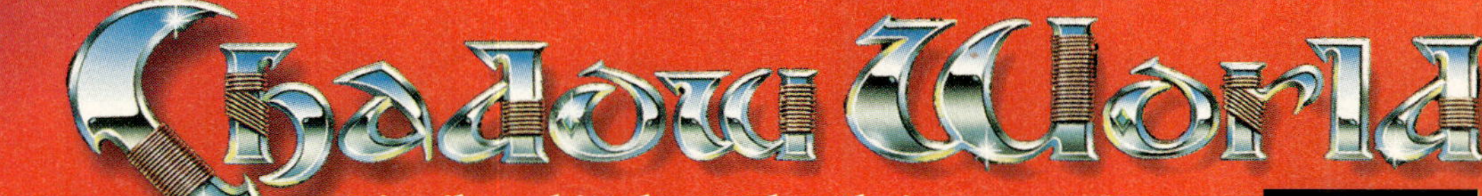

Distributed in the UK by Chris Harvey Games,
P.O. Box 38 Bath St., Walsall WS1 3BY
Phone: 44-922-28-181 FAX: 44-922-721644

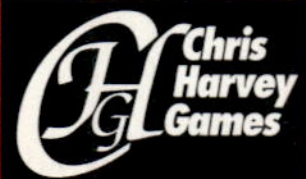

Get Ready, Get Set, GO!

Mr. Sulu, virtual reality, and Marvel at the 1993 GEN CON® Game Fair

by Tom McLaughlin

In just two months, convention planners at TSR will give the world's biggest game fair the green light. If you haven't made plans to come to the 1993 GEN CON® Game Fair, get going. It's one show you don't want to miss!

Highlighting this year's Game Fair are tons of brand new events, including cutting-edge virtual reality games from Dream Park Corporation and Virtual World Entertainment. Another first is Sci-ence Fiction Saturday, with special *Star Trek* events and guest of honor George Takei. And, for all of you comic-book fans, we're unleashing our first-ever Marvel Comics Mini-Con!

Held August 19-22 at the MECCA Center in Milwaukee, this huge event (sponsored by TSR, Inc.) features four days of gaming in almost a dozen categories. It boasts more than 1,000 computer, video, arcade, virtual reality, multiplayer network, mili-tary, strategy, board, role-playing, and miniatures games.

The list of author and artist celebrities is huge, too. You can meet: R. A. Salvatore, Robh Ruppel, Frank Kelly-Freas, Jeff Easley, Larry Bond, Tracy Hickman, Margaret Weis, Brom, Ed Greenwood, Fred Fields, Doug Niles, Frank Chadwick, Greg Farshtey, and many others!

In last month's DRAGON® Magazine, we described the convention's role-playing,

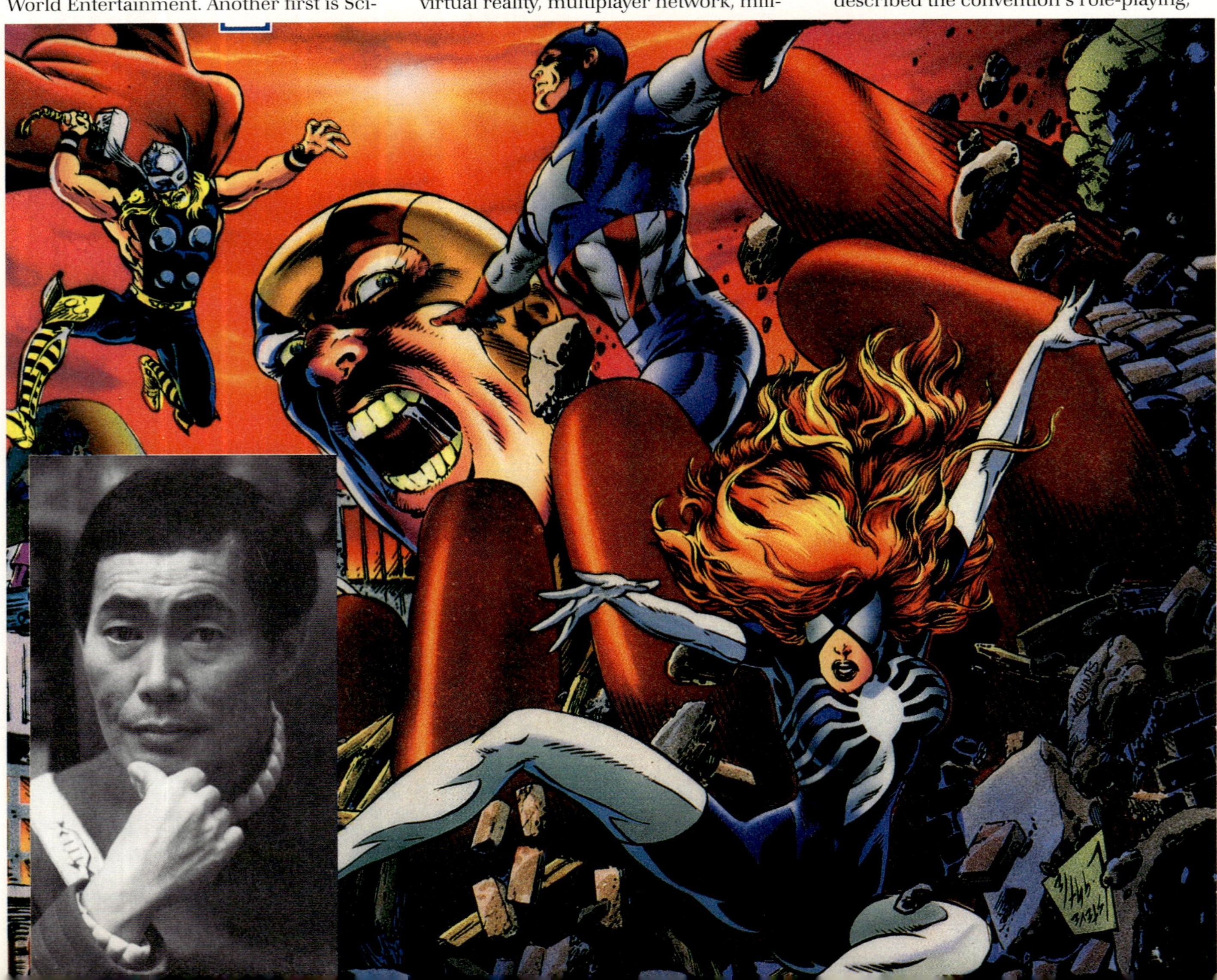

miniatures, and strategy game events. Here's the low-down on more activities.

Arcade and virtual-reality games

Get wired! The new virtual reality games from Dream Park Corporation and Virtual World Entertainment are just a tiny part of over 100 high-tech networked computer, video, and arcade games coming to Milwaukee. What can you do?

• Climb into a BATTLETECH* cockpit for the 'MechWarrior fight of your life;

• Experience Larry Niven's Ringworld in Virtual Ringworld;

• Try new computer games like *Revenge of the Patriarch* and the *Mythos Engine*, and test your skill in the Virtual Parlor;

• Compete in the hottest computer and video games, including *MidiMaze, Lemmings, Ultima, Risk, Batman Returns, Black Crypt, M.U.L.E., Sonic, Falcon*, and others; and

• Try some old favorite arcade games, such as *Tetris, Joust, Rampage, Double Dragon, Xybots, Tempest, Space Harrier, Quix, Centipede, I-Robot, Phoenix*, and *Black Tiger*.

Meet George "Sulu" Takei

Another convention first is the August 21 Science Fiction Saturday, with special *Star Trek* events and guest George Takei. The star who played Mr. Sulu in over 70 TV episodes and six movies in the amazing *Star Trek* series will meet fans, give seminars, and sign autographs all day long.

Science Fiction Saturday features dozens of celebrities and events like:

• *Star Trek* novel authors Gene DeWeese and Leah Rewolinski;

• A *Star Trek* costume contest—judged by George Takei;

• STAR FLEET BATTLES*, STAR TREK: THE ROLE-PLAYING GAME*, STAR FLEET MISSIONS*, TRAVELLER*, STAR WARS*, and Star Trek Trivia game tournaments;

• A fantastic Hollywood-style Star Fleet model display;

• TSR's brand-new BUCK ROGERS™ and AMAZING ENGINE™ games;

• Movie hits like *Star Trek II, Fantastic Planet*, and *20 Million Miles to Earth*; and

• The $1 million science-fiction and fantasy art show and memorabilia exhibit hall.

Marvel artist & comics, too

The world's biggest comic-book company, Marvel, is coming to the Game Fair. And the hottest comic magazine in the country, *Wizard*, is right behind them. This is the first time we're unveiling a comic track at the game fair. This two-day mini-con, August 20-21, is packed with events like these:

• Meet and get a free autographed poster from Steve Lightle, Marvel's top *Avengers* artist;

• Check out the reels from the animated *X-Men Adventures* series;

• Meet the pros and get free copies of the newest *Wizard* magazine;

• See the newest and hottest comic projects from Les Dorscheid, Jeff Butler, John Statema, Mike Machlan, Tony Harris, Doug Gregory, and a dozen other artists;

• Bring your art portfolio and talk to the pros at great seminars like "Breaking into the Business";

• Get a behind-the-scenes look at how your favorite comics are made;

• Score tons of great freebies like limited edition trading cards and comics;

• Play dozens of adventures in the CHAMPIONS*, MARVEL SUPER HEROES™, DC HEROES*, VILLAINS & VIGILANTES*, JUDGE DREDD*, and TEENAGE MUTANT NINJA TURTLES* games; and

• Meet surprise costumed super-heroes—and villains!

And play games!

The 1993 GEN CON Game Fair will feature hundreds of game tournaments and is giving away over $10,000 in prizes. The biggest tournaments are the Avalon Hill Classics Open, RPGA™ Network events, MidiMaze, MONOPOLY*, and the BATTLETECH Miniatures Open tournaments. And don't miss the Puffing Billy, *Games* Magazine Triathalon, Mythos Virtual Reality Shootout, and Rubout tournaments, or the 13th Annual Miniatures Painting Competition.

The convention also has its famous art show; an expanded strategy board-game track with special guest Rich Berg; and a line-up of incredible historical, science-fiction, and fantasy miniatures and board-game events.

The 1993 GEN CON Game Fair is *the* multi-media game event of the year! Grab your friends and come see it all; there's something for everyone. Daily fees are just $5 for spectators and $10 for players.

Registration

To register, send your name and address before June 1st to: Registration Dept., 1993 GEN CON Game Fair, P.O. Box 756, Lake Geneva WI 53147, U.S.A. After June 1, 1993, call Sandy Kinney at: (414) 248-3625, ext. 424. Ω

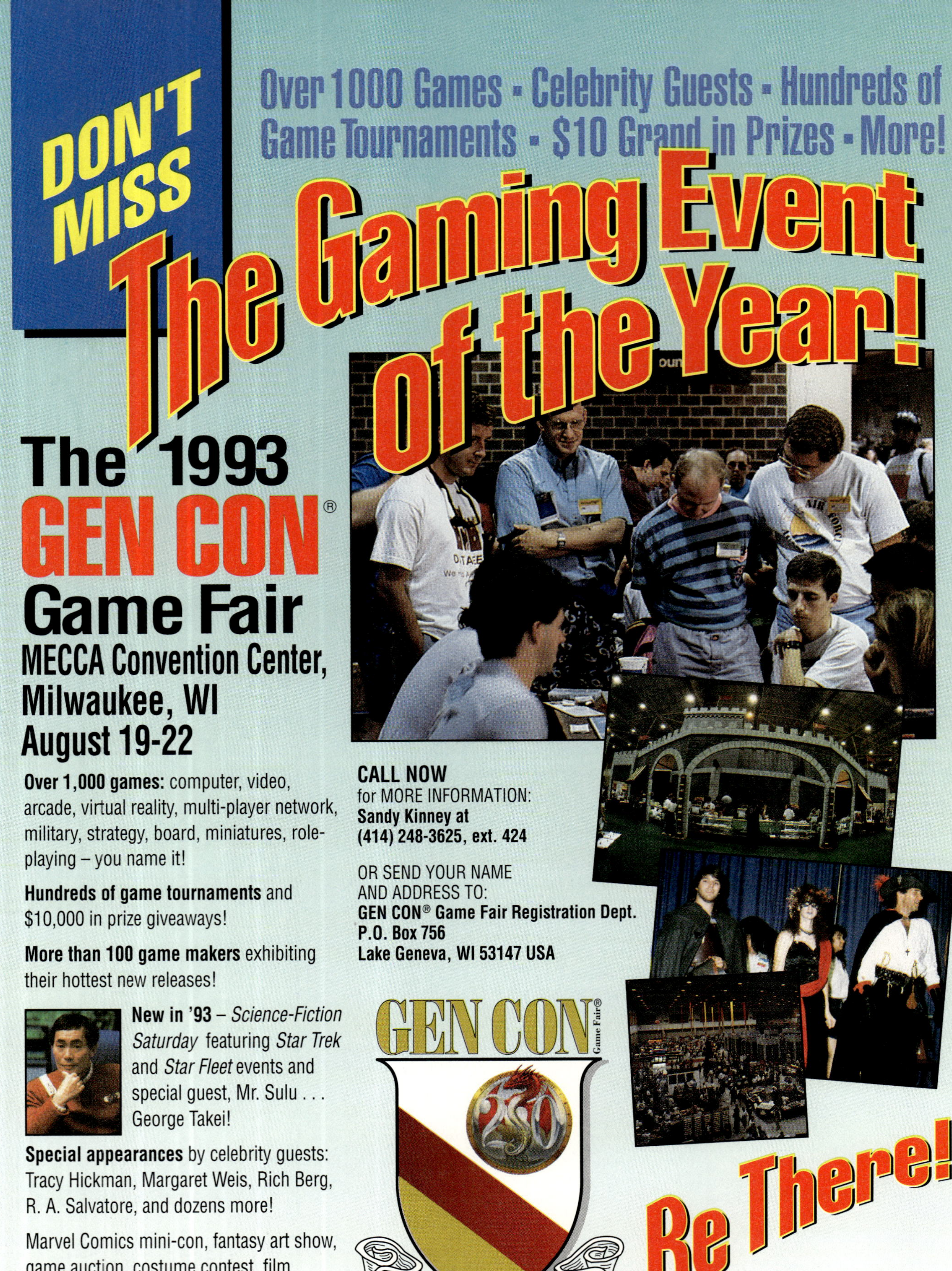
DON'T MISS

Over 1000 Games · Celebrity Guests · Hundreds of
Game Tournaments · $10 Grand in Prizes · More!

The Gaming Event of the Year!

The 1993
GEN CON®
Game Fair
MECCA Convention Center,
Milwaukee, WI
August 19-22

Over 1,000 games: computer, video,
arcade, virtual reality, multi-player network,
military, strategy, board, miniatures, role-
playing – you name it!

Hundreds of game tournaments and
$10,000 in prize giveaways!

More than 100 game makers exhibiting
their hottest new releases!

New in '93 – Science-Fiction
Saturday featuring Star Trek
and Star Fleet events and
special guest, Mr. Sulu . . .
George Takei!

Special appearances by celebrity guests:
Tracy Hickman, Margaret Weis, Rich Berg,
R. A. Salvatore, and dozens more!

Marvel Comics mini-con, fantasy art show,
game auction, costume contest, film
festival – and for the 18,000 gamers
attending, that's just the beginning!

CALL NOW
for MORE INFORMATION:
Sandy Kinney at
(414) 248-3625, ext. 424

OR SEND YOUR NAME
AND ADDRESS TO:
GEN CON® Game Fair Registration Dept.
P.O. Box 756
Lake Geneva, WI 53147 USA

GEN CON Game Fair

Celebrating the 20th Anniversary
of the DUNGEONS & DRAGONS® Game!

Be There!

GEN CON and DUNGEONS & DRAGONS are registered trademarks owned by TSR, Inc. ©1993 TSR, Inc. All Rights Reserved.

MAKE ONLY ONE VOTE IN EACH CATEGORY. ONLY THIS FORM MAY BE USED TO VOTE. YOU MAY WRITE-IN A DIFFERENT PRODUCT.

1991 Calendar Year Releases

ORIGINS™ AWARDS FINAL BALLOT

RESPOND BY JUNE 20!
BALLOT MUST BE RECEIVED BY JUNE 25. PHOTOCOPY & DISTRIBUTE FREELY

1. Best Historical Figure Series, 1991
- ☐ Adler 6mm Napoleonics (Stone Mtn.)
- ☐ American Civil War 15mm (Old Glory)
- ☐ English Civil War 15mm (Essex)
- ☐ Franco-Prussian 15mm (Rank & File)
- ☐ Pendragon Knight & Lady Sets (Lance & Laser)
- ☐ Title________________ Company________

2. Best Fantasy/Science Fiction Figure Series, 1991
- ☐ 25mm Dioramas by Tom Meier (Thunderbolt Mtn.)
- ☐ AD&D Boxed Sets (Ral Partha)
- ☐ Call of Cthulhu (RAFM)
- ☐ Pendragon (Lance & Laser)
- ☐ Shadowrun (Ral Partha)
- ☐ Title________________ Company________

3. Best Vehicular Figure Series, 1991
- ☐ BattleTech Aerospace Fighters (Ral Partha)
- ☐ BattleTech Mechs & Vehicles (Ral Partha)
- ☐ Black Guard (ICE)
- ☐ GHQ Micro Armour 1/285 (GHQ)
- ☐ Houstons 1/1200 Ironclads (Stone Mtn.)
- ☐ Title________________ Company________

4. Best Miniature Accessory Series, 1991
- ☐ Battlescapes (Geo-Hex)
- ☐ Castles (Minifigs)
- ☐ Dungeon Works (Dungeon Works)
- ☐ Flex Terrain (Editions Brokaw)
- ☐ Hovels 25mm Spanish Village (Stone Mtn.)
- ☐ Tiny Terrain 1/300 (Simtac)
- ☐ Title________________ Company________

5. Best Miniatures Rules, 1991
- ☐ BattleSystem Skirmish Rules (TSR Inc.)
- ☐ Harpoon: South Atlantic War (GDW)
- ☐ Princess Ryan's Space Marines (Simtac)
- ☐ Star Wars Miniatures Rules (West End)
- ☐ Tactica Ancients (Quantum Printing)
- ☐ Warfare in the Age of Reason (Emperor's HQ)
- ☐ Title________________ Company________

6. Best Role-Playing Rules, 1991
- ☐ Amber Diceless Role-Playing (Phage Press)
- ☐ Dark Conspiracy (GDW)
- ☐ Dungeons & Dragons Basic Rules (TSR Inc.)
- ☐ Dungeons & Dragons Cyclopedia (TSR Inc.)
- ☐ Vampire: The Masquerade (White Wolf)
- ☐ Title________________ Company________

7. Best Role-Playing Adventure, 1991
- ☐ AD&D: DS1 Freedom (TSR Inc.)
- ☐ AD&D: FA1 Nightmare Keep (TSR Inc.)
- ☐ Call of Cthulhu: Horror on the Orient Express (Chaosium)
- ☐ GURPS: Space Adventures (Steve Jackson Games)
- ☐ Ravenloft RA2: Ship of Horror (TSR Inc.)
- ☐ Title________________ Company________

8. Best Role-Playing Supplement, 1991
- ☐ AD&D: FOR2 Drow of the Underdark (TSR Inc.)
- ☐ AD&D: HR1 Vikings (TSR Inc.)
- ☐ GURPS: Time Travel (Steve Jackson Games)
- ☐ Shadowrun: Virtual Realities
- ☐ Vampire: Players Guide (White Wolf)
- ☐ Title________________ Company________

10. Best Pre-20th Century Boardgame, 1991
- ☐ 1835 (Mayfair)
- ☐ Blackbeard (Avalon Hill)
- ☐ Great Battles of Alexander (GMT)
- ☐ High Ground (Crown Tactics)
- ☐ Peloponnesian Wars (Victory/Avalon Hill)
- ☐ Title________________ Company________

11. Best Modern-Day Boardgame, 1991
- ☐ Black Sea Fleet 1914-1918 (Pacific Rim)
- ☐ EastFront (Columbia)
- ☐ Express (Mayfair)
- ☐ The Legend Begins (Rhino)
- ☐ Line in the Sand (TSR Inc.)
- ☐ WWII Pacific Theater of Operations (TSR Inc.)
- ☐ Title________________ Company________

12. Best Fantasy or Science Fiction Boardgame, 1991
- ☐ Cosmic Encounter (Mayfair)
- ☐ Greyhawk Wars (TSR Inc.)
- ☐ HeroQuest (Milton Bradley)
- ☐ Silent Death (ICE)
- ☐ Star Fleet Battles: Captains Rules (Task Force)
- ☐ Title________________ Company________

14. Best Play-By-Mail Game, 1991
- ☐ Belter (Classified Information)
- ☐ Hyborian War (Reality Simulations Inc.)
- ☐ Illuminati (Flying Buffalo)
- ☐ StarWeb (Flying Buffalo)
- ☐ World Wide Battle Plan (Flying Buffalo)
- ☐ Title________________ Company________

15. Best New Play-By-Mail Game, 1991
- ☐ Buck Rogers (TSR Inc.)
- ☐ El Mythico (Graaf Simulations)
- ☐ Middle Earth (Game Systems Inc.)
- ☐ The Realms of Fantasy (Graaf Simulations)
- ☐ Title________________ Company________

16. Best Fantasy/Science Fiction Computer Game, 1991
- ☐ Death Knights of Krynn (SSI)
- ☐ Eye of the Beholder (SSI)
- ☐ Might & Magic III (New World)
- ☐ Pool of Darkness (SSI)
- ☐ Secret of Monkey Island (LucasArts)
- ☐ Wing Commander II (Origin Systems)
- ☐ Title________________ Company________

17. Best Military or Strategy Computer Game, 1991
- ☐ Castles (Interplay)
- ☐ Civilization (Microprose)
- ☐ Red Baron (Dynamix)
- ☐ Warlords (SSG)
- ☐ Title________________ Company________

18. Best Professional Adventure Gaming Magazine, 1991
- ☐ Challenge (GDW)
- ☐ Command (XTR)
- ☐ Computer Gaming World (Golden Empire Publishing)
- ☐ Dungeon Adventures (TSR Inc.)
- ☐ White Wolf (White Wolf)
- ☐ Title________________ Company________

19. Best Amateur Adventure Gaming Magazine, 1991
- ☐ Alarums & Excursions
- ☐ Berg's Review of Games
- ☐ ETO
- ☐ MWAN- Midwest Wargamers Association Newsletter
- ☐ The Zouave
- ☐ Title________________ Company________

Voter Name_______________________________________

Address____

City_________________________ **State**______ **Zip**___________

Signature_________________________ **Phone** (____)___________

BALLOTS WITHOUT CURRENT PHONE NUMBER, OR IN ANY FORMAT BUT THIS ONE, WILL BE DISALLOWED.

Note that Categories 9, 13, and 20 are for Academy Membership Vote Only, thus do not appear on this ballot.

Send your Final Ballot to the following address by the deadline, June 20, 1993 (postmark).

BALLOTS RECEIVED AFTER JUNE 25 WILL NOT BE VALID

ORIGINS™ Awards
5575D Arapahoe Rd.
Boulder, CO 80303

For More Information:
Phone 303-786-9727
Fax 303-786-9797

See Other Side for your 1992 Ballot!

MAKE ONLY ONE VOTE IN EACH CATEGORY. ONLY THIS FORM MAY BE USED TO VOTE. YOU MAY WRITE-IN A DIFFERENT PRODUCT.

1992 Calendar Year Releases

ORIGINS™ AWARDS FINAL BALLOT

RESPOND BY JUNE 20!
BALLOT MUST BE RECEIVED BY JUNE 25. PHOTOCOPY & DISTRIBUTE FREELY

1. Best Historical Figure Series, 1992
- [ ] Adler 6mm Napoleonics (Stone Mtn.)
- [ ] Chariot 15mm Romans (Stone Mtn.)
- [ ] Hyksos- Ancient Biblical (Ral Partha)
- [ ] Napoleonic- Austrians (Emperor's HQ)
- [ ] Revolutionary French (Emperor's HQ)
- [ ] Title_______________Company_______

2. Best Fantasy/Science Fiction Figure Series, 1992
- [ ] Hot 15mm Dwarfs (Alternative Armies)
- [ ] Le Morte D'Arthur (Thunderbolt Mtn.)
- [ ] Pendragon (Lance & Laser)
- [ ] Ravenloft (Ral Partha)
- [ ] Star Wars (West End Games)
- [ ] Title_______________Company_______

3. Best Vehicular Figure Series, 1992
- [ ] 15mm WWII (Quality Castings)
- [ ] BattleTech Aerospace Fighters (Ral Partha)
- [ ] BattleTech Mechs & Vehicles (Ral Partha)
- [ ] Houstons Ships 1/1200 Dreadnoughts (Stone Mtn.)
- [ ] Mekton (RAFM)
- [ ] Ogre (Ral Partha)
- [ ] Title_______________Company_______

4. Best Miniature Accessory Series, 1992
- [ ] Precision Details 15mm ACW Buildings (Stone Mtn.)
- [ ] Spanish Buildings (The Drum)
- [ ] Tiny Terrain 15mm Fantasy (Simtac)
- [ ] Title_______________Company_______

5. Best Miniatures Rules, 1992
- [ ] Command Decision II (GDW)
- [ ] Ogre Miniatures (Steve Jackson Games)
- [ ] Red Baron (Emperor's HQ)
- [ ] Toy Wars (Crunchy Frog)
- [ ] Warhammer (Games Workshop)
- [ ] Title_______________Company_______

6. Best Role-Playing Rules, 1992
- [ ] Al Qadim (TSR Inc.)
- [ ] Call of Cthulhu 5th Edition (Chaosium)
- [ ] Dream Park (R. Talsorian)
- [ ] Shadowrun 2nd Edition (FASA)
- [ ] Werewolf (White Wolf)
- [ ] Title_______________Company_______

7. Best Role-Playing Adventure, 1992
- [ ] Any: Grimtooth's Dungeon of Doom (Flying Buffalo)
- [ ] AD&D Forgotten Realms: Haunted Halls of Evenstar (TSR Inc.)
- [ ] AD&D Ravenloft: Thoughts of Darkness (TSR Inc.)
- [ ] Call of Cthulhu: Blood Brothers II (Chaosium)
- [ ] GURPS: Cyberpunk Adventures (Steve Jackson Games)
- [ ] Title_______________Company_______

8. Best Role-Playing Supplement, 1992
- [ ] Any: City Book VI (Flying Buffalo)
- [ ] Any: Grimtooth's Traps Lite (Flying Buffalo)
- [ ] AD&D: Ravenloft Forbidden Lore (TSR Inc.)
- [ ] AD&D: Forgotten Realms Menzoberranzan (TSR Inc.)
- [ ] AD&D: Dragonlance Tales of the Lance (TSR Inc.)
- [ ] GURPS Illuminati (Steve Jackson Games)
- [ ] Title_______________Company_______

10. Best Pre-20th Century Boardgame, 1992
- [ ] Across Five Aprils (Avalon Hill)
- [ ] Bloody Roads South (The Gamers)
- [ ] Four Battles of the Ancient World (Decision Games)
- [ ] Franco-Prussian War (Decision Games)
- [ ] Russo-Turkish War (Decision Games)
- [ ] SPQR (GMT)
- [ ] Title_______________Company_______

11. Best Modern-Day Boardgame, 1992
- [ ] Advanced Third Reich (Avalon Hill)
- [ ] A Winter War (Games Research/Design)
- [ ] Bloody Kasserine (GDW)
- [ ] Guderian's Blitzkrieg (The Gamers)
- [ ] Hacker (Steve Jackson Games)
- [ ] Nippon Rails (Mayfair)
- [ ] Title_______________Company_______

12. Best Fantasy or Science Fiction Boardgame, 1992
- [ ] BattleTech 3rd Edition (FASA)
- [ ] BattleTech Technical Readout 3055 (FASA)
- [ ] Minion Hunter (GDW)
- [ ] More Cosmic Encounter (Mayfair)
- [ ] Nuclear Proliferation (Flying Buffalo)
- [ ] Uncle Al's Catalog From Hell (Steve Jackson Games)
- [ ] Title_______________Company_______

14. Best Play-By-Mail Game, 1992
- [ ] Continental Rails (Graaf Simulations)
- [ ] Illuminati (Flying Buffalo)
- [ ] Middle Earth (Game Systems Inc.)
- [ ] Starweb (Flying Buffalo)
- [ ] State of War (Game Systems Inc.)
- [ ] Title_______________Company_______

15. Best New Play-By-Mail Game, 1992
- [ ] Lords of Destiny (Maelstrom)
- [ ] Isle of Crowns (Adventures By Mail)
- [ ] Galactic Overlord (Gem Games)
- [ ] Darkness of Silverfall (Ark Royal Games)
- [ ] Star Queen (Deltax Gaming)
- [ ] Title_______________Company_______

16. Best Fantasy/Science Fiction Computer Game, 1992
- [ ] Wizardry VII- Crusaders of the Dark Savant (Sir-Tech)
- [ ] Ultima 7 (Origin Systems)
- [ ] Ultima Underworld (Origin Systems)
- [ ] Might & Magic: Clouds of Xeen (New World Computing)
- [ ] Title_______________Company_______

17. Best Military or Strategy Computer Game, 1992
- [ ] Carriers At War (SSG)
- [ ] Computer EastFront (Columbia)
- [ ] V for Victory (Three-Sixty Pacific)
- [ ] Hellcats Over the Pacific (Graphic Simulations)
- [ ] A Line in the Sand (SSI)
- [ ] Title_______________Company_______

18. Best Professional Adventure Gaming Magazine, 1992
- [ ] Challenge (GDW)
- [ ] Command (XTR)
- [ ] Dungeon Adventures (TSR Inc.)
- [ ] The Gamer (InPrint/The Gamer)
- [ ] Vortext (Vortext Publishing)
- [ ] White Wolf (White Wolf)
- [ ] Title_______________Company_______

19. Best Amateur Adventure Gaming Magazine, 1992
- [ ] Alarums & Excursions
- [ ] Berg's Review of Games
- [ ] ETO
- [ ] MWAN- Midwest Wargamers Association Newsletter
- [ ] The Zouave
- [ ] Title_______________Company_______

Voter Name_______________________________

Address_______________________________

City_______________**State**_____**Zip**_______

Signature_______________**Phone_(___)**_______

BALLOTS WITHOUT CURRENT PHONE NUMBER, OR IN ANY FORMAT BUT THIS ONE, WILL BE DISALLOWED.

Note that Categories 9, 13, and 20 are for Academy Membership Vote Only, thus do not appear on this ballot.

Send your Final Ballot to the following address by the deadline, June 20, 1993 (postmark).

BALLOTS RECEIVED AFTER JUNE 25 WILL NOT BE VALID

ORIGINS™ Awards
5575D Arapahoe Rd.
Boulder, CO 80303

For More Information:
Phone 303-786-9727
Fax 303-786-9797

See Other Side for your 1991 Ballot!

Sage Advice

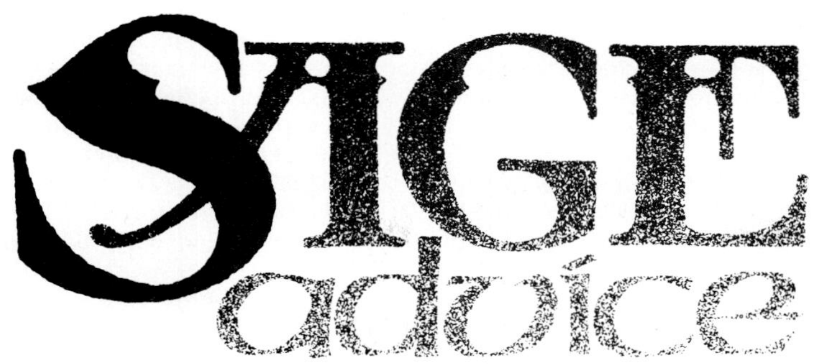

By Skip Williams

Rary's Fortress Upper Level 3: Map 10

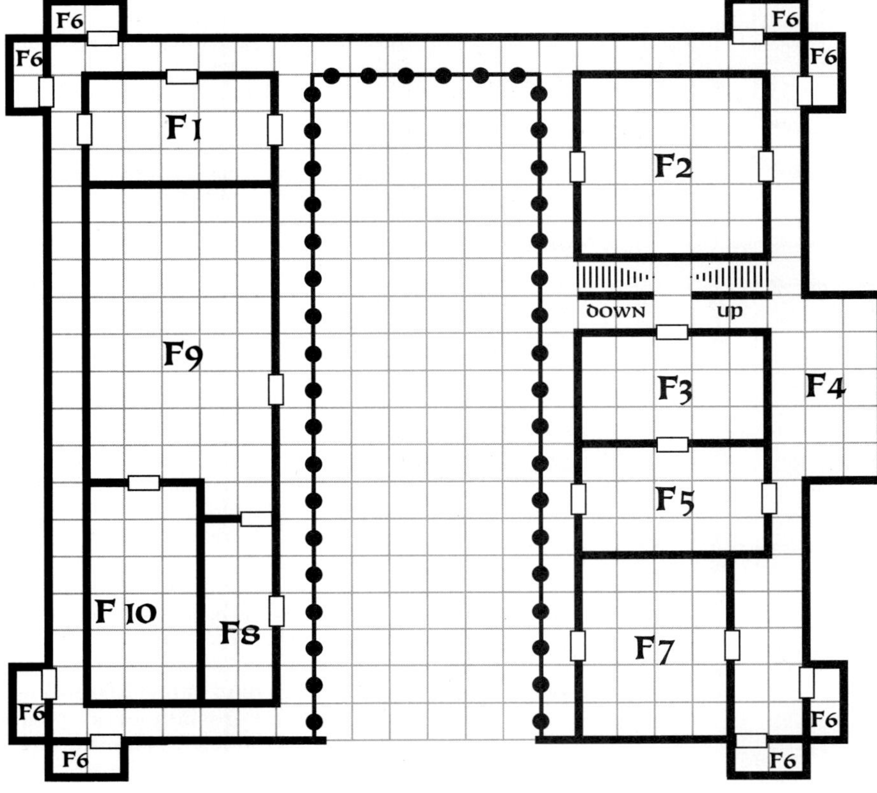

If you have any questions on the games produced by TSR, Inc., "Sage Advice" will answer them. In the United States and Canada, write to: Sage Advice, DRAGON® Magazine, P.O. Box 111, Lake Geneva WI 53147, U.S.A. In Europe, write to: Sage Advice, DRAGON Magazine, TSR Ltd., 120 Church End, Cherry Hinton, Cambridge CB1 3LB, United Kingdom. We are no longer able to make personal replies; please send no SASEs with your questions (SASEs are being returned with writer's guidelines for the magazine).

This month, "Sage Advice" looks at a potpourri of topics, all straight out of the mailbag. This particular batch of letters contained a lot of questions about the various settings for the AD&D® game, so this particular column has a theme in spite of itself. We start with the case of the missing maps. . . .

Hey, what happened to the maps in the AD&D GREYHAWK® Adventures module, WGR3 *Rary the Traitor*? Aren't a few of them missing?

Yes—maps 10, 11, and 12, which depict sections of Rary's fortress, are missing. I'll skip the whole sordid story of how they came to be that way and direct you to the missing maps, which are presented in this very column for your erudition and use.

Do thief abilities such as hide in shadows and move silently work on undead in the D&D® game?

Generally, yes. This also is the case in both editions of the AD&D game, too.

Unless the monster description states otherwise, undead have no special ability to detect creatures that are invisible, hidden, silent, or otherwise concealed. Note that undead have infravision, which can detect creatures hiding in shadows if there is no infrared (heat) source creating "infravisional shadows" in the area.

I have encountered campaigns that assume undead creatures can somehow sense living creatures. The reasoning goes something like this: Undead have no functioning sense organs—their eyes, ears, etc.—have rotted away. Since they can detect neither light nor sound, their "senses" operate in some arcane manner that makes invisibility or silence irrelevant. This house rule can add a new dimension to undead, even to lowly creatures such as skeletons and zombies; however, the published rules assume that undead somehow really do see, hear, etc. If you decide to adopt an undead "sense life" rule, increase each undead monster's experience value to reflect this special ability to see invisible creatures. Also, you'll need to decide on a number of other parameters for the ability, such as its range and what, if anything, blocks or disrupts it.

Could a wizard on Athas make a living just selling *walls of iron* for scrap?

How many ceramic pieces would a *wall of iron* be worth? Could the iron be used for weapons, armor, and tools? If the wizard kept a piece of a *wall of iron*, could she use it as the material components for more spells? Would this also be true for *wall of stone* or *wall of ice*?

Iron is worth one gold piece (100 ceramic pieces) per pound in DARK SUN® campaigns (see *Dune Trader*, page 72). A *wall of iron* contains a minimum of 12,403 lbs. of iron (about 25 cubic feet at 490 pounds per cubic foot). However, in DARK SUN campaigns, a *wall of iron* spell has a duration of one turn per caster level (see the DARK SUN rule book, page 93). A wizard might be able to sell a few chunks of iron as a scam, but the practice will catch up with her if she tries it too often.

While the material in a *wall of iron* functions as normal iron in most respects, there is no reason why a Dungeon Master has to assume it can be worked as regular metal can. For example, the DM might decide that iron from a *wall of iron* contains certain impurities that cause it to form useless lumps of slag if heated and worked, and that it simply flakes apart if worked cold. Note also that, regardless of its duration, metal from a *wall of iron* radiates magic and can be dispelled. Even if it could be used to manufacture items, those items can be destroyed by *dispel magic* effects.

Having material components for spells is an optional rule. I don't know any DM who uses this rule and also lets his players get around it by using magically created material components—this is a question of game balance. From the standpoint of game logic, the dweomer that maintains the *wall of iron* or other magically created material either interferes with the spellcasting process or unravels during the process. First, attempts to cast spells using a magically created object as a material component are disrupted. Second, the magically created material component ceases to be and it just isn't available to complete the spell. In either case. the attempted spell fails. Some exceptions exist. Generally, items brought into being by a *wish* work fine as material components, at least if the component is not rare or valuable; and a *Zagyg's spell component case* (from *Unearthed Arcana*) always produces usable material components.

How would the Veiled Alliance interact with advanced beings such as dragons, elementals, and avangions?

The same way everybody else does: with great circumspection. This would take the form of admiration and civility in the case of elementals and avangions, and fear and loathing in the case of dragons. Since avangions are high-level preservers, it's a pretty good bet that they work pretty closely with any local branch of the Veiled Alliance—in fact, they probably are former members of one Veiled Alliance or another.

***Dragon Kings* says that avangions attract followers. Where are the charts for this?**

There aren't any. The appearance of an avangion is a momentous event in any campaign, and its affect on the game has to be carefully considered, then played out. The first thing the DM has to do is identify the most notable and powerful good-aligned NPCs in the game; such characters are certain to make overtures to an avangion when they learn that such a creature exists. Likewise, most neutral and good folk who meet an adventuring avangion are going to take a liking to the character (unless the player controlling it is a complete idiot). This is what the rules are referring to when they mention allies.

Do avangions eat and sleep?

This is up to the DM. Judging from my conversations with Tim Brown, *Dragon Kings* author, advanced beings obey all the rules for spellcasting (see "Sage Advice," issue #189), which means they must sleep to regain spells. Otherwise, the DM is free to assume that avangions never rest. Since the rules say that an avangion's mouth begins to disappear as its form evolves, it would be reasonable to assume that avangions of 25th level or higher either don't eat at all or eat unusual materials, such as the silver linings of clouds, moonlight reflected off cactus spines, or the like. Perhaps only fully transformed avangions are completely self-contained. Lower-level avangions who still have basically human forms probably have to eat, but this, too, is up to the DM.

Can avangions of level 26 and up use the Prolific Forestation and Prolific Vegetation psionic enchantments? These spells not only require the use of hands (to carve a staff), but also require the caster to walk, not run, fly, or levitate. Since high-level avangions

RARy's FORTRESS UppER LEVEL 4: Map II

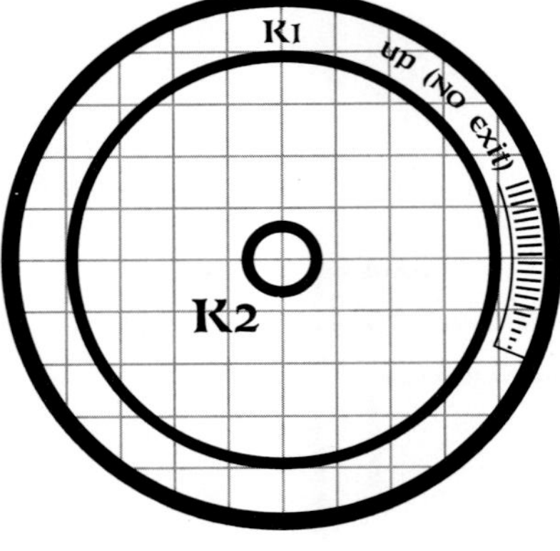

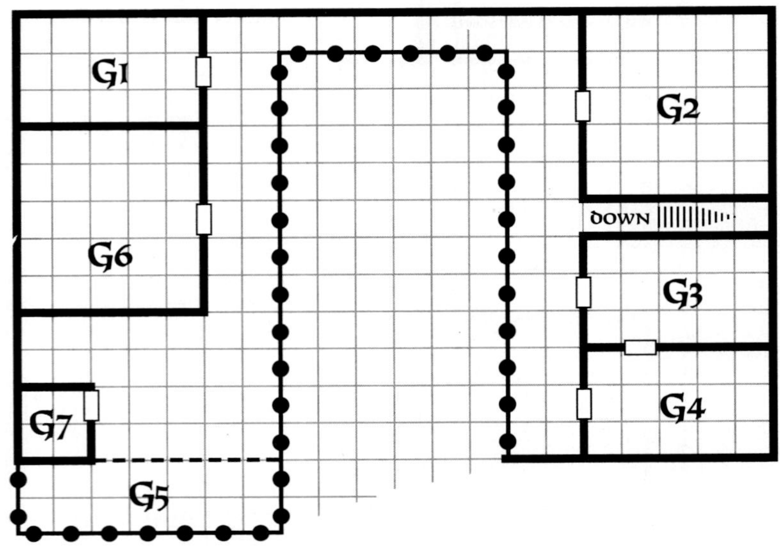

I SQUARE   IO fEET

must fly only, they would have a hard time meeting this requirement.

Yes, avangions can use these spells. Nevertheless, the caster must *walk*. While avangions of 26th level and above cannot walk in their natural forms, nothing prevents them from using spells or psionics to change into something that *can* walk. A simple *polymorph self* spell or Metamorphosis psionic power are only two examples of things that can do the trick. Note that the avangion can stop and renew a spell if he needs to, so long as the Prolific Forestation or Prolific Vegetation spell is not interrupted for more than a full round.

The *Player's Handbook* states that elves routinely live up to 1,200 years. Given this, I cannot fathom why elves suffer a –1 Constitution penalty. The rules do say that elves are not as "sturdy" as humans, but this is illogical. If anything, elves should get a +1 bonus to Constitution due to their hardiness and longevity.

Longevity is not necessarily synonymous with hardiness. A parrot lives a lot longer than a horse, but horses have much better Constitution scores than parrots do. Still, play balance in your campaign probably won't suffer if you fiddle with demihuman racial modifiers a bit. If you want to give elves a Constitution bonus, just eliminate the Dexterity bonus and assign a penalty to some other ability score; elves in your campaign might have lower Wisdom scores since their long years tend to make them a bit frivolous and impulsive.

The notes about grey elves on page 17 of *The Complete Book of Elves* says that only the Conjuration, Enchantment, and Greater Divination schools of magic are open to elven mages. However, the chapter on the magic of the elves in the same book contradicts this by including an Alteration spell, *camouflage*. Where did this rule come from? I can't find anything like it in any of the other books.

The passage on page 17 is erroneous. It refers to Table 22, Wizard Specialist Requirements, in the *PH* (page 31). It should read: "Because the only wizard specialties available to elves are Diviner and Enchanter, grey elves usually do not become specialist wizards."

Elven mages (nonspecialized wizards) can use any kind of spell, just as mages of any other race can. Note that page 17 mentions Conjuration, but Conjurers must be human or half-elven. Note also that elves also can become wild mages, but *The Complete Book of Elves* author Colin McComb suggests that this specialization, too, is rare among grey elves.

Since plants take in carbon dioxide and give off oxygen, what effect do they have on spelljammers? Since elven ships are made from living plants, do their air envelopes last indefinitely?

Individual plants produce only minuscule amounts of oxygen. They also actually *consume* some oxygen when metabolizing the sugars they manufacture during photosynthesis. Healthy plants also require lots of water, soil, and 12-18 hours of sunlight each day. Note that some darkness also is essential for healthy plants. These limitations make them impractical for spelljammers. The only reason plants can help maintain planetary atmospheres is because they vastly outnumber the animals.

The various "live" elven ships do not produce enough oxygen to affect their own air envelopes—though I suppose a derelict wild ship that is badly overgrown might have a fresh envelope when found. Elves can produce breathable atmospheres from old armada-style ships (see *Lorebook of the Void*, page 56), but only when several of these large ships are linked together in a large ring and allowed to grow into a solid, immobile mass.

Can a riddlemaster (a kit from *The Complete Bard's Handbook*) use his probable path ability to choose a specific card from a *deck of many things*?

No. The probable path ability depends upon clues that the riddlemaster can comprehend and analyze. A *deck of many things* provides no such clues. Ω

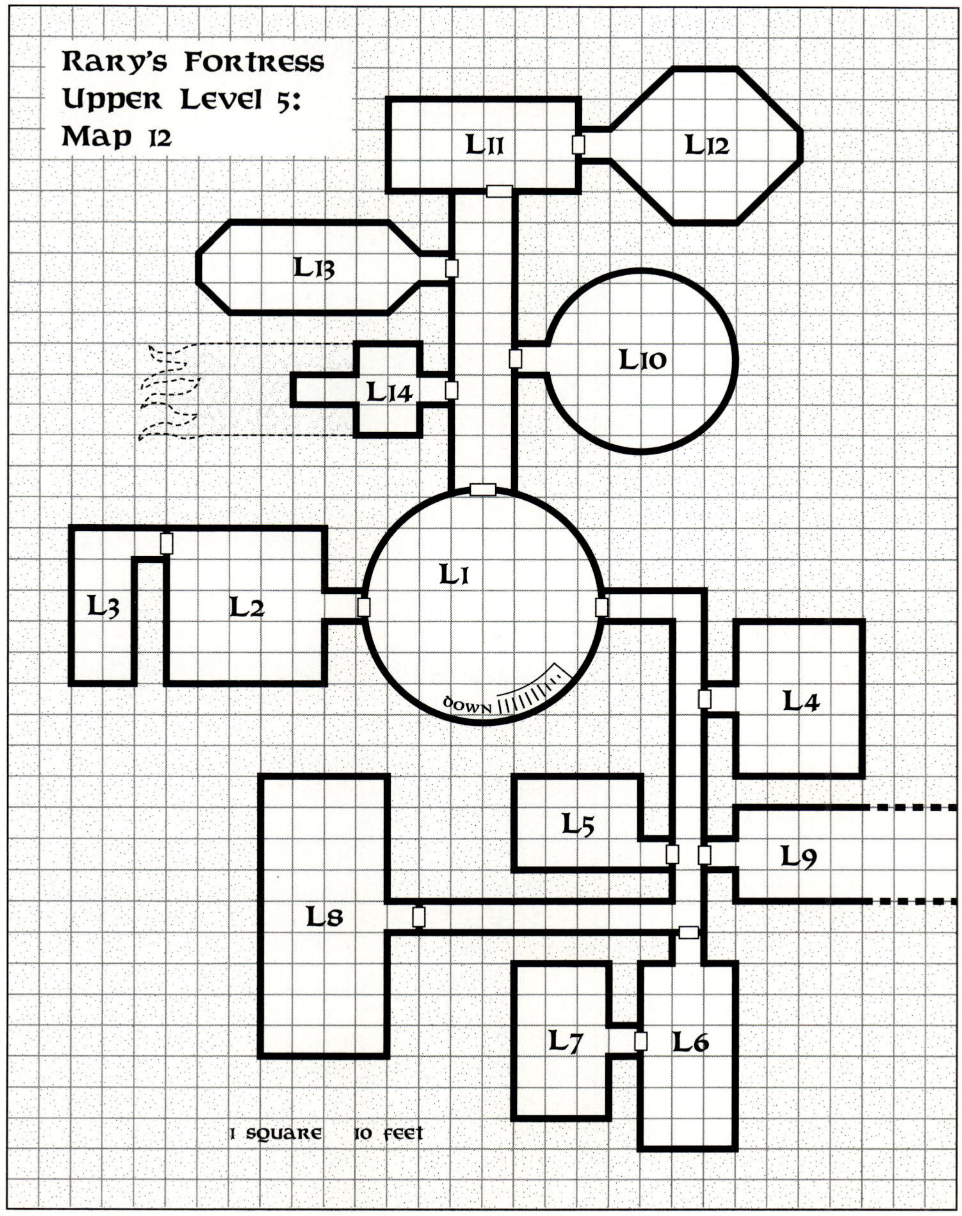

If you've ever said, "Give me the chance, and I'll create the greatest fantasy game of all."

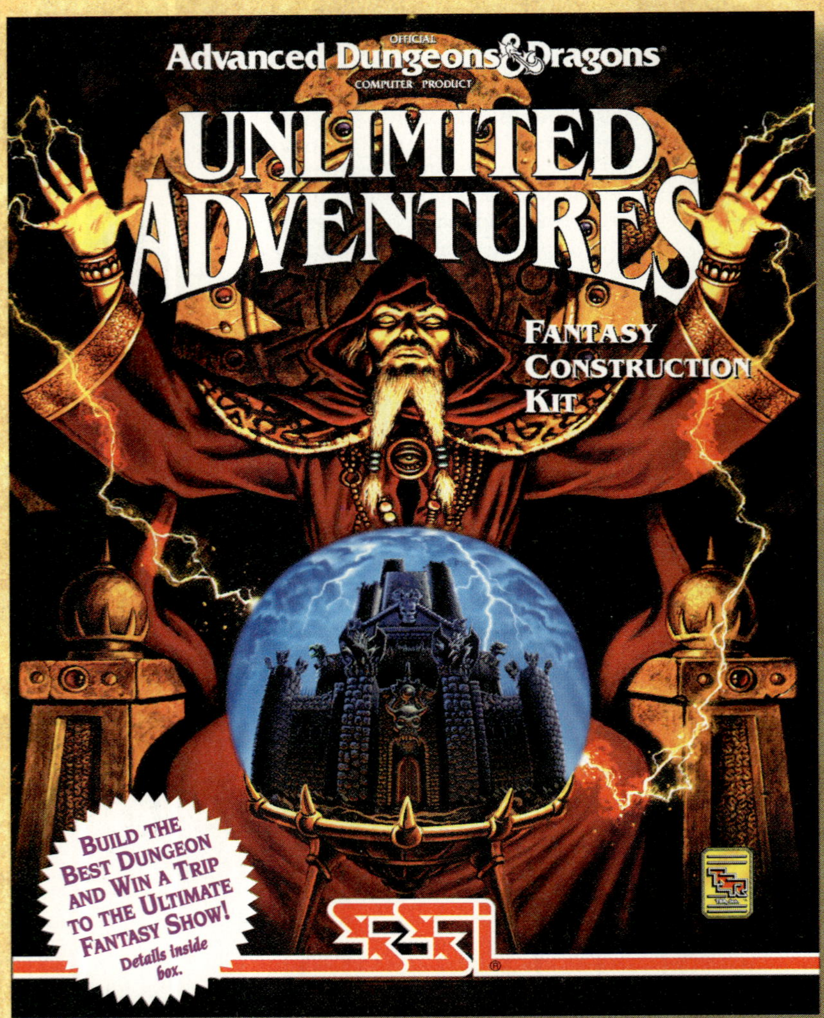

STOP FANTASIZING AND DO IT!

This is your chance to break the chains and create your own AD&D® adventure scenarios in the incredible FORGOTTEN REALMS® world. Your tools: More than 200 classic art images from AD&D Gold Box games of the past. Digitized illustrations from the pen-and-paper AD&D game. And original art drawn especially for your creation. Your only limitation is the size of your hard drive.

You'll build maps with the easy-to-use grid screen and link them with teleporters, doorways and stairwells. You'll choose from the massive bank of 112 monsters and multiple non-player characters. You'll design the dungeons of your dreams and test them as you go with a point-and-click interface that makes errors gone forever — at the touch of a button!

The 3-D views are drawn directly from popular SSI titles.

The strategic over-head-view phased combat scenarios feature easy-to-use commands. And you can back it all up for later play on your or a friend's machine.

Test your mettle by playing the pre-created scenario *"The Heirs to Skull Crag"*, with its four huge areas, a killer plot and four separate quests to solve. If you choose, you can even modify this ready-to-go adventure.

To make a long story short, if you've discovered just about every other AD&D adventure limits your imagination, you'll find UNLIMITED ADVENTURES, in a word, fantastic!

IBM (286 or greater)
MACINTOSH

TO ORDER:
Visit your retailer or call 1-800-245-4525 (in USA & Canada) with VISA/MC.

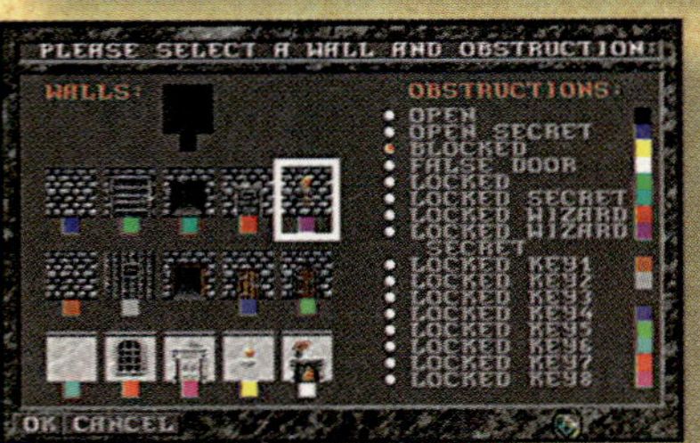
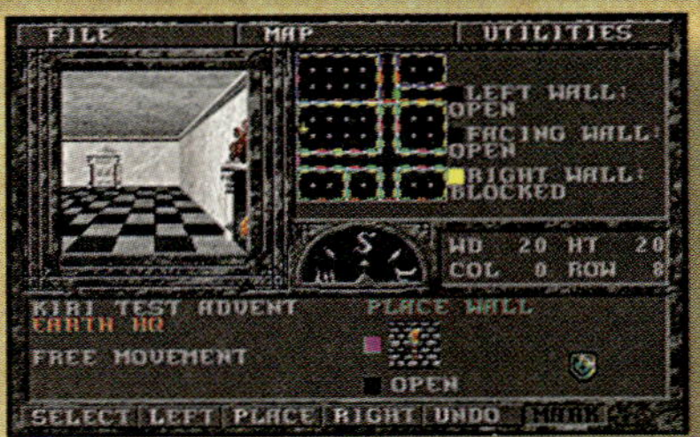
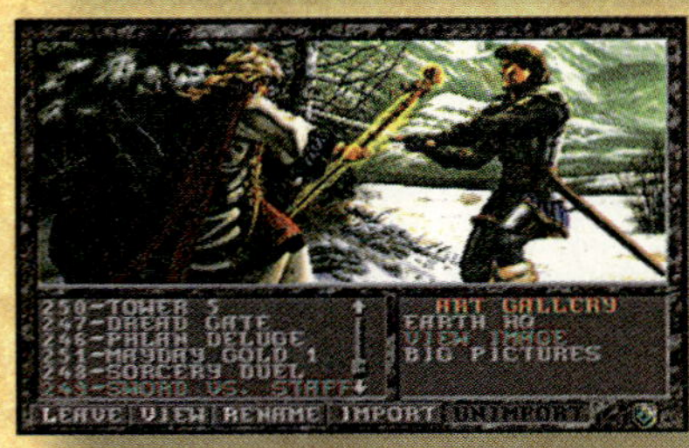
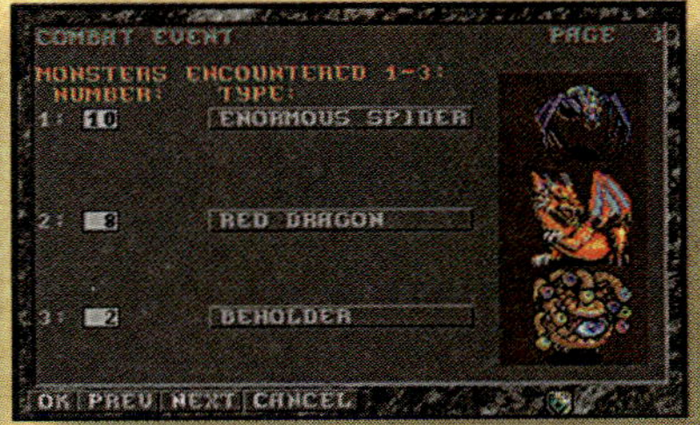

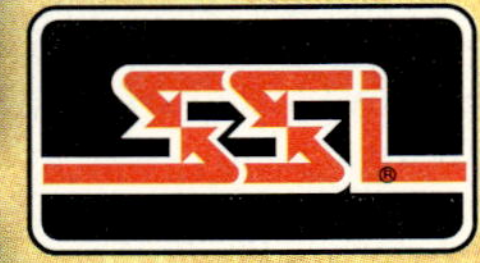

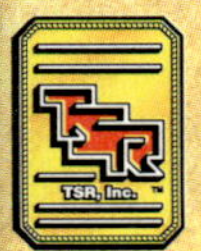

SCREENS SHOWN: IBM 256-COLOR VGA.

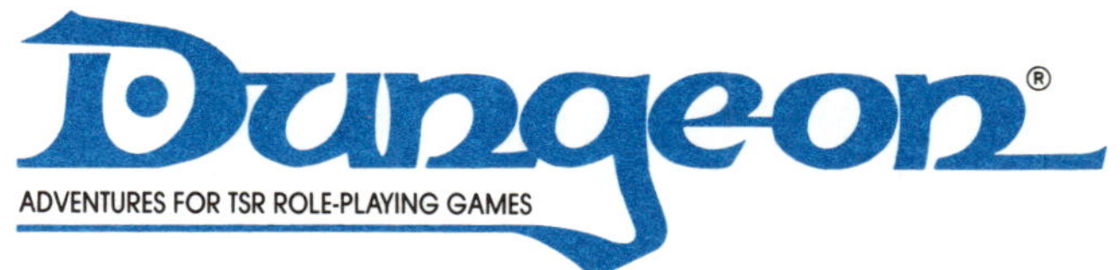

DUNGEON® Adventures is available to our readers in the UK and EUROPE on annual subscription: £21 for 6 issues, mailed to any address in the UK; or £28 for 6 issues, mailed to any address in Europe. (Prices include postage and packing).

To ensure your regular copy of DUNGEON Adventures send for your subscription now!

Simply enclose a cheque or postal order made payable to DUNGEON Adventures, and send it to: DUNGEON Magazine Subscriptions Dept., PO Box 500, Leicester, LE99 0AA, United Kingdom. For payment by Access or VISA, telephone: +44 (0)858 410510 and ask for DUNGEON Magazine subscriptions.

Dungeon

ADVENTURES FOR TSR ROLE-PLAYING GAMES

EUROPEAN SUBSCRIPTIONS ONLY

How to Order:

Simply fill in the coupon and send to DUNGEON® Adventures Subscriptions Dept., PO Box 500, Leicester, LE99 0AA, **OR** telephone +44 (0)858 410510 and quote your credit card number.

Amount of Payment (UK Funds Only!)

☐ 6 issues to UK address for £21.00

☐ 6 issues to European (non-UK) address for £28.00

All subscriptions will start with the next available issue.

Mr/Mrs/Miss _______ Initials _________ Surname _______________________

Street

Town

County

Post Code

Country

Payment

1. Cheque: I enclose my cheque/postal order for £ .... (Payable to DUNGEON Magazine)

2. Credit Cards: Please charge £ .... to my Access/Visa Account

Card Number:

Expiry Date: ..../.....................

Signature: .... Date: ....

Please tick here if you do **NOT** wish to receive details of any special offer or new products ☐

©1993 by Hartley, Patricia, and Kirk Lesser

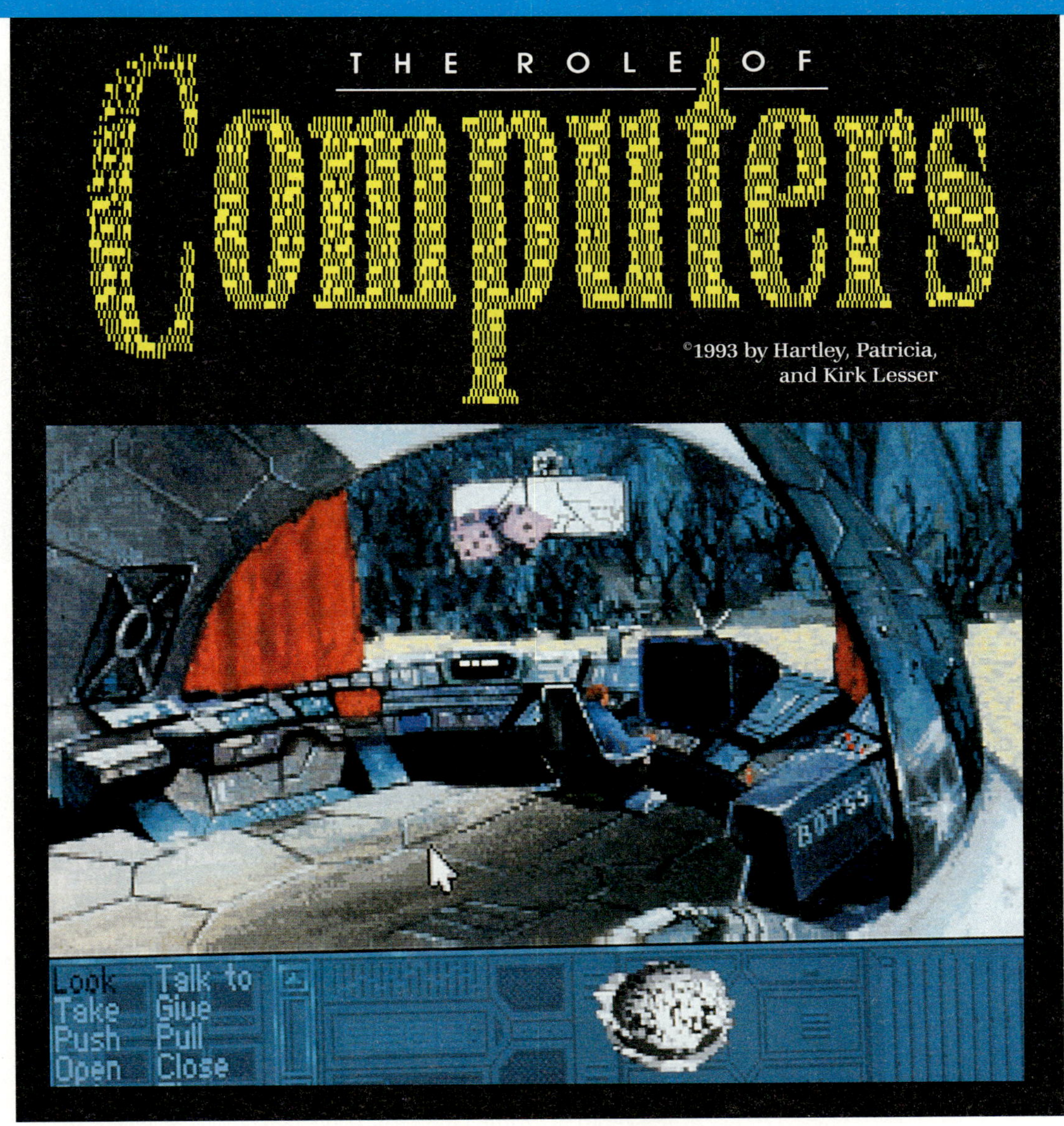

Rex Nebular and the Cosmic Gender Bender (MicroProse)

Back to the wars in fantasy land

Knightline

Sierra has signed ex-police chief Daryl Gates, L.A.P.D., to author the company's next Police Quest installment. Gates stated, "I want to give computer users the opportunity to see what it's like to be a cop in L.A. I want to show the day-to-day pressures officers face and provide an accurate picture of the dangers and difficulties they encounter in trying to solve a crime."

UBI Soft, the publisher of *Koshan Conspiracy*, has told us that some gamers have a problem running the PC/MS-DOS versions of that game. When the game starts, the screen with GAME and CREATION pops up. In a few seconds, the game defaults to the opening credits or, in some instance, to the first screen of the game. If the game defaults to the credits, you can leave that screen by holding down the left mouse button for a few seconds.

This returns you to the GAME/CREATION screen. When you get here, press the left mouse button and the game starts. If you press the right mouse button, you're switched to the CREATION option. Press the left mouse button, and the CREATION process is activated. If you have any additional problems, you can contact UBI Soft's technical support hotline at (415) 332-5011.

One of our favorite on-line services in addition to The Sierra Network is America Online (AOL). If you are a Macintosh

Computer games' ratings	
X	Not recommended
*	Poor
**	Fair
***	Good
****	Excellent
*****	Superb

gamer, we recommend you head for that service's game forum and download *Darkwood 1.2.* It's in a compressed file that will de-archive when you log off. This extremely simple game lets you select a character and get involved in arena combat. A variety of creatures are offered for you to fight, each worth a reward in gold pieces. The tougher your opponent, the more gold you can win. To improve your chances in the arena, use your gold to buy better weapons and armor; you can obtain healing at the local inn. Save your game after each successful combat and learn the individual strengths and weaknesses of the hostiles you'll face. It takes about three minutes to learn how to play, but you'll be surprised at the entertainment value this small game offers. The author of the game, Robert Chancellor, requests a $10 shareware fee if you enjoy the game. For such a small price, *Dark-*

wood is definitely worth the approximately 40-minute download (at 2400 baud).

H.E.L.P.

"In *Knights of Legend,* by Origin, how do you solve Lieutenant Trimrose's problem of his missing heirloom? [Also,] in response to Dale Ketcherside's query in your column in issue #189: First, you may find the Shard of Cowardice in the underworld that can be accessed through the Dungeon Hythloth. Make certain to bring gems and 'Blink' spells. You'll also want to get the 'Mystic Arms and Armor' located there. Second, the jewels Sir Simon refers to are the Crown Jewels of Lord British: the Sceptre, the Crown, and the Amulet. There are only three items, not four."
—Andrew Webb, Columbia, Mo.

"I have a Deathspider ship with an 11th-level mage as captain, and am infamous in reputation. I wish to improve the reputation and also figure out a way to have Melcar the Wise, a wizard and my helmsman, remember spells—he always forgets them. This is very irritating when engaged in boarding combat. Any help with either of these issues would be appreciated."
—Paul Rosin, Houston, Tex.

"I am in need of help or a hint for *Pools of Darkness,* from SSI. I am presently in Moander's Heart and have literally cleared out the entire Heart about 20 times. I am almost at the 22nd level. Here is the clincher: I have already mixed the potions, as stated by the Watcher. But every time I enter the left ventricle to confront Tanetai, the Scepter of Bane is grabbed, the walls contract, and I'm thrown into another section of the Heart. Is there a way to confront Tanetai without being hurled away?" —Sydney Arcand, Quebec

Anthony Caniano of Massapequa Park, N.Y., comes to the assistance of Brad Aufderheide, whose H.E.L.P. request for SSI's *Eye of the Beholder* was published in issue #190. "The special quest of level 7 is completed this way: Find the room in which there are five portals. On the south wall are three niches. Remove all of the items from these niches. In the easternmost niche, place the stone medallion. In the center niche, place the stone dagger. In the westernmost niche, place the stone necklace. Notice that the stone implements you placed correspond to the portals in the north wall.

"The special quest of level 12 is quite difficult. Make your way to the door of Xanathar's chamber. Cast Invisibility 10' Radius, and read the Wand of Silvias. Enter, and Xanathar attacks. Use the Wand of Silvias to force Xanathar back and prevent him from destroying you. Force him back into his chamber east, then south, past the traps that your invisibility prevents from activating, into a small room. In the southern end of this room is a spike pit. Force Xanathar into this pit using the

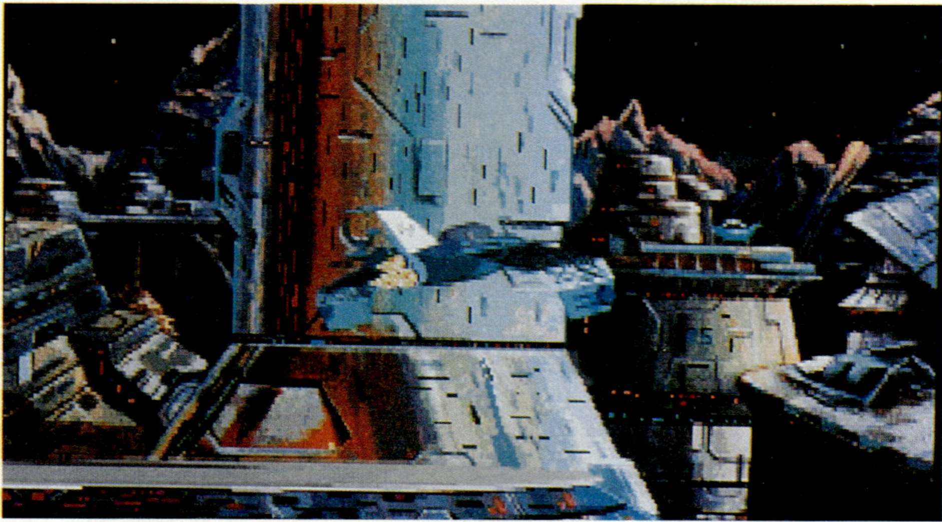

Rex Nebular and the Cosmic Gender Bender (MicroProse)

wand."

Anthony also has a question regarding *Eye of the Beholder*: "Can anyone tell me how to complete the special quests for levels 8, 10, and 11? They are the only ones I cannot discover, despite my best efforts."

Christopher Carter of Brooklyn, N.Y., also answered Brad's plea. His hints are basically the same as Anthony's, but he adds that the special wand you need to complete level 12 is the wand given to you by the dwarves on level 5 as a reward for bringing them the dwarven healing potion. He also recommends you save your game after you become invisible and tackle Xanathar the Beholder. As far as level 7 is concerned, when you place the stone items in the niches, scrolls appear. Clues are received by reading the scrolls.

Derek Bruff posed a question in our column in issue #190 regarding SSI's *Champions of Krynn* Confusion spell bug. D. Millheim of Tallevast, Fla., writes, "When a character has a Confusion spell cast on him, that character temporarily becomes an NPC, run by the computer. When Derek saved his game, the character was still an NPC. Once the game is saved, the bug prevented the computer from recognizing the Confused character as a player character again. If he had allowed the Confusion spell to wear off before saving his game, Pellinore wouldn't be in such a bind. To the best of my knowledge, the bug is permanent. Derek will most likely need to create a new character to replace Pellinore."

However, Ned Martell of Delta, B.C., believes he has a solution to this problem. He writes, "What Derek should do is during the next combat (possibly a random encounter, if there are any left) is to cast Hold Person, Stinking Cloud, or other similar magic on Pellinore to render him 'helpless,' then attack him with one of his other characters until he is reduced to

zero hit points. When combat is over, his cleric can heal him with healing spells, and during the next combat, Pellinore should be on the correct side again. As a side note, the extra references in the Adventurer's Journal to which Derek refers (Sir Era, gully dwarves, etc.) are red herrings. I would encourage Derek to purchase *Curse of the Azure Bonds*, since I think he will find it more challenging and more difficult than the DRAGONLANCE® game series."

Reviews

Conquered Kingdoms   ****
Quantum Quality Productions, PC/MS-DOS

This is a must-buy for all fantasy strategist gamers. With a many scenarios, a wide variety of military units, and the need to increase production during play, *Conquered Kingdoms* (CK) is a great game that begs for continued play. Hundreds of hours of play are built into this game, and your time is well spent as you move from scenario to scenario, learning how to take advantage of each unit's strengths and weaknesses. CK's graphics, sound effects, and soundtrack are not as crisp as other games like it, but you'll soon be absorbed in the geographical conquests presented.

Selecting either the basic or advanced play mode, you command human and fantasy units and seize territory. You gain points for occupying towns, acquiring castles, and defeating enemy units. You must also locate and use resources such as coal, gold, and lumber. Without resources, you can't build additional units, and without castle acquisition, you can't obtain replacement units. The first thing you must do is locate a castle, then try to occupy it immediately! Resources abound and are designated with icons. On some maps, strategic points are acquired

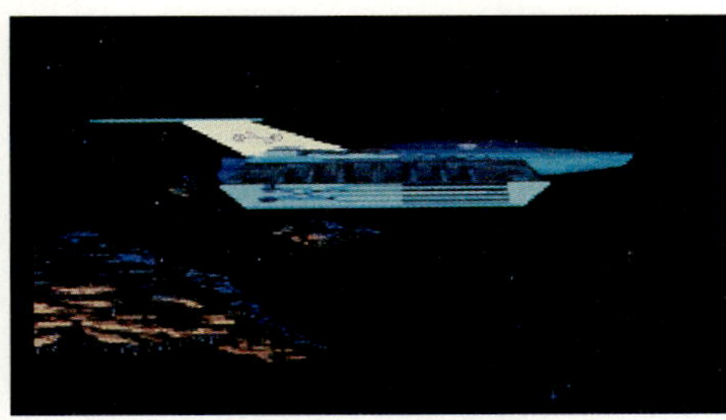

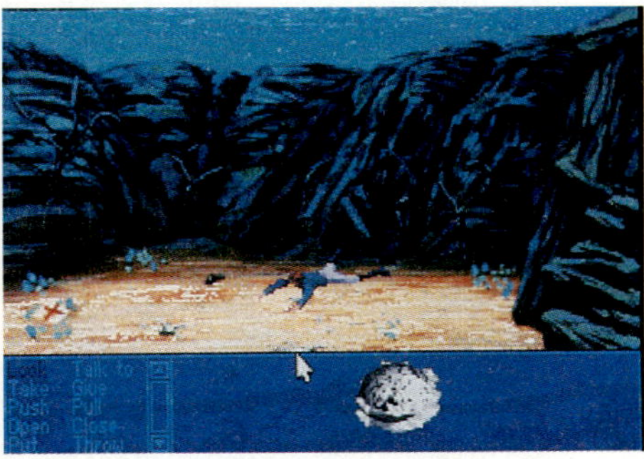

Rex Nebular and the Cosmic Gender Bender (MicroProse)

should you conquer a specific location.

Once you decide where to start your first scenario, you purchase troops by spending points. These troops range from the powerful knight units to your most exotic unit, the spy. The latter can move quickly and can't be observed by enemy units unless they're in the same square he's in. We found the spy perfect for acquiring new towns, resources, and assassinations! Some of the fantasy units include gargoyles, which can fly over anything (great for acquiring uninhabited castles), wizards, and dragons. Wizards can bombard enemy units with fireballs, while a dragon can bombard castles and enemy troops (it also has a high hit-point attribute, making it hard to defeat).

How you combine your units and use them against the enemy is the key to success. For example, if you're confronted by several units of enemy cavalry, you should bring your lancers forward, as they can ruin a cavalry unit quickly. You must protect your wizards and those units best suited for dragon defense. You also can build ships, which are great for transporting archer units across water. However, even the water isn't a safe place, as creatures called rogs love the water and attack units there.

Once you acquire resources, you'll spend time in the resources screen, where you designate what units will be built based upon your stored materials. You highlight the unit you wish to build, then left-click your mouse button (you can cancel your selection with a right button click). Units can be built by spending either gold alone or a combination of gold, coal, and wood. You can always find the number of resource units you currently possess by viewing the information at the top of the screen. At the bottom of

the screen, you're informed as to the number of resource units you are receiving each turn. This helps in planning to build the more costly units, such as dragons and wizards at 20 points each.

If you'd like to take on an opposing king in a tournament, you can select the Cascatia mode of play. The object is to capture 60% of the counties on the map. Special squares contain free resources, such as gold or a wizard or dragon. Since you can randomly select provinces, games are never repeated!

Another great feature of CK is modem play. One computer becomes the controller, then the game is on. The F1 key sends messages between players. A special modem-save-game toggle temporarily saves your current game when the controller's turn arrives; this prevents annoyance when a connection might be lost due to line noise and the like.

CK is a highly enjoyable strategy offering. With additional features such as modem play, the less-than-perfect graphics are quite forgivable. Learning the capabilities of your units and forging toward world domination is a great deal of fun. This game rates highly on our dollar-to-play ratio, as the number of different scenarios and the randomness availability allow you to play hour after hour without repetition. We think you should take a look at this offering at your local retailer—we're betting it finds a place in your software library. We would also like to see CK offered for the Macintosh and Amiga.

Lure of the Temptress   ★★★★
Konami, PC/MS-DOS

Get set to take on Selena, an enchantress who has seized the once-peaceful land of Turnvale. Using what the company calls "Virtual Theatre," Konami's graphic-fantasy game is top-notch. The interface uses a simple click-and-point directional command. When your character, Diermot, moves to an area you've clicked on, a clock icon appears when the repositioning is completed. When you see a movie icon on-screen, an animation sequence is about to take place (such as a door opening). The animation is quite smooth, and the sound effects are really good.

You're never obligated to run your mouse cursor to the top of the screen to reveal hidden command menus, except for those that deal with game operations like saving or loading games. If you click the right button on your mouse anywhere on-screen away from characters or objects, you receive a general action pop-up menu with commands such as Look, Status, Examine, or Drink. You can set up some combination commands as well, such as ordering others to complete a set of actions, all through the pop-up menu structures and your two mouse buttons. For example, you could tell a companion

to go somewhere and complete an action, then return to your location. If you wish to look at something, your on-screen cursor turns into a crosshair that you place over the item you wish to examine. Exits from the screen are located by moving your cursor around; when it turns into a solid arrow pointing in a direction, that is an exit. All of the command structures are easy to learn and become instinctive as you progress through the game.

Conversations with others are indicated by moving your cursor over an individual. When the crosshair appears, press the right button (the left button would bring up the Examine menu); a talk menu then appears. When an NPC is engaged in conversation, a word balloon appears above his head, and the text of that conversation is presented in a window as though typed in. To continue the conversation, you move your cursor over the character's name at the top of the dialog window and press either button. You'll be given a choice of questions or statements at the top of the screen, from which you select what you wish to say to the NPC. Then press your left button. Unfortunately, although you've already highlighted the text you wish to say, it appears as though typewritten in a dialog box above your on-screen character's head. This slows down the interaction and is repetitive—there's really no need for this.

Combat is a treat, though it does take a few encounters to learn how best to attack and defend. Three icons must be watched for: an Advance or Retreat arrow, and the Axe. These represent attack and defense positions. To attack, you press the mouse button nearest to the target. To defend, you press the button the farthest from the enemy.

Don't expect NPCs you've seen in specific locations to be there later! Time moves on, and so do NPCs. Some good ideas to keep in mind during play include: You can Bribe others (if you have cash); peeking through objects is quite informative; and talk to everyone you encounter.

One other problem we noted revolved around a funny fellow we rescued form the dungeon. When not assigned a task or allowed to follow us from one screen to another, he wandered about aimlessly. Additionally, this fellow blocked Diermot's movement through a narrow passageway. There was no immediate way for you to move past him. You must order the NPC out of your way by having him do something, which seems a little absurd as the "friend" must know that he's blocking your progress. We also found a bottle early in the game that was quite useful; two scenes later, the bottle was suddenly broken glass, with no indication of how that happened!

We feel Konami has published a good graphic adventure, despite a few problem areas. The story is interesting, the puzzles are not overly difficult, and the interface is easy to learn. *Lure of the Temptress* easily fits into our software library as one of those adventures we'd play again.

Realms

***½

Virgin Games, PC/MS-DOS

It's quite exciting to face off against an enemy as intent of ridding the world of your presence as you are his. This game is much like *Castles* and *Conquered Kingdoms*, but this time it's not a question merely of combat and who can out-think the other—you've also got to keep your populace happy. A discontent citizenry coughs up few taxes, and without the cash to spur your economy, you can't buy grain to feed your citizens, you can't train cavalry or armies, and you can't equip your troops well enough to ensure their success in battle.

The graphic interface in this game requires some getting used to. It's not simply point-and-click; you've got to move the various screens by interacting with on screen icons, some of them not necessarily self-explanatory.

There are eight realms within which you can adventure, each populated by various races. For example, the Three Kingdoms finds orcs, dwarves, and elves all in the race for supremacy. The Great Divide finds barbarians, orcs, dwarves, and elves in an area where an inland sea divides two continents. Other scenarios contain Vikings and amazons as well.

The first screen you encounter is within your fortress. From this point, you control the action around the known world. Markers, like stick pins, are stuck into a relief map of the world. Yellow markers indicate your cities, red markers enemy cities, and blue markers friendly cities. The largest marker is the capital. All realms have at least one city and a capital. Taxes flow from your cities to your capital. Should a tax route be broken by an enemy unit, you'll have to figure out another way for that money to get to the capital. You can select alternate routes, but they are not usually the best routes, so it takes more time for the cash to get to the capital.

You adjust the tax rate from inside your fortress. A scale shows if you have enough cash to pay your armies. Simultaneously, you want to decide how best to grow your cities (definitely consider building stone walls when you have the money to do so). And don't forget to buy grain! Without it, your citizens starve, their health declines, they become despondent and vulnerable to other ideas, and that's not good for you!

When you view the Playfield, time starts. You can focus in on individual army units to determine overall strengths. There is also a crystal ball in this screen. If it sparkles, a message is awaiting to be read. Should crossed swords appear in it, it's time for battle. Simply click on the crystal ball and you enter the Battle Screen.

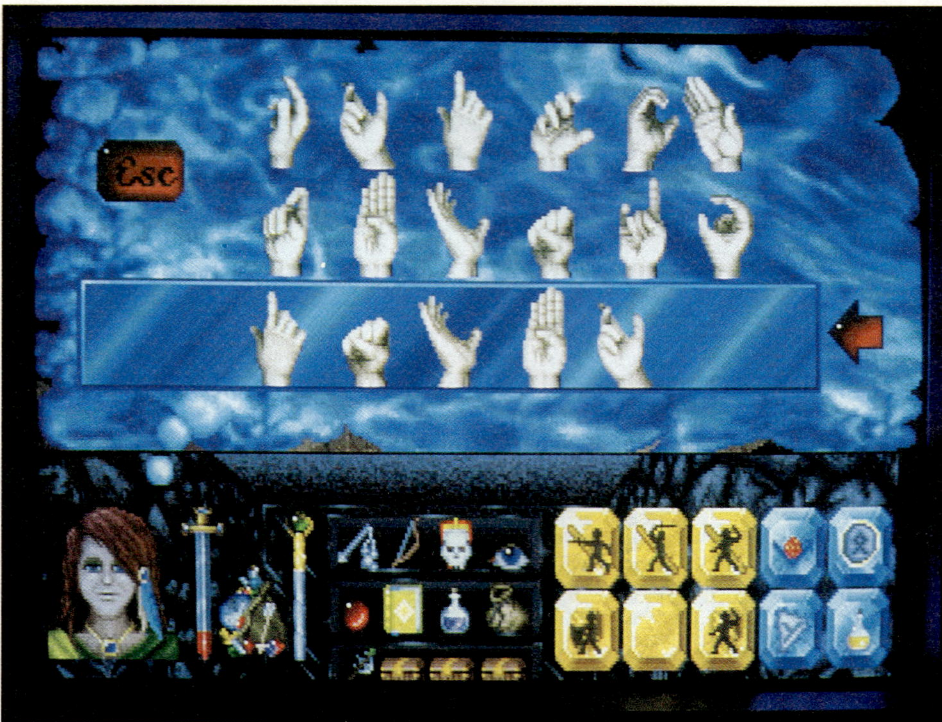

The Summoning (SSI)

On the Battle Screen, your army and the enemy army march onto the field. Your heaviest troops are in the center of your formation, the lighter troops on the flanks. Note where the high ground is; you may have to march away from an enemy unit simply to seize the high ground, but a troop of heavily armed warriors with spears in a defensive position could probably hold out against a larger but lighter force of enemy warriors or cavalry from such a location. By taking advantage of terrain features, we managed to cut enemy forces nearly in half with a smaller army, and thereby lifted a siege of our capital on more than one occasion.

Flags in either corner of the screen reveal the morale of the armies engaged in combat. The lower the flag, the lower the morale. Units that break because of low morale sometimes cause others within their army to rout as well. You command your various armies by clicking on the unit flag, then clicking on the icon that represents the command you wish followed. You can change formations from wedge (best for attacking) to square (best for defense). Or, you may rotate units in any direction you wish. For your missile-equipped armies, you select the unit you wish to fire, then select the fire missile icon, then select the enemy unit you wish struck by your fire. You can also retreat, if necessary. The best way to fight enemy units is to break up their formations; draw out units one at a time and try to avoid direct, frontal assaults. If you have bowmen, use them right away. Once enemy units start approaching, there's little time for missile melee.

One lesson we learned early was to ensure that all of our core cities (those you first start with) were consolidated with plenty of armies and great citizen morale. When playing against more than one opponent, we really enjoyed having them fight one another over territory and weakening themselves before we initiated our own conquests.

Realms is a highly enjoyable, real-time, strategic fantasy game. Once you've become comfortable with the interface, you should be prepared for hours of fun. Certainly, *Realms* should be one of the games you investigate at your software retailer to become part of your library.

Rex Nebular and the Cosmic Gender Bender

*****

MicroProse, PC/MS-DOS

MicroProse has successfully combined the humor of the *The Hitchhiker's Guide to the Galaxy*, the lusty good times of *Leather Goddesses of Phobos*, and the graphics and high adventure value of *Monkey Island* into one of the best graphic adventure games on the market: *Rex Nebular and the Cosmic Gender Bender*.

As Rex, you've been given the task of finding a vase for an eccentric trillionaire. The problem lies with that the planet where the vase was last seen has disappeared. When Rex finally finds the invisible planet, he runs into the natives—who happen to be female and not too happy that an outsider has found their planet. Rex's ship is blown up, and he is stranded on the surface of the cloaked world. It's your task to successfully guide Rex off the planet with the vase, perhaps even negoti-

LEGENDS  FANTASY LITERATURE

PRAISE A LEGENDARY NEW GAME

ROGER ZELAZNY
Author of *The Prince of Chaos*

"A rousing and engaging game where the well-honed edge cuts well—Betrayal at Krondor."

ANDRE NORTON
Author of *Witchworld*

"The idea of combining your game with a book seems to me to be enriching and I most heartily endorse it."

RAYMOND E. FEIST
Author of *The King's Buccaneer*

"I feel great pride and satisfaction that this beautiful piece of computer fiction was based upon my work."

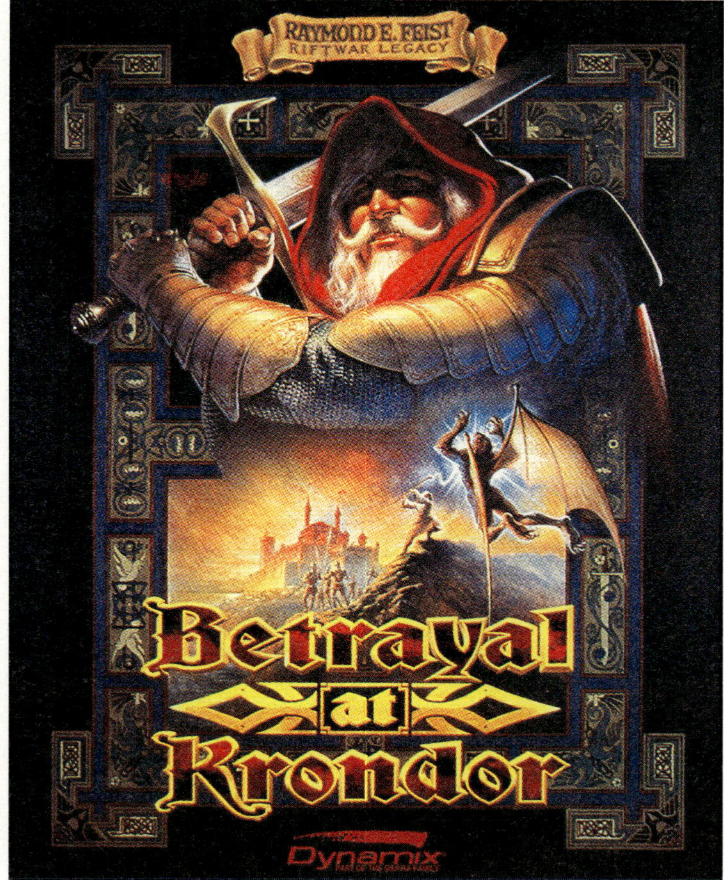

EXPERIENCE the cinematic intensity of *Betrayal at Krondor*, a revolutionary fantasy role-playing game based on the *New York Times* best-selling *Riftwar Legacy* books by Raymond E. Feist. *Betrayal at Krondor* launches all-new legends of Midkemia, a breathtaking mystical land. Elegant story-telling and revolutionary 3Space visuals immerse you in the most realistic, detailed fantasy ever created.

ENDURE savage enemy combat. Opponents not only act but *think* using revolutionary artificial intelligence.

SEE the wonders of Midkemia for the first time as over 2,500 frames of rotoscoped animation, exquisite hand-painted backgrounds and Dynamix's 3Space technology combine to create a "virtual" fantasy.

WIELD more than sixty unusual spells that unleash superhuman magical powers.

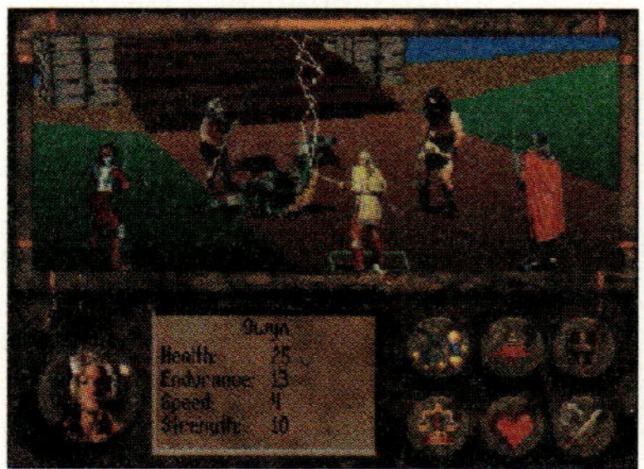
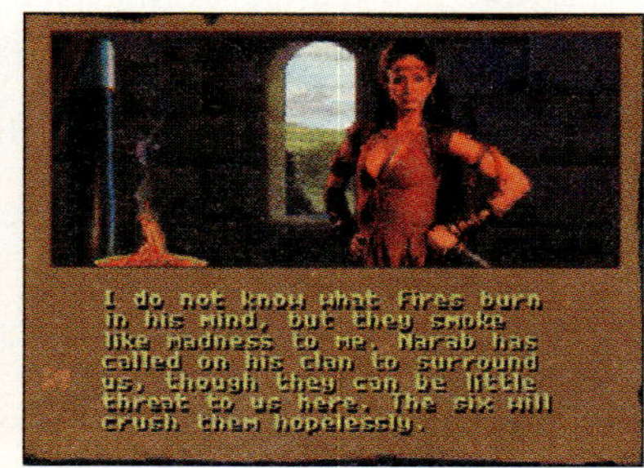

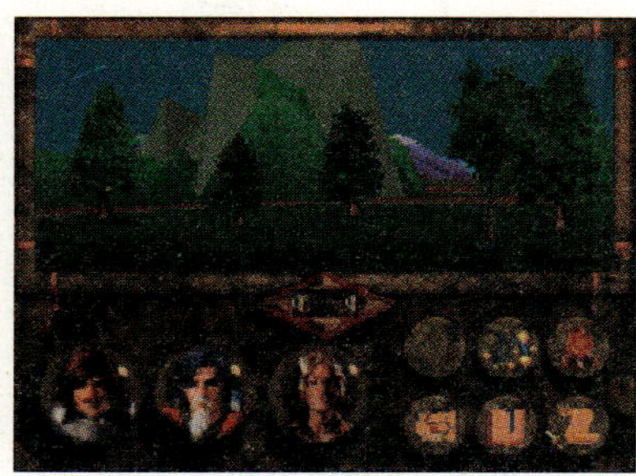

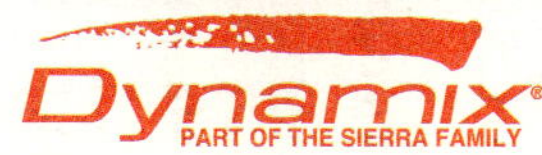

Visit your local software retailer or call **(800) 326-6654** to order.

ating with the hostile beauties who inhabit the planet.

The game uses a command structure similar to LucasArts adventure games. Actions are accomplished by selecting a command for Rex from a list at the bottom of the screen, then selecting the object, person, or inventory item to complete the process. The commands Look, Take, Push, Open, Pull, Put, Talk, Give, Close, and Throw are present. When an item is picked up, you are shown the object (if you have enough memory within your computer, the object revolves in three dimensions!), and a list of special commands are shown that can be used for that object only. For example, by having Rex pick up a pair of binoculars, the two new commands of Look At and Disassemble appear in the command set.

The animation and backgrounds are extraordinary, taking advantage of rotoscoping techniques. The music and sound are absolutely fabulous, as is the speech in the introduction (for those who have Soundblaster cards). Even the introduction itself is good, setting up the game's background in a highly entertaining manner. The only problem we ran into with the game is the amount of space it consumes, both in RAM and hard disk space. The game consumed 20+ megabytes on our hard drive, and even with 4 MB of RAM, we still had to turn off a special feature or two. It is recommended on the game box that the game be played on at least a 30386 machine at 20 MHz, and we wholeheartedly agree. For those who can meet these hardware demands, *Rex Nebular* is a fun and challenging game with three different, difficulty levels.

Rex Nebular has both "nice" and "naughty" capabilities. The "naughty" setting includes nudity and many double-entendres. You have the ability to switch the content of the game from "naughty" to "nice" when curious, young eyes are watching the game. One setting allows you to keep the game fixed at "nice" until a password is typed in to unlock the "naughty" feature.

In our opinion, the *Rex Nebular* team at MicroProse deserves a round of applause for this great adult offering. We eagerly await future adventure games from this company.

The Summoning
SSI, PC/MS-DOS   *****

The Summoning is great entertainment and adventure rolled into a huge labyrinth controlled by the Shadow Weaver. With more than 40 levels of action, with many NPCs, creatures, weapons, magical items, pits, and teleporters, *The Summoning* provides the gamer one of the highest dollar-to-play ratios we've experienced. In *The Summoning,* your hero is not treated very well within the corridors and subterranean passages that abound in the

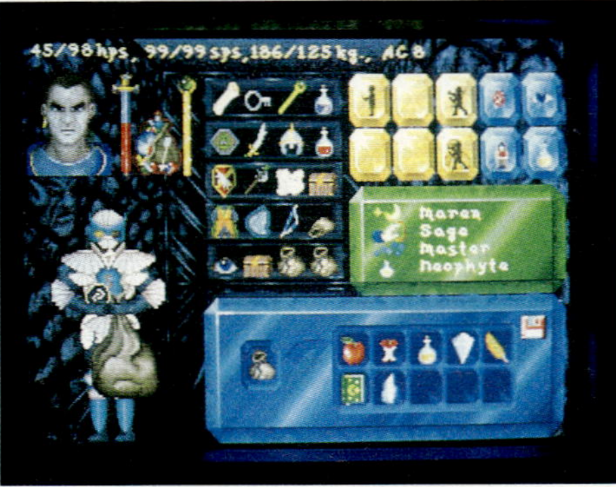

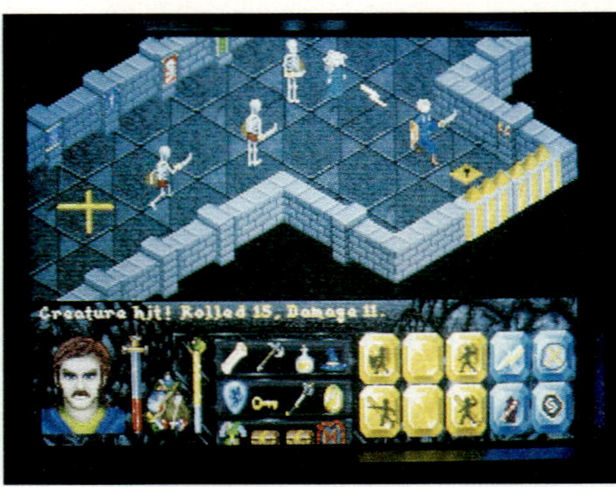

The Summoning (SSI)

labyrinth. Only through your experience and numerous saved games will you be able to master the Shadow Weaver.

At first, the interface may leave you somewhat confused. You observe a three-dimensional overhead map occupying approximately two-thirds of your screen. Below the overhead screen is the top one-third of the character screen. It shows your portrait, a sword that fills with red as you suffer hits, your encumbrance, your spell point status, your right- and left-hand action icons, and the spells you currently have memorized. To see the remaining portion of the character screen, you need to drag this window up and over the overhead view screen. Now you can easily view your inventory: a full-body view of what armor you are wearing and what weapons you have equipped, rating statistics for everything from magic to attributes, and at the bottom a status block that reveals your current experience points and a disk icon for saving and loading saved games. Once you get the hang of using this screen, it doesn't interfere with game play.

You can easily equip your hero with the character screen at its lowest position simply by picking up an item and depositing it on your character portrait. When you retrieve something, either from the three-quarter perspective view screen or from your inventory, your cursor turns into an image of that item. If your character had an item in his right hand, the cursor becomes that item and you can deposit it in your inventory or throw it

away. However, some actions require the screen be brought up immediately. Let's say you're in combat (which you'll be involved in quite a bit) and your falchion breaks. Unless there happens to be another weapon lying on the ground that you can grab and use, you've got to pull up the screen and switch items from your inventory to the right or left hand of your character's body presentation. While you do this, you're taking hits! It's called real-time adventuring, and it works very well.

Magic is impressive. Hand movements are required to cast spells. The higher your experience with the various magic skills, the more hand movements become available to you. This is the one time during the game—when you are channeling a spell—that game play halts, thank goodness! When you enter the spell memorization screen, you select from an assortment of hand positions to cast your spell. Multiple spells can be created; however, overtax yourself and you might find yourself losing a spell. Keep an eye on your spell points indicator. Multiple spells are designated by a small number within the appropriate spell icon area.

There are four types of spells: wizardry, sorcery, enchantment, and healing. You determine at the opening of the game which area you wish to specialize in, as well as which weapon skill is your base skill. Rowena of the Council will supply you with all of the background information you require regarding the Shadow Weaver and the threat he presents. There are also rune stones within the labyrinth. Different stones offer unique magicks: For example, Perth randomly increments a magic skill by one level, Dagaz casts a Spell of Slaying, and Hagalaz casts a Spellfire spell. There are 24 different Rune Stones (good luck finding all of them).

Once you're in the labyrinth, you're on your own except for whatever information you can retrieve from Magic Mouths, NPCs, and other documents. You've got a long way to go before success can be claimed. We found a combination of mouse and numeric keypad use was the best way to maneuver through the game. We used the numeric keypad for character movement, as far more precise positioning is available this way. When you're confronted by pits, surrounded by creatures that are pounding you with sharp weapons, or trying to avoid rolling balls that tend to leave you a little less than you were before you met them, you want to make certain your character is correctly aligned to counter the opposition. A mouse click simply doesn't offer the precise control needed. However, the mouse is best used for all other game requirements, such as inventory switching, selecting options from the various submenus, and for dragging the character screen up and down.

You can always tell how well (or how

badly) your character is doing by viewing his hit point and spell point status. The foes that run amok throughout the labyrinth are varied and quite combative. Thankfully, you can save the game at any time you wish, so you can always be prepared to recall your last activity should your current one end in your demise. There is automapping through the use of an object called a palimpsest. Plus, *The Summoning* offers a feature we wish other fantasy role-playing games would offer: You can print the layout of the level your character is currently exploring! You can also print the text of the many NPC interactions your character experiences.

The Summoning is top-notch stuff and will provide gamers with hundreds of hours of adventuring. There isn't room this month to discuss some of its finer points. We do expect to offer some hints and tips in future columns. Although the graphics and animation are not "photorealistic" (the latest buzzword), they are standard for VGA screen visuals. We have not yet completed our adventure and are loathe to leave *The Summoning* to start other game reviews—that's how much we enjoyed this adventure. You absolutely must consider *The Summoning* as a more-than-worthwhile addition to your software library!

Clue corner

Dark Queen of Krynn (SSI)

With this trick, you can create a knight that has 255 hp. First, use Modify mode on the knight that you wish to give higher hit points. If his/her Constitution is 15 or higher, lower it to 14 or less. Now, lower his/her hit points until the character has 0 hp. All you do now is subtract one more hit point, and the character now has 255 hp.

Adam Di Carlo
Homewood IL

Pirates of Realmspace (SSI)

1. To get the crew under your control, use the quick option in boarding combat and click on the crew icons. This way, they actually help instead of get in the way.

2. After using the above trick, sometimes the computer automatically switches the crew over to short bows instead of keeping their cutlasses. Since they have such limited ammunition for the bows, this can be a major pain. To pass this option up, move the crew next to the enemy you wish to attack and switch them to computer control. When you want to move them to a new position, take control as in #1 above and move them to the new spot.

3. In ship-to-ship combat, a good way to hit the enemy ship without being hit yourself is to find the right speed that keeps the enemy ship about two or three millimeters from the edge of the radar screen. Have the enemy ship centered in the main view screen, and pound them with your weapons. If you are running away and want to hit them, use the same maneuver.

Paul Rosin
Houston TX

Curse of the Azure Bonds (SSI)

1. In the Tilverton sewers, you may come across a room filled with a dozen otyughs and a half-dozen neo-otyughs. If you win, you gain about 30,000 xp and gain four gems plus a piece of jewelry. The gems are cheap (25 to 50 gp value), but the jewelry is worth 3,000 gp.

2. When adventuring, drop all coins. Don't worry, you can always clone magical items like Bracers of Defense (AC 4), which are worth 9,000 gp. Rings of Wizardry are worth 25,000 gp!

3. When fighting the "Bits of Moander," lightning and fire attacks are useless, but cold does affect them. Also, the spell Charm Monster works, too.

4. When entering Yulash, ask permission to get in. When you're in the waiting room and the Zhentil spies run by, fight them. When you chat with the Commander, parlay "nice." He will order his men to leave you alone. Also, when you encounter dirty-looking people, use the Flee option; trying to parlay with them gets you into a fight.

5. This is for Yulash and the drow caves outside Hap: When moving around, turn off the Search option to reduce the number of encounters.

6. Don't underestimate the usefulness of the magical item, Dart of the Hornet's Nest. It is particularly useful against any drow elf or monster with magic resistance.

7. If you are in Hap, fight with the drow patrols before entering the barn. If you wish to avoid them, do not allow Akabar to join your party; he always stirs up trouble.

8. If you are going to let an NPC join your party, make sure you have extra magical armor and weapons to give the NPC. If you don't give NPCs these items, they are pretty much useless except as cannon-fodder.

9. After defeating Dracandros, get out quick. There are still salamanders and dark elves about in the courtyard.

10. When entering Zhentil Keep, don't open doors that have no writing above them. If you do, all you'll gain is a battle and a mark against your record.

Matthew Appleyard
Coldwater, Ontario

Write and tell us what you want to see reviewed. Your hints and tips for fellow gamers are tremendously important. Mail them to: Clue Corner, c/o The Lessers, 521 Czerny Street, Tracy CA 95376. Until next month, game on!

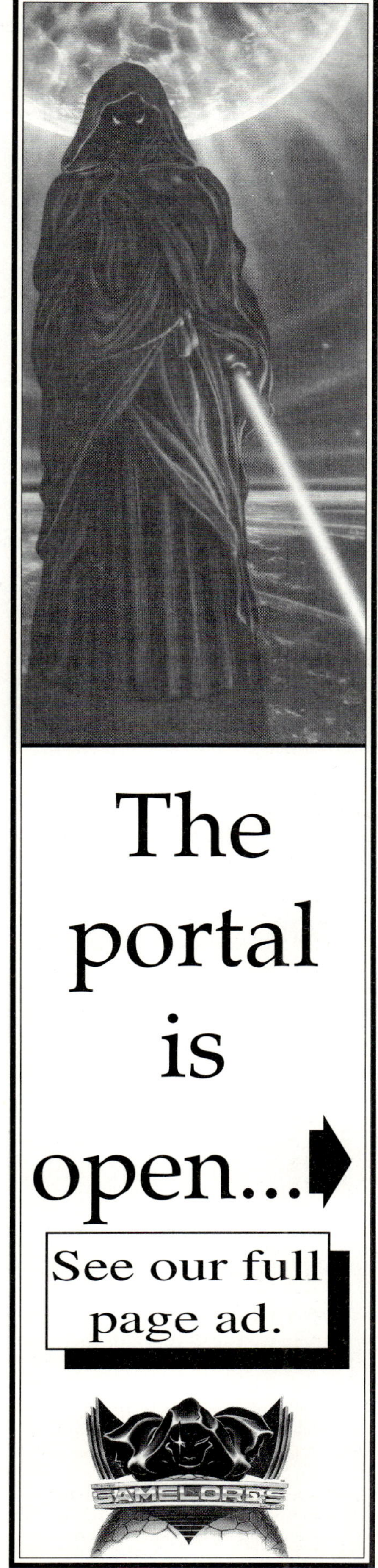

Gamma Terra Revisited

Create even more bizarre GAMMA WORLD® game mutants with these new mutations

by Kim Eastland

Artwork by Tom Baxa

Now that TSR has unleashed the GAMMA WORLD® 4th Edition game on the gaming public, players once again can enjoy that marvelous class of character abilities: mutations. Oh, sure, there are pure strain humans and robots on Gamma Terra, but the vast majority of GAMMA WORLD game players like to play mutated humans, animals, and even plants. Why? Because the combination of mutations generated for a GAMMA WORLD player character is unique to each individual. Characters do not usually belong to "races," so no other character has that singular mix of mutations, skills, and now—in the 4th Edition game—character classes.

Creating new mutations is also one of the big kicks for GAMMA WORLD game masters. It is always enjoyable to see a player's eyes go wide when she rolls a mutation she has never heard of or hears how a previously known mutation is now slightly different.

This article is an expansion of the Physical Mutations table on page 18 of the GAMMA WORLD rulebook and incorporates new and altered physical mutations. Some mutations have been expanded to include more options within their original definitions, while others are completely new. By perusing this list of new powers, a GM may learn how to combine existing mutations and devise new ones to suit his own particular campaign. GMs should feel free to reassign the percentages listed here if any of the mutations are inappropriate for the campaign.

In any case, there is more variety in this new list due to the additions and redefinitions, which ultimately means more mutants roaming the strange and savage lands of Gamma Terra.

Mutation descriptions

Anti-Necrobiosis
Physical; Automatic, no MP

The mutant undergoes necrobiosis, the natural death of tissues caused by wear or aging, at an incredibly slow rate. The character ages so slowly that his natural lifespan is 500+1d100 years. The mutant with this power is *not* immortal; she can be killed in an accident or combat. Aging effects of any kind—natural, mutational, magical, or by device—age the character only 20% of the normal effect. Furthermore, this mutation allows the character an additional +3 bonus on any Health rolls vs. disease, poisons, or radiation.

Darkness Creation
Physical; Activated, MP 4d6-L

The mutant's body can absorb light, with a radius of 5+(MP modifier) meters. The effect lasts for 1d10+(MP modifier) rounds. This darkness blocks all illumination into the area up to an intensity equal to that of a glow cube. All other brighter lights, such as floodlights, arc lamps, the Photogeneration mutation, etc., have their intensities and their ranges halved. A PC mutant cannot see in his own area of darkness, but it is rumored that some creatures with this mutation can see in it as if it were daylight. Lowlight amplification mutations and devices do not work in a Darkness Creation area, though infravision and ultravision do work. Once activated, this darkness exists until either the mutant switches it off or the duration ends, even if the character is unconscious or dead.

Defects
Physical; Varied

Most of the physical defects have been gathered under this heading in the master table. Roll 1d12 and consult the subtable to see which defect the character has. Remember, no PC can have more than one physical defect. Most of these defects can be found in the rulebook, but the Phased Out and Uncontrollable Power Wave defects are new and explained here.

Phased Out (*Physical; GM Activated, MP 4d6-L*): The GM rolls this defective version of the new Phasing mutation once per day. First, roll a hi/low die and 1d12. This will determine what hour of the day, starting at midnight, the defect will occur. Second, the GM rolls to activate the defect; a +2 modifier is allowed if the character is involved in stressful activity, such as combat. Third, the GM rolls 1d10+10 for the number of rounds the defective mutant will be Phased Out.

Uncontrollable Power Wave (*Physical; GM Activated, MP 4d6-L*): The GM rolls this defective version of the new Power Wave mutation once per day. When the character is created, the GM must consult the Power Wave mutation for range, damage, and so on, then roll on the revised Hands of Power mutation subtable to see what kind of power is emitted. Next, he rolls a hi/low die and 1d12 to find at what hour of the day, starting at midnight, the defect occurs. Finally, at the appointed time, the GM rolls to activate the defect; a +2 modifier is allowed if the character is involved in stressful activity, such as combat. The Uncontrollable Power Wave mutation causes tremors within the player character that he can feel, occurring 1d4+2 rounds before the actual explosion of energy.

Since this is an extremely difficult defect for the character to play with, the GM may wish to grant the player character an additional "saving throw" when the defect activates. Whenever the character starts trembling, the player can be allowed a MS+IN modifier roll to keep the explosion from occurring—a willpower attempt made by the character to contain his explosive nature.

Flight
Physical; varied
The mutant can fly by a specific means that is rolled on the Flight subtable using 1d6. When maneuvering while flying, the MP Score is used instead of the DX Attribute. Details on each new type of flight follow (some have been changed from the rulebook):

Gas Bags (*Plant; Activated, MP 4d6-L*): See the rulebook, page 32.

Wings (*Automatic, MP 4d6-L*): See the rulebook, page 47.

Air Sail (*Automatic, MP 4d6-L*): See the rulebook, pages 26-27.

Whirling (*Activated, MP 4d6-L*): The character can spin his body and whirl his arms at great speeds. While doing this, he can fly or hover in place like a helicopter. He has a flying speed of 10+(MP modifier). A spinning character can maneuver in the air as well as one with wings, but he does tire more quickly and so can only whirl for a number of minutes equal to this MP score. Once on the ground, he cannot fly for at least an hour.

While whirling, he has a +1 bonus to his AC, and no one with less than a PS of 40 and a DX of 30 can grasp or wrestle him. While whirling, the mutant can still make an unarmed attack as a physical combat action, with a +2 THAC and +1 damage bonus. However, a spinning character can perform no other action except this attack or flying. He cannot dive or perform mental mutations unless he has the Dual Brain mutation.

Energy Release (*Activated, MP 4d6-L*): The mutant can focus and expel a certain type of energy about herself; when directed below and behind her, this energy propels her through the air. The type of energy is up to the character when she is created. Heat, sonics, gravitic waves, and magnetic pulses are the most common types. The energy surrounding her also grants her a +2 AC bonus. The air speed for this type of flight mode is 20+(MP modifier), but *never* slower than half of that. This energy release is so powerful that a –2 modifier is applied for the purpose of maneuvering. A character can fly this way for 1d6+2+(MP modifier) rounds before she must land. She need not rest, but she must build up the energy again for three hours.

The mutant can do little else than fly when this mutation is activated, but she can use this flight to attack. She does this by flying into the target, using her body as a powerful ram. This causes (2+MP modifier) × 1d6 bludgeon damage to the target, with damage to the flyer equaling 2+(MP modifier). The mutant can control or emit this energy in no other way.

Note: If the mutant has one of the power attack mutations and it is the same type as the energy release mutation she uses to fly, she is allowed this power attack while flying.

Gas Generation
Use the Gas Generation mutation in the rulebook on page 33, but roll 1d10 on the appropriate subtable on the Revised Physical Mutation List. The first six types of gas are described in the rulebook; the others are detailed here.

Partial Nerve Damage: Treat as the Diminished Sense: Touch defect while the gas lasts.

Extreme Irritation: Treat as the Doubled Pain defect while the gas lasts.

Molecular Agitation: Treat as Pyrokinesis to everyone in the area, building up damage per round as per the mutation.

Molecular Insulation: Treat as Cryokinesis to everyone in the area, building up damage per round as per the mutation.

Hands of Power
This expands and slightly revises the existing mutation, given in the rulebook on page 33. The mutation's description is the same, but roll 1d12 on the expanded subtable to determine the type of energy released. Energy types are detailed here:

Zapping Hands: Bolts of electricity.

Hot Hands: Microwave heat.

Laser Hands: Short-range laser beams; player's choice of what kind.

Gamma Hands: Deteriorating radiation causing 3d6 damage only; no other checks need be made.

Cold Hands: Shimmering waves of arctic cold; can even freeze liquids.

Weed-Whacker Hands: Defoliating waves of sonics that damage only plant life.

Blaster Hands: White flash and a bang,

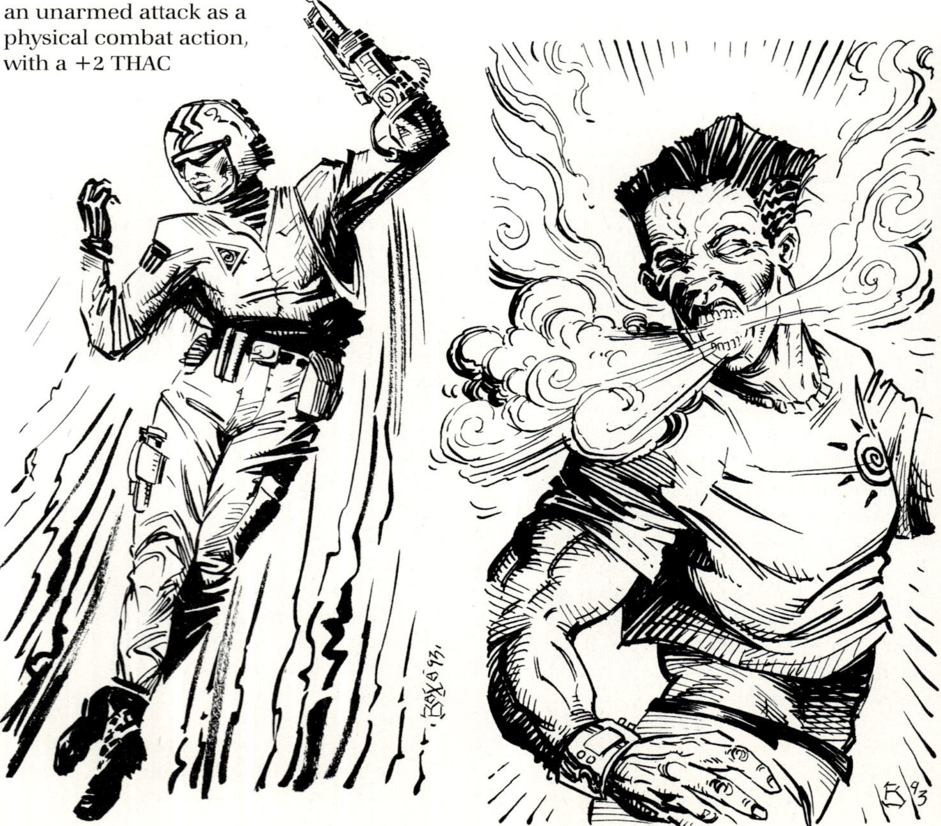

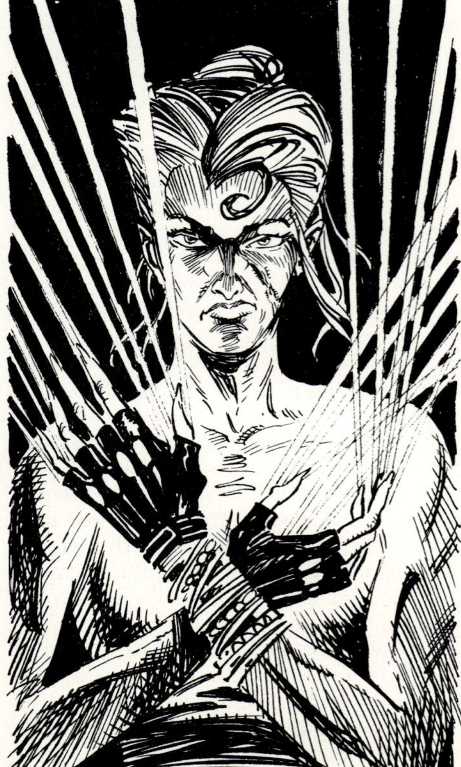

just like the blaster weapons.

Disrupter Dukes: Accelerated charged particles fired; damage is increased to 3d8+(MP modifier).

Gravitic Pulse Paws: No damage, but halves target's movement rate and numbers of actions performed by increasing the gravity around it.

Fluctuating Fists: Hands emit alternating heat waves and cold blasts, damaging like Hot and Cold Hands to living targets, but causing double damage to materials susceptible to expansion and contraction: concrete, metal, plastics, etc.

Stun Mitts: A magnetic pulse that does no damage but acts as a stun ray pistol.

Alternating Emissions: Roll 1d10 on this chart each time the mutation is used to see what energy is emitted (Stun Mitts cannot be generated with this form of the mutation).

Improved Vision

Physical; Automatic, No MP

This mutation entry simply combines similar, existing mutations.

Insomnus

Physical; Permanent, No MP

The mutant has little or no need for sleep. Roll 1d6 and consult the table below to see what sleep the mutant may require:

1d6	Sleep needs
01-03	Mutant needs four hours of sleep every 24 hours
04-05	Mutant needs two hours of sleep every 24 hours
06	Mutant needs no sleep at all

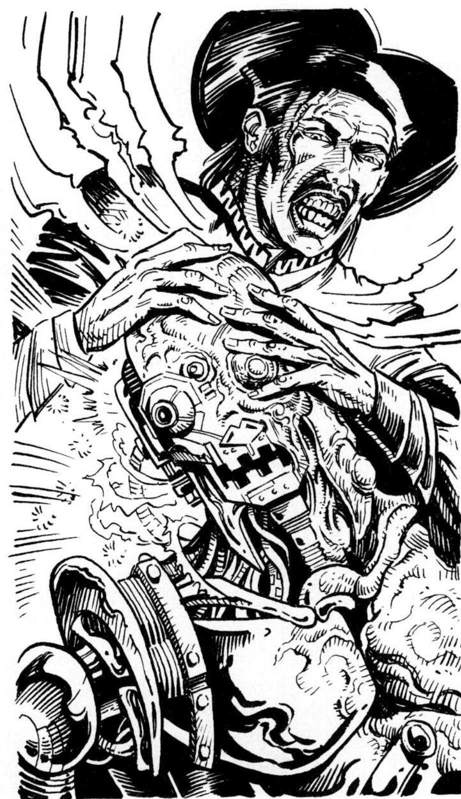

Material Transformation

Physical; Activated, MP 4d6-L

The mutant is able to touch a certain type of material and transform it into another material. The area affected is the item touched, plus any amount of the same material connected to it within a 1-meter radius. If dealing with a large area like a wall, the depth of the material transformed is 30 cm (about a foot). The materials affected are established upon the creation of the character and never change. An example of this mutation is the hoop's ability to transform metal into rubber. The transformation is permanent until someone with the reverse Material Transformation power changes it back. The mutant must roll 1d12 to determine what material is affected and 1d6 to determine what material results. Any duplication, such as wood into wood, must be rerolled.

Material touched (roll 1d12)
1. Duralloy
2. Leather
3. Plastic
4. Stone or rock
5. Wood
6. Synthetics (e.g., nylon)
7. Rubber
8. Bone
9. Cloth
10. Glass
11. Pottery or ceramics

Revised Physical Mutation List

1d100	Mutation
01	Anti-Life Leech
02	Anti-Necrobiosis (N)
03	Bodily Control*
04-05	Carapace*
06	Chameleon Power*
07	Darkness Creation* (N)
08-11	Defects (C)
01	Achilles Heel (D)
02	Allergy (D)
03	Attraction Odor (D)
04	Chemical Susceptibility (D)
05	Diminished Sense (D)
06	Doubled Pain (D)
07	Energy Sensitivity (D)
08	Fadeout (D)
09	Nocturnal (D)
10	Photodependent (D)
11	Phased Out* (D,N)
12	Uncontrollable Power Wave (D,N)
12	Density Control (Self)*
13-14	Dual Brain
15	Energy Absorption*
16	Energy Metamorphosis*
17-18	Flight*
01	Gas Bags*
02-03	Wings*
04	Air Sail*
05	Whirling (N)
06	Energy Release (N)
19	Gas Generation*
01	Stench
02	Blinding
03	Poison, Debilitative
04	Hallucinogenic
05	Paralytic
06	Burning
07	Partial Nerve Damage (N)
08	Extreme Irritation (N)
09	Molecular Agitation (N)
10	Molecular Insulation (N)
20-21	Hands of Power*
01	Zapping
02	Hot
03	Laser
04	Gamma
05	Cold (N)
06	Defoliating (N)
07	Blaster (N)
08	Disruption (N)
09	Gravity Pulse (N)
10	Fluctuating (N)
11	Stun (N)
12	Alternating Emissions (N)
22	Heightened Balance
23-26	Heightened Physical Attribute
27	Heightened Precision
28-29	Heightened Sense
30	Heightened Speed*
31-32	Immunity
33-34	Improved Vision (C)
01-02	Infravision*
03-04	Night Vision*
05-06	Ultravision*
35	Insomnus (N)
36	Kinetic Absorption*
37	Material Transformation* (N)
38-39	Multiple Limbs
40-69	New Body Parts (C)
70	Phasing* (N)
71	Photogeneration*
72	Plasma Spheres* (N)
73	Poison*
74	Power Touch* (N)
75	Power Wave* (N)
76-77	Regeneration*
78	Shapechange*
79	Shapechange Into Object* (N)
80	Silence Field* (N)
81-83	Size Change
84-85	Sonar
86	Sonic Blast*
87	Sonic Roar* (N)
88	Sound Imitation
89-91	Transfusion*
92	Vocal Imitation
93-94	Zip Healing* (N)
95-96	New GM-created mutation
97-99	Roll two mutations, rerolling this result
00	Player chooses one mutation

* Mutation has a power score; roll 4d6-L
(C) The new mutation selection combines previously separated mutations under one heading
(D) Defect
(N) New or altered mutation

12. Metal (roll a hi/low die for soft or hard metal)

Resultant material (roll 1d6)
1. Fleshlike, organic, living substance
2. Rubber
3. Wood
4. Leaflike fiber
5. Glass
6. Metal (roll a high/low die for soft or hard metal)

New Body Parts
Physical; Automatic, No MP

This mutation is similar to that found in the rulebook on page 39, but combines all the unusual body parts under this heading. These include such standards as Photosynthetic Skin, Gills, Horns and Antlers, Poor Dual Brain (D), Poor Respiration (D), Quills or Spines, Skeletal Enhancement, and so on, along with any new ones the GM wishes to add. Once this selection is rolled, the player has a 10% chance for a defective new or altered body part. Otherwise, he should select a beneficial mutation, with the GM's guidance.

Phasing
Physical; Activated, MP 4d6-L

Once per day, the mutant can vibrate the molecules of her body (and all items she is wearing and carrying) so that she moves "out of phase" with the world around her. This does not affect the status of anyone else, but it allows the mutant to travel through any substance except a force field at a movement rate of 3. While phased, the character still requires nor-

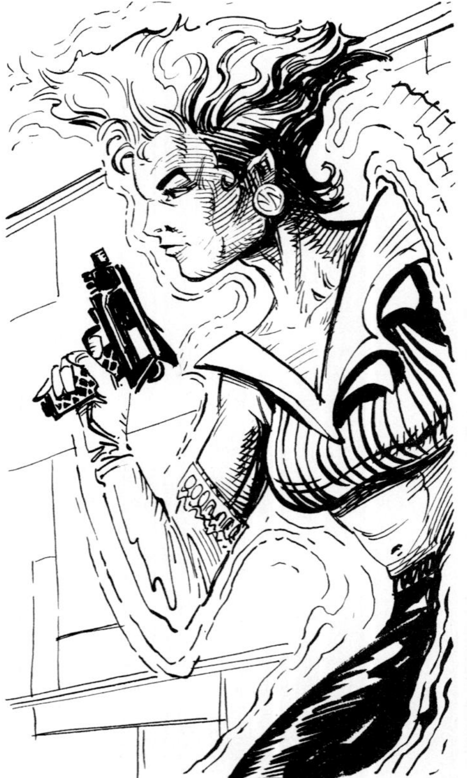

mal light to see but appears to others as a ghostlike form not easily recognizable. She cannot affect nonphased creatures in any way, nor can they affect her without being Phased themselves. Phased characters can react to each other normally, as if on the same plane of existence.

The duration of this mutation is 20+(MP modifier) rounds. The character can phase back into real time/space either through her own desire or because the mutation's duration has lapsed normally. If a mutant, for any reason, suddenly Phases back to her normal state while an object intersects her body in any way, she suffers terrible damage equal to half her normal available hit points (not her current total, but her normal maximum) if less than half her body intersects the object. If more than half of her body is interrupted by solid matter, instant death results. In either case, she loses whatever body parts were molecularly bonded with other materials.

Plasma Spheres
Physical; Activated, MP 4d6-L

By activating this mutation, the character can create a sphere of invisible, stable, low-grade plasma by merely touching a surface. The sphere is 1 cm in diameter and can be seen by only the mutant producing it and anyone with Ultravision or the proper detection equipment (which is extremely rare). The sphere remains wherever the mutant creates it, whether on a path, an item, in a doorway, etc. If anyone else touches the sphere, it explodes immediately in a 2-meter radius for 1d8+(MP modifier) damage. A force field touching the sphere will not detonate it, so it is possible for someone with a working force field to step on a sphere and not detonate it. This mutation generates an unusual plasma energy that is *not* included in the standard Energy Absorption, Reflection, or Conversion mutations. The mutant can create 4+(MP modifier)

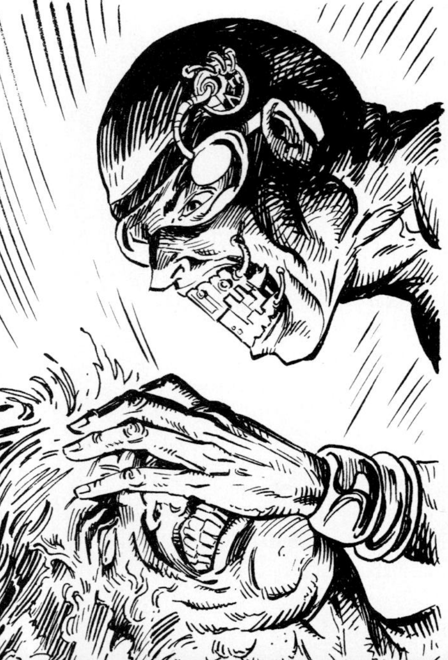

spheres per day. Untouched spheres fade away after 1+(MP modifier) hours.

Power Touch
Physical; Activated, MP 4d6-L

This mutation is similar to Hands of Power, and the type of energy emitted is rolled on the table under that mutation. This mutation differs from the latter, though, in that: a) the mutant must *touch* his target to cause damage (make a successful Unarmed Combat attack if target is unwilling); b) the damage is 1d6+(MP modifier); c) the mutant can store 10+(MP modifier) blasts; and, d) one blast is regenerated every hour.

Power Waves
Physical; Activated, MP 4d6-L

The mutant has the power to emit special energies from his body, somewhat like the Hands of Power mutation. However, the blast affects a 15-meter-radius area from the user, plus 1 meter per MP modifier. The damage is still 3d6+(MP modifier), but it radiates out in waves from the mutant for 2+(MP modifier) continuous rounds, even if he moves or performs other actions. Once started, it stops only if the mutant loses consciousness or dies. The mutant is completely immune to the effects of this power, no

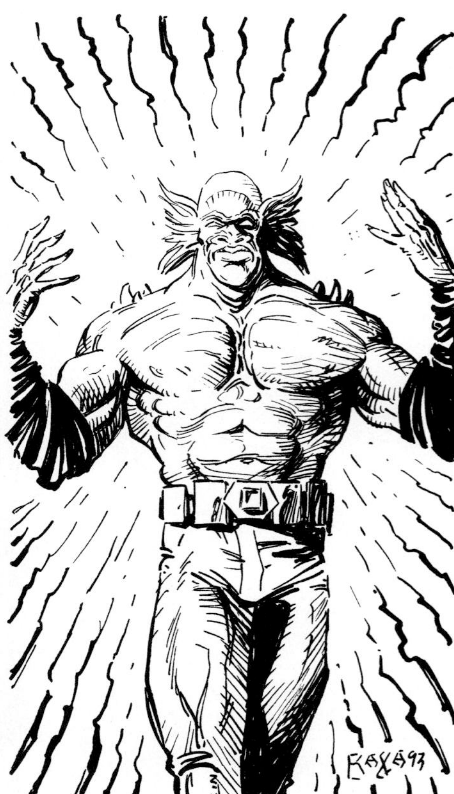

matter what the source. Once the waves stop, two hours are required to regenerate another blast. Roll on the expanded Hands of Power mutation subtable for the type of energy emitted.

Shapechange Into Object

Physical; Activated, MP 4d6-L

The mutant can assume the shape of any item or nonsentient geographic feature (such as a normal tree, a boulder, etc.) that she has touched for at least two consecutive turns. A Difficulty rating modifier may be assigned by the GM based on how different the size and shape is from the being's original form. This change allows the mutant to duplicate any of the natural physical abilities of the assumed form, such as a sword's edge and, thus, its damage, but does not duplicate the inner mechanical or energy workings, or magical or mutational abilities, such as a laser beam (though she could look like a laser pistol), an internal combustion engine's ability to burn gasoline and run, etc. It takes one turn to transform. Unlike the other Shapechange mutation, all the being's gear or clothing

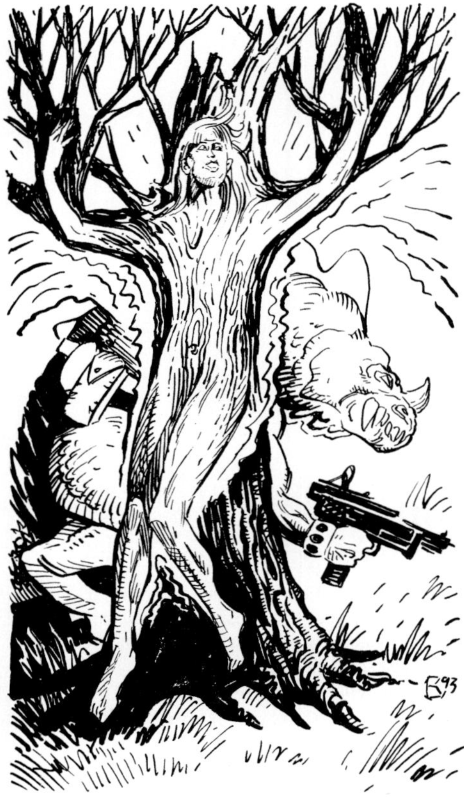

transform with her, as long as she is not heavily encumbered.

While changed, the character retains her mental mutations and awareness (IN, MS, a Perception of 4, and her own personality), but is immobile (the mutant cannot transform into any device as complicated as any type of functional vehicle). It is up to the GM to determine what physical mutations she keeps, if any, when the mutant changes.

The duration of this mutation is much shorter than the normal Shapechange mutation, being (5+(MP modifier)) × 10 rounds.

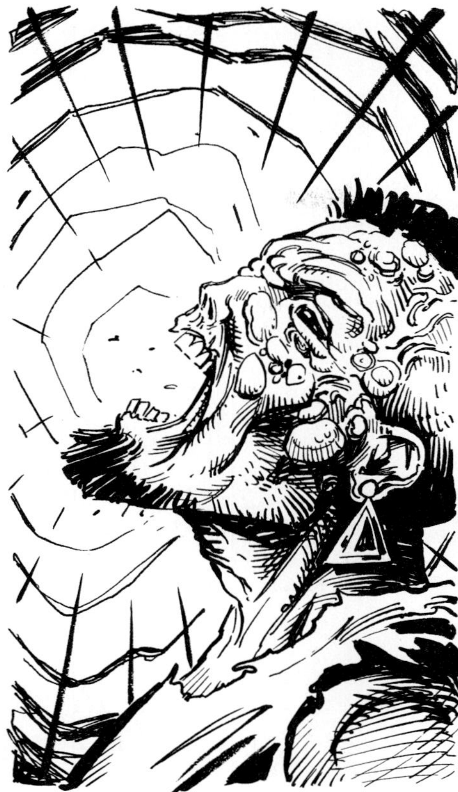

Silence Field

Physical; Activated, MP 4d6-L

The mutant can generate a field of silence around himself that extends in a globe with a radius of 2+(MP modifier) meters. Once activated, the field lasts for 10+(MP modifier) rounds, whether or not the mutant loses consciousness. The mutant can store enough energy to create 1+(MP modifier) silence fields. It takes four hours to regenerate a field. The field completely negates all sound within it, including sonic attacks. Anyone in this field during a sonic attack is also exempt from its damage. The player characters cannot talk with anyone within the field, as no sound can be heard at all, including pleas of help beyond the party's line of sight. A silence field grants the user a +4 to any Stealth or Surprise roll he must make.

Sonic Radar

Physical; Activated, 4d6-L

This mutation is similar to the Sonic Blast mutation, with two important exceptions: a) it is not a projected sonic beam, but an area-effect attack with a radius of 10+(MP modifier) meters; and, b) the mutant can use this attack once every 10-(MP modifier) rounds.

Zip Healing

Physical; Activated, 4d6-L

This mutation differs from Total Healing, so it has been moved to the physical mutation list. This mutation reflects the body's recuperative powers, not a mental attempt to override pain or talk the body into something. (The faster,

greatly increased healing is an attempt to make the game more playable in extremely tough situations. Other mutations, such as Transfusion, may also be altered like this.)

Replace the first paragraph of the Total Healing mutation, found in the rulebook on page 47, with: "The character can completely heal himself of all his lost hit points once per 24-hour period. He can do this up to (MP modifier)-1 times per week, but never less than once per week. It takes 4-(MP modifier) rounds for all these hit points to return, but always at least one round. The GM can figure out what percent of the lost hit points return every turn if necessary. The healing mutant may do nothing more than stand or lie down while he heals. He must consume three times the normal food and water rations each day that he uses this mutation."

The second paragraph of the Total Healing mutation stands unaltered except for the last sentence, which should read, "One attempt can be made at the end of every round of healing, if the healing mutant has uninterrupted concentration."

Ω

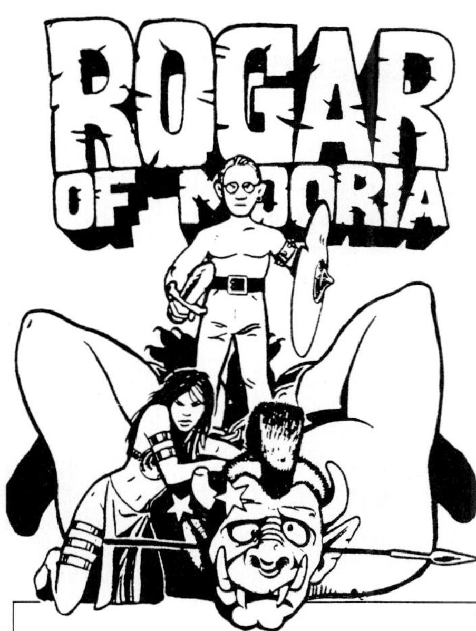

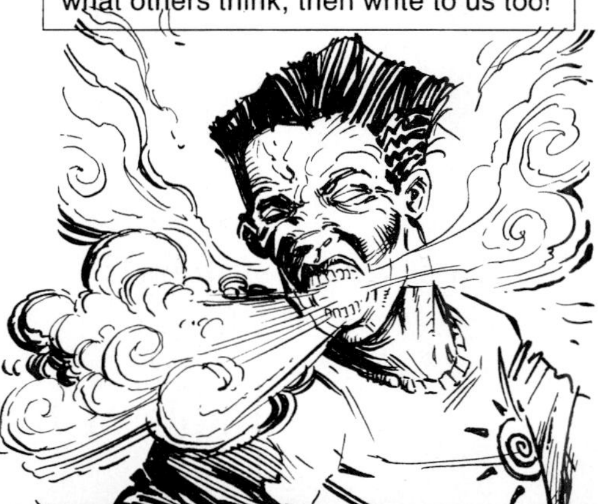

Macross II™
The Role-Playing Game

A new role-playing game based on the Japanese mini-series, **Macross II.**

The Zentraedi have returned with a deadly ally, the savage Marduk. Together they plan to crush the Earth into submission and add it to their intergalactic empire.

The book will be a complete role-playing game and uses Palladium's famous *mega-damage* combat system, making it compatible with **Rifts, The Mechanoids** and the entire Palladium Megaverse.

Tons of spectacular artwork, front, side and back views, cut-aways, close-ups and detail drawings based upon the original animation model sheets, including new transformable robots, battle armor, vehicles, equipment, alien invaders and spacecraft.

Highlights Includes:
- **Five transformable Valkyries.**
- **Spaceships and satellites.**
- **Vehicles, weapons, equipment and war machines.**
- **Marduk and Zentraedi battle suits and vehicles.**
- **Many cut-aways, detail drawings and close-ups.**
- **Stats on major characters from the animated series.**
- **Compatible with Rifts and all of Palladium's M.D.C. games.**
- **Cover by Kevin Long. Interior art by Newton Ewell, Wayne Breaux and Thomas Miller.**
- **Written by Kevin Siembieda.**
- **Approx. 100 pages — $11.95**
- **Available July 1993!**

Macross II
Sourcebook One™

More good stuff. The powerful robot juggernauts that compose the ground troops, experimental valkyries, more characters and complete details and floor plans on the U.N. Spacy's Battle Fortress.

Highlights Include:
- **Compatible with Rifts and all of Palladium's M.D.C. games.**
- **Artwork Kevin Long, Newton Ewell, and Wayne Breaux.**
- **Written by Kevin Siembieda.**
- **48 pages — $7.95**
- **Available October 1993!**

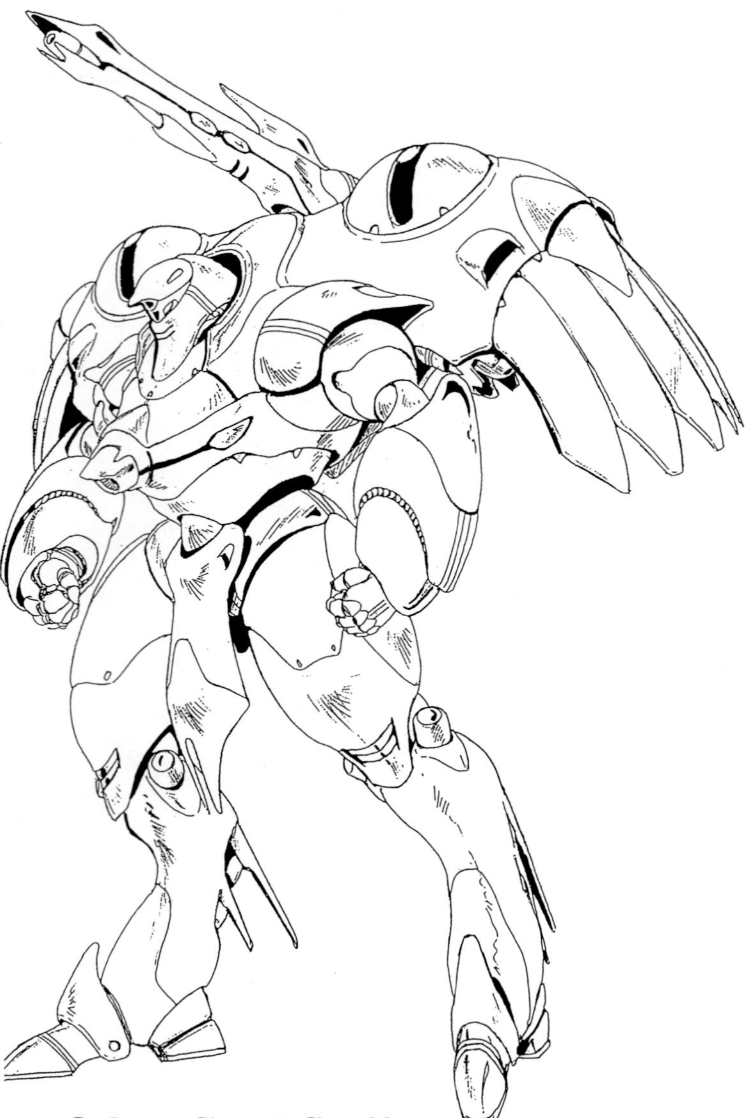

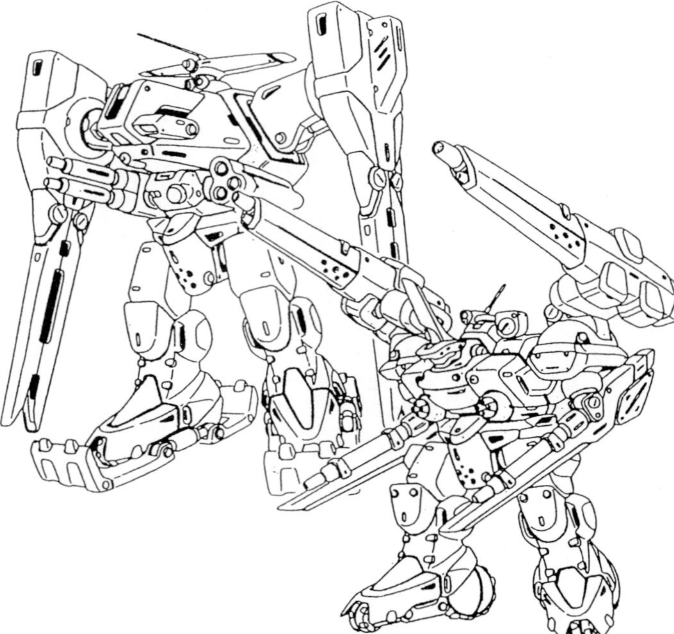

One basic game system...
A Megaverse® of Adventure!

Other Good Stuff
Compendium of Modern Weapons™

Those of you who remember and loved our little 48 page weapon compendium haven't seen anything yet! Over 300 weapons, plus experimental weapons, multi-round shotguns, incendiary devices, grenades and explosives, light artillery, body armor, scopes, and much more!

A compatible reference for RECON®, Heroes Unlimited™, Ninjas & Superspies™, Mystic China™, Beyond the Supernatural™, Rifts®and just about **any** game system that uses modern weapons.

Highlights Include:
- **Over 300 weapons, plus knives, body armor, and accessories with complete statistical data and all fully illustrated!**
- **Explosives and incendiary devices**
- **Body armor and special equipment.**
- **Everything illustrated, with much new art and many cut-aways and detailed illustrations by Siembieda, Long, Gustovich and introducing Steve Stalter.**
- **Written By Maryann Siembieda.**
- **180 + pages — $19.95**
- **Available in August.**

Palladium Books®
Dept. D
12455 Universal Drive
Taylor, Mi. 48180

Available at hobby shops and comic stores everywhere!

Slave Hunters and Silt Sailors

Character kits in a DARK SUN™ Campaign

by L. Richard Baker III

Artwork by Brom

The world of Athas is filled with dangers and perils unknown in the other worlds of the AD&D® game. Evil sorcerer-kings, ambitious templars, fierce thri-kreen, and deadly new monsters such as the silt horror or the braxat all set the DARK SUN™ world apart from the traditional fantasy campaign. While the uniqueness of the setting makes for an outstanding campaign, it also makes it very hard for a Dungeon Master to use material from sources like the various "complete character handbooks" in his own DARK SUN campaign.

The character kits introduced in the PHBR series are archetypes built around the literary and historical examples of heroic adventurers. Unfortunately, a DARK SUN campaign can't draw on very much of this material. Swashbucklers? Cavaliers? Pacifists? Many of the best character kits of the AD&D game do not work in a DARK SUN setting. Obviously, it is going to take a little tinkering with some of the tried and true player-character types to come up with a set of stereotypes that belong in an Athasian setting.

Using existing kits

Let's begin by taking a look at some of the kits of the AD&D game. While a number have to be dropped entirely, we can adapt several of the player-character types to a DARK SUN campaign without too much trouble. Note that items like required equipment, weapon selection, or nonweapon proficiencies may have to be tailored to a DARK SUN setting.

Warrior kits
  Amazon
  Barbarian (human, dwarf, or elf herds-
men of the Tablelands)
  Beast-rider (crodlus, kanks, pterrans,
or inixes)
  Myrmidon
  Savage (halflings and thri-kreen)
  Wilderness warrior (elves or thri-
kreen)

Wizard kits
  Amazon sorceress
  Militant wizard
  Mystic (preservers only)
  Patrician

Priest kits
  Amazon priestess
  Barbarian priest (no templars)
  Nobleman priest (no druids)

Thief kits
  Assassin
  Bandit
  Beggar
  Bounty hunter
  Cutpurse
  Fence
  Scout
  Spy

Bard kits
  Blade
  Charlatan
  Herald
  Jongleur

New DARK SUN™ kits

The following section describes several
character kits unique to the DARK SUN
game world. Two kits for each character
group—warrior, wizard, priest, rogue
(thief and bard), and psionicist—are presented. If you do not want a kit in your
campaign, delete it.

All kits are presented in the following
format:

Description: This paragraph presents
a thumbnail sketch of the character's general appearance, manner, and background. It includes any requirements
necessary for a character to take the kit.

Role: The character's place in his society is discussed in this paragraph. There is
a world of difference between the role of a
sycophant bard and a slave warrior
fighter.

Secondary skills are omitted from the
kit descriptions. The DARK SUN campaign
world relies on the use of nonweapon
proficiencies to describe a character's talents and skills.

Weapon proficiencies: Some kits
require the character to use specific
weapons that are associated with his origin.

Nonweapon proficiencies: Each
character kit includes a few bonus nonweapon proficiencies that the character
gains without expending nonweapon proficiency slots. In addition, a few recom-

mended proficiencies are included.

Equipment: Any special requirements
for character equipment are listed here.
These are generally not hard-and-fast
restrictions, but a player who insists on
using equipment specifically barred by his
character's kit is not doing a good job of
role-playing and may need to consider
abandoning the kit.

Special benefits: Most kits enjoy a
special benefit or two. These may be reaction bonuses, special rights in the character's society, or attack or defense bonuses.

Special hindrances: Most kits also
suffer from a special disadvantage of some
kind. The character may be a hunted outlaw or may have a reaction penalty with
certain kinds of people.

Wealth options: A few kits have special
rules regarding their beginning wealth
and the amount of treasure they can
retain.

Warrior kits

Slave warrior

Description: The majority of the noble
and merchant houses of Athas field a
force of armed guards to protect their
properties and caravans. A number of
these are free mercenaries, but almost all
of these forces include fanatical slave warriors—people born into slavery and raised
from a very early age to be loyal body-
guards and enforcers. Player-character
slave warriors may either be free of their
patron houses or may elect to retain some
ties with the houses they were born to
fight for.

The slave warrior is one of the most
highly skilled fighters on Athas. From
early childhood, he has survived a brutal
regime of exercise, training, and indoctri-
nation designed to make him into a mind-
less killing machine who would sacrifice
his own life for the sake of his owners.
Almost all slave warriors are visibly
branded or tattooed with the emblem of
their owning houses. They are the only
slaves who are ever armed outside the
arena.

Fighters and gladiators may take the
slave warrior kit. Rangers require a less
urban background to learn their survival
skills. Muls, dwarves, and half-giants are
ideal for this kit; thri-kreen and halflings
are very difficult to indoctrinate and are
rarely used in this way. In addition to all
other requirements, a slave warrior must
have a minimum Strength and Constitution of 13.

Role: The first decision the player of a
slave warrior must make is whether or
not the PC is still owned by his patron.
Enslaved characters represent the elite of
Athas's slaves; they are well fed, receive
good quarters, and are equipped with the
finest gear money can buy. A PC slave
warrior who is enslaved is assumed to go
adventuring on the orders of his patron
and may be recalled at any time for

assignment to different duties.

Free slave warriors may have simply
escaped or have won their freedom
through some great act of courage. Of
course, escaped characters must always
watch for templars or slave hunters.
Freed characters may occasionally be
mistaken for escapees and attacked as
well. In either case, the free slave warrior
no longer has the resources and wealth of
a noble or merchant house to aid him.

Weapon proficiencies: Required:
choice of spear, crossbow, or pole arm,
and also a specialization in an unarmed
combat style (not required for gladiator
characters.) The slave warrior receives a
bonus proficiency slot which may be used
to specialize in any melee weapon.

Nonweapon proficiencies: Bonus:
Endurance, Heraldry. Recommended:
Animal Handling, Animal Training, Blind-
fighting, Gaming, Land-based Riding,
Reading Lips.

Equipment: A slave warrior receives
one set of any nonmetallic armor and a
nonmetallic melee weapon of his choice
for free. In addition, enslaved characters
are completely equipped (including supplies and a mount, if appropriate) by their
patron houses at no cost to the characters. There is a 5% chance per level that a
character's patron house supplies him
with a metallic weapon of his choice.

Special benefits: Slave warriors are
well-known as powerful, single-minded
fighters. They gain a +3 reaction bonus with
any civilized NPC they encounter, since few
people wish to fight a slave warrior.

Enslaved slave warriors gain a bonus of
+1 to attack rolls, +1 to damage, and a +1
bonus on saving throws when fighting in
the direct defense of their patrons. Free
characters lose this benefit.

Special hindrances: Enslaved characters are not their own masters and must
obey the orders of their owners. PC slave
warriors are assumed to have earned a
great deal of trust and responsibility, but
are still required to spend one-third of
their time on guard over some activity of
their patrons. Characters who desire an
extended reprieve from this requirement
must demonstrate to their patron that the
adventure will bring some tangible
reward to the house. The DM should play
this to great effect—after all, what's the
use of training an elite bodyguard if you
just let him wander off into the desert all
the time?

Free characters have lived as slaves all
their lives and suffer a -3 reaction penalty
in dealing with non-slave civilized characters. Escaped characters are suspicious
and paranoid, and legitimately free characters still carry the social stigma of a
slave's birth.

Wealth options: Enslaved characters
begin with only 1d4 × 10 cp, while free
characters begin with the normal 5d4 × 30
cp. Enslaved characters must return 90%
of any treasure to their patrons, including

any gems, jewelry, or magical items. However, the patrons may often reward such characters for their loyalty.

Raider

Description: The deserts of Athas are home to countless raiding tribes, desperate bands of cutthroats and criminals who take what they can from those weaker than themselves. The raider is a hard, cruel character who is the ultimate survivalist. He depends on no one but himself, takes what he needs, and guards what little wealth he gains with his life.

Raiding tribes are of all sizes and descriptions. Some are bands of escaped slaves who know no other way to survive. Some are peasants and villagers whose homes were destroyed by another raiding clan, forcing them into the outlaw's life. Others are swift elven clans who have been raiding together for hundreds of years, passing down the tactics and traditions from one generation to the next. When a PC chooses this kit, it is important for the DM to sit down with the player and work out the details of the raiding tribe the character calls home.

Fighters and rangers are most appropriate for this kit, although a gladiator who is also a war-leader or tribal champion is not too far-fetched. Since some raiding tribes are nothing more than collections of escaped slaves, any PC race is appropriate. Raider characters are almost always neutral or evil in alignment; a good character would have to insist on taking only from those who can share their wealth, such as the forces of the sorcerer-kings or rich merchants. There are no special ability requirements to be a raider.

Role: The raider is an outlaw, hated and feared by most of the common folk of Athas. He responds to this universal loathing with violence and fierce self-reliance. The raider long ago decided that the end justifies the means, and he is a pragmatic survivalist. He plays to win.

In a campaign, raiders are villainous characters who are known for fighting hard and dirty. They consort with the worst kind of criminals and represent a chaotic force that threatens the fabric of Athasian civilization. Almost the only place a raider is welcome is in the company of his own tribe. Even then, most raiding tribes recognize the strongest fighter as their leader.

Weapon proficiencies: Raiders must spend one weapon proficiency slot on a weapon suitable for close combat—a knife, dagger, hand axe, or unarmed combat style specialization.

Nonweapon proficiencies: Bonus: Direction Sense, Heat Protection, and either Running or Land-based Riding. Recommended: Appraising, Bowyer/Fletcher, Endurance, Fire-building, Gaming, Hunting, Intimidation, Navigation, Survival, Water Find.

Equipment: Raiders believe in the

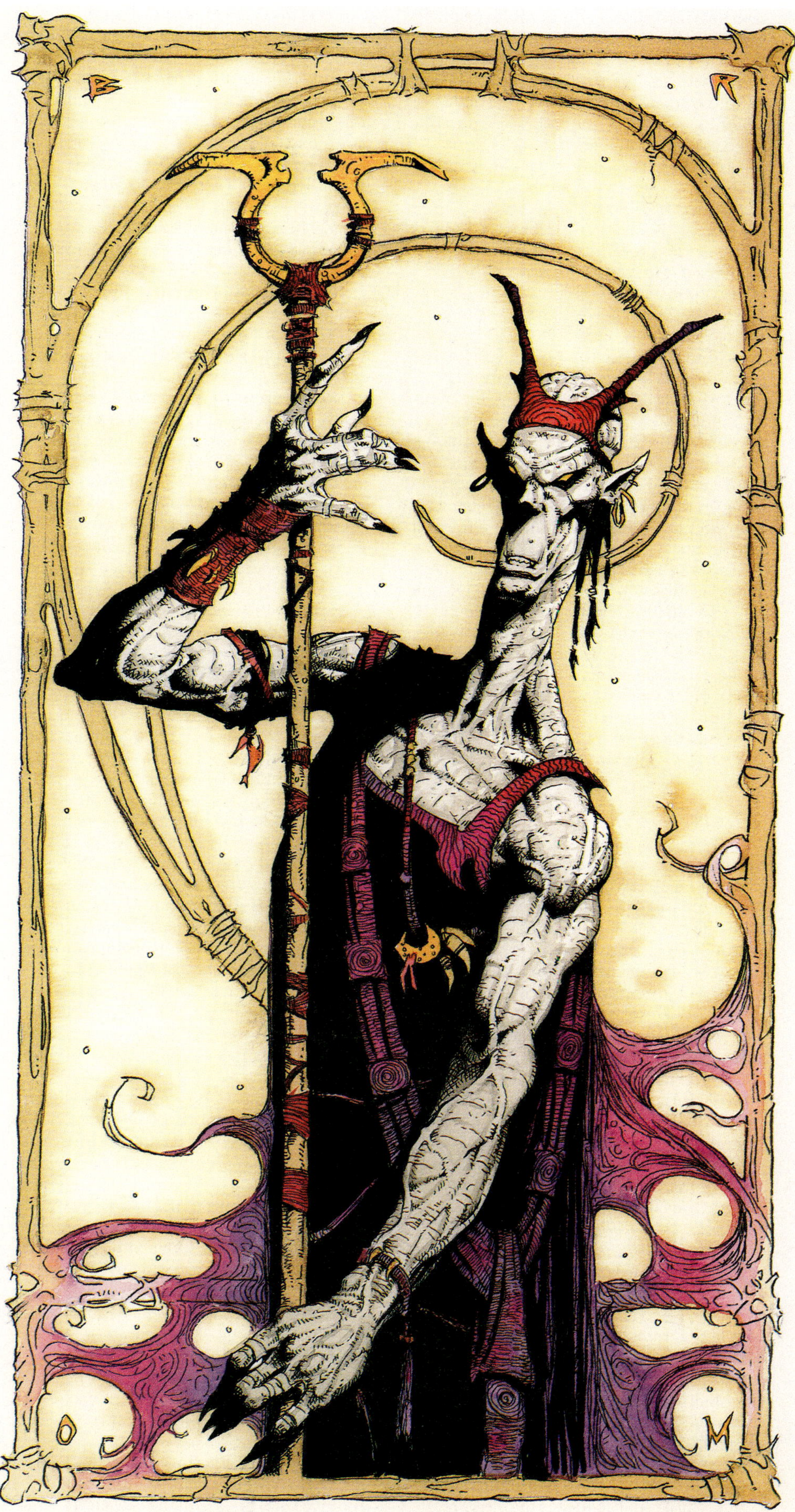

value of moving fast and do not wear armor that could slow them down. A raider never voluntarily carries so much equipment that he becomes encumbered, although he may exceed this restriction when he carries loot. In addition, a raider must purchase at least three weapons when he begins play—raiders are famous for being armed to the teeth.

Special benefits: Experts at lying in wait and striking swiftly from concealment, raiders have the ability to *prepare ambushes*. The raider must spot the enemy before they spot anyone in his party and have at least 10 minutes to get ready. Optionally, the raider can prepare an ambush at a site that is likely to be traveled, such as an oasis or a commonly used road. If the raider has time to set up, his side imposes a -4 on the opponents' surprise roll when the ambush is sprung.

Raiders are also at home dealing with criminals and cutthroats. The former gain a +3 on their reaction checks when approaching such characters in a neutral setting, such as a tavern.

Special hindrances: Raiders are generally despised by all other people except their own tribes. They suffer a -3 reaction check penalty when dealing with townspeople, villagers, templars, or merchants. In addition, if a raider becomes known to the templars of a city, they make every effort to arrest him on sight.

Wealth options: Raiders start with 5d4 ×30 ceramic pieces.

Wizard kits

Veiled One

Description: A loyal member of the Veiled Alliance, the Veiled One has learned all he knows of magic from his contacts within the organization. He is part of a network of preservers and psionicists who assist each other and carry out a secret agenda of working for change on Athas. The Veiled One is an urban character, skilled in intrigue and espionage.

Veiled Ones often adopt disguises, aliases, and other diversionary measures to maintain their secrecy. Wizards are feared and despised all over Athas, and many lose their lives to the angry reactions of the common people. Above all, Veiled Ones fear the sorcerer-king and his templars. In addition to all other requirements, a character must have a Wisdom of 13 or better to show the common sense and willpower to be a Veiled One.

Role: The Veiled One is a revolutionary in a brutal police state. Above all, he maintains his secrecy. Second to the goal of survival, he tries to advance the agenda of the Alliance. The Veiled Alliances of the cities each vary in their organization, strength, and aggressiveness; some are so powerful they barely disguise their movements, and others have been decimated by the strikes of the local king's templars.

The DM must carefully develop the scenario for the PC's chapter of the Alliance, as well as contacts for the PC in the Alliance. The DARK SUN campaign accessory *Veiled Alliance* contains a wealth of information on running a Veiled Alliance campaign.

Preferred schools: All schools of magic are welcomed into an alliance, provided the wizard is a preserver and not a defiler. Illusionists, diviners, transmuters, and enchanters are particularly valuable for the subtlety of their spells.

Weapon proficiencies: Small, easily concealable weapons are preferred by Veiled Ones. They may choose from the following: blowgun, knife, dagger, sling, wrist razor.

Nonweapon proficiencies: Bonus: Reading/Writing, Disguise, Somatic Concealment. Recommended: Ancient History, Spellcraft, Local History, Reading Lips, Sign Language. Veiled Ones are required to select at least one craft proficiency relative to their cover identity. These include nonweapon proficiencies such as carpentry, cobbling, leatherworking, pottery, or bargaining.

Equipment: Veiled Ones are required to purchase any equipment necessary to their cover identity. A wizard posing as a potter should have a wheel, clay, and a workshop; a wizard posing as a carpenter needs a set of tools, etc. The DM should decide on the amount of equipment necessary to establish a cover.

Special benefits: There are several benefits to being a member of the Veiled Alliance. First and foremost, the wizard enjoys access to the spells and research of other wizards. He has tutors available to instruct him when he advances in level, he can obtain spell components, and he can pass along his own findings to other wizards in need. Every time a Veiled One gains a level, he may automatically add one new spell to his spellbook, just as if he were a specialist wizard. This is cumulative with the specialist's bonus, so specialist wizards gain two spells when they gain a level.

The Veiled One has a network of information gatherers and accomplices in place through which he can arrange for safe houses or similar assistance. No matter how much trouble he is in, the character can hide for up to three days with no possibility of the sorcerer-king's forces finding him. For each day after the third that he holes up, there is a 10% chance that the character's whereabouts are discovered. To effectively hide, a character must not leave his haven or attempt to contact anyone outside of his shelter. Doing so increases the chance of his being spotted to 50% per day. The character can include one companion per three levels in his hiding place.

Instead of holing up, the character can leave the city. Arranging transport requires 1d3 days, during which the char

acter hides; then the Veiled One may be smuggled out of the city. There is a base 80% chance of success, but the DM may modify this for the intensity of the search and other similar factors.

Last but not least, the character has a cover identity that allows him to move around the city and interact with others as a law-abiding citizen. The cover is complete unless the character casts a spell in the sight of others or takes some other action that would arouse suspicion.

Special hindrances: As noted above, the character has a cover identity that must be carefully maintained. As a rule of thumb, the character must spend half of his time playing the part of his cover— making pots, buying and selling goods, or whatever. A character who neglects his cover (poor potters taking long trips and returning with great wealth, merchants missing opportunities to purchase goods cheaply, etc.) runs the serious risk of becoming outlawed.

Outlawed wizards are among the most sought-after of criminals in any city-state. There is a 50% chance per day that the law comes so close to the character that he must hole up or leave the city. Failure to do so guarantees an encounter with a templar sweep for the character. It requires 2d4 months to re-establish a cover after one has been blown.

The character must also honor requests for assistance by his fellow Veiled Ones. From time to time, the character is called upon to perform jail breaks, to test prospective new members for hints of defiler magic, or to hunt down and kill wizards attempting to leave the Alliance. Again, the DM should develop these as very real commitments to the character and give the resolution of these matters a lot of attention. A wizard may not like the idea of blowing his comfortable cover by participating in a prison break, but as long as the wizard is in the Alliance, he has to be prepared to obey orders.

Wealth options: Wealth is as normal for a wizard. However, the character may derive a steady income from a well-developed cover profession.

Arcanamach

Description: Each of the sorcerer-monarchs selects an elite few to study and learn magic under his protection. These hated creatures are arcanamachs— defilers sponsored by the sorcerer-king and loyal to him. Acting as his emissaries and spies, the arcanamachs are the only wizards of Athas who freely and openly practice their art. Only the protection of the sorcerer-king himself keeps an arcanamach from an ugly death at a mob's hands.

Only defilers may choose to be arcanamachs, and only the best and brightest of potential students are selected. The arcanamach must possess a Wisdom of 13 or better, an Intelligence of 17 or better, and a Charisma of 15 or better to qualify as an arcanamach. Some arcanamachs begin as neutral characters, but at some point in their careers they must wholly give themselves over to the service of their king and assume an evil alignment.

Role: Arcanamachs are some of the most powerful characters in a campaign. Even the dreaded templars dare not trouble the arcanamachs for fear of the sorcerer-king's wrath. The lifestyle of the arcanamachs varies from city to city, but they generally have any materials or luxuries they could want and guarded carefully. Arcanamachs enjoy the favor of their kings, and their fortunes rise or fall with the sorcerer-monarchs.

Arcanamachs are known by different names in different cities. In Draj, they are known as Lawgivers; in Nibenay, they are called Hands of Shadow. In the free city of Tyr, Kalak's arcanamachs are now wanted criminals. Most have fled the city, although there are rumors that a few have sworn allegiance to Tithian.

Preferred schools: Each of the schools of magic has its uses to a sorcerer-king, and a wide variety of specialists is recruited to serve as in the ranks of the arcanamachs.

Weapon proficiencies: Arcanamachs are occasionally required to serve with the sorcerer-king's armies. They may choose from the following weapons: staff, dagger, sling, short bow, short sword, dart, javelin.

Nonweapon proficiencies: Bonus: Ancient History, Reading/Writing, and Spellcraft. Recommended: Land-based Riding, Etiquette, Herbalism, Engineering, Bureaucracy.

Special abilities: Arcanamachs are the only wizards of Athas who can openly practice their art. Their access to the excellent libraries of the sorcerer-kings provides them with the ability to automatically learn one spell of their choosing whenever they gain a level. Specialists may learn two. In addition, there is a 5% chance per level of the character that the sorcerer-king takes personal notice of the character's studies and allows him to immediately add 1d4 spells to his spell repertoire. Characters who enjoy the sorcerer-king's notice can also research spells or manufacture magical items at no cost to themselves, although they must still take time to arrange for the correct materials to be brought to them.

Arcanamachs can requisition all sorts of magical items from the sorcerer-king's hoard, and they begin play with 1,500 xp worth of magical items already in their possession. When the arcanamach gains a level, he can request another 1,500 xp worth of items. There is a 5% chance per level of the wizard that his request is granted.

Within the domain of their sorcerer-king, arcanamachs will not be arrested or interfered with by the king's templars or guards, within reason. An arcanamach caught in a treasonous act is in just as much danger as anyone else. Arcanamachs can request guards at any time after they reach 5th level; usually a pair of 3rd-level fighters are assigned for up to a month, but the numbers and skill of the guards are increased as the arcanamach gains levels. The DM should be careful to ration the arcanamach's use of this power; an arcanamach whose guards consistently die during their assignments eventually finds no guards willing to serve him.

Special hindrances: The arcanamach is a marked man. He has enemies everywhere—the Veiled Alliance, jealous nobles and templars, and even his ambitious peers—and only one friend: the sorcerer-king. In return for the favor showered upon the arcanamach, the sorcerer-king expects absolute loyalty. The arcanamach must vigorously pursue his sorcerer-king's interests or risk disfavor.

Anytime the arcanamach wishes to pursue his own studies, go on an adventure, or even just take a vacation, there is a base 50% chance that the sorcerer-king's demands interfere. The character may be assigned as part of a diplomatic party to another city-state, he may be "asked" to accompany a military force to battle, or he may even be loaned out to a powerful noble or templar to assist in their enterprise. The DM should play this carefully; if the player has been playing his character well, his arcanamach might not be bothered quite so often. If the player has been abusing his character's perks, however, it's a good sign that the wizard is leaning heavily on the sorcerer-king and is in the monarch's thoughts.

Then, too, the arcanamach is very often the target of the sorcerer-king's enemies. There is a 25% chance per month that someone moves against the arcanamach. The Veiled Alliance may attempt to assassinate him, or a templar may attempt to discredit the arcanamach in the sorcerer-king's eyes by planting evidence or similar tactics. The arcanamach must be eternally vigilant for the machinations of his many enemies.

Wealth options: The arcanamach begins with the standard amount of money for a wizard character. However, he always has free lodging available to him in the sorcerer-king's palace.

Priest kits

Chronicler

Description: The chronicler is a priest who seeks wisdom in the lost records of the past. He knows more about the forgotten history of Athas than any other character, and he tries to use the ancient secrets in pursuit of his own goals in modern Athas. The chronicler is not just a tomb-robber or archaeologist; he is also a histo-

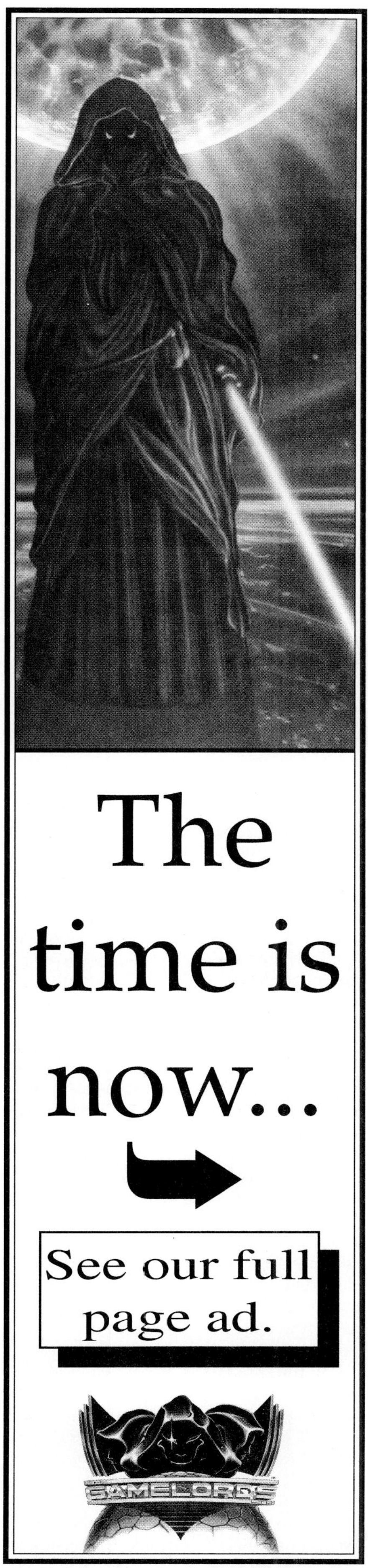

rian who makes painstaking efforts to record current events and pass on his own knowledge to future generations.

Both templars and clerics may be chroniclers; druids have too many pressing cares in the immediate present to care much about lost secrets and lore. The long lifespans of elves and dwarves make them particularly appropriate for this kit, but priests of any race may choose to be chroniclers. Chroniclers may be of any lawful alignment, and require an Intelligence of 13 in addition to all other prerequisites.

Weapon proficiencies: There are no special weapon requirements for chroniclers.

Nonweapon proficiencies: Bonus: Ancient History, Reading/Writing, Astrology. Recommended: Etiquette, Land-based Riding, Heraldry, Ancient Language, Religion.

Equipment: Chroniclers may use any weapons or armor appropriate for their class. They are required to purchase astrological charts, histories, journals, pen and ink, and papyrus. These materials cost a total of 20 cp multiplied by the priest's level.

Special benefits: Chroniclers gain the thief's ability to read unknown or ancient languages. This skill begins at a percentage chance equal to the chronicler's Intelligence score, and increases by 5% per level that the character advances. Chroniclers also have a 5% chance per level to identify the general purpose and function of ancient magical items, tomes, or texts, just as a bard. The chronicler can identify only those items with some historical significance; a bone *sword +1* wielded 30 years ago by a common outlaw would not qualify, but a *sword +1* wielded by an ancient warlord 700 years ago would.

Chroniclers also are known for their extraordinary memories. Athasian scholars must deal with extensive oral histories and epic poems, and they rigorously train themselves to remember incredibly long texts or songs. Once a chronicler reads or hears anything, he can commit it to memory and remember it to the word forever. This process takes 1d4 turns plus the time of reading or listening. The character can also memorize maps, faces, or conversations. In many cities, the chronicler's memory is considerable admissible as evidence in a trial.

The game effect of this ability is to allow the player controlling the chronicler character to confer with the DM and recall the exact wording of instructions, directions, or bargains made with NPCs. The character also carries around a map of the Tyr Region in his head; the DM can allow the player to refer to any nonkeyed map relevant to the situation at any time. This ability gives the character a +1 bonus on Intelligence checks and nonweapon proficiency checks for navigation, direction sense, survival, bargaining, and any other proficiency the DM allows.

Special hindrances: The chronicler must attempt to recover any item of ancient work he knows of and return it to his school or library. A templar chronicler who finds a steel *long sword +3*, or a suit of plate mail, or even a rare and expensive book will go to any lengths to either purchase or steal the item and return it to his sorcerer-king. Chronicler clerics have similar responsibilities to a library, museum, or hidden temple. The Dungeon Master should be reasonable with this requirement; the chronicler will not attack his teammates over one rusty steel sword, but if his fellow adventurers came across an ancient artifact or book, the chronicler should insist on its return and study.

Chroniclers may keep only magical items that have no historical significance. All others must be returned to their organizations.

Wealth options: The chronicler begins with the standard starting money for a priest character.

Tribal priest

Description: The struggle for survival in the badlands outside the city-states of Athas is fierce and terrible. Thousands of tribes wander the wastes; each year hundreds of these are slaughtered, enslaved, or simply starve. One of the most vital edges a tribe can possess over its competitors is access to the magic of a druid or cleric, whose spells can mean the difference between life and death for the tribesmen.

Templars cannot be tribal priests—their power lies in the domains of the sorcerer-kings. Tribal priests may be of any alignment and race. Clerics are most often found as tribal priests, since they are not tied to one place and can accompany their tribe in its travels. On occasion, a druid will be found as the patron of a tribe that spends a lot of time in the druid's guarded lands. Tribal priests have to be able to survive the rigorous life of a tribesman before they become a priest; a character must have a Constitution score of 13 or better to qualify as a tribal priest.

Role: The tribal priest is a character with a heavy burden to bear—the survival of his family and friends. He is often one of the most respected and feared members of the tribe, and his words are extremely influential. PC tribal priests are assumed to come from a tribe that can spare them for the occasional adventure; otherwise, the character would spend all of his time creating water, quelling squabbles, and healing the tribe's warriors. The DM can explain this freedom in two ways: Either the priest character is only a student or shaman-in-training with an NPC tribal priest who remains with the tribe, or the tribe is successful and stable enough that the PC can leave them to fend for themselves from time to time.

The tribal priest kit is especially effective in a campaign built around the raiders and nomads of the wastes. A tribal priest who spends most of his time associating with urban characters from Athas's city-states is playing the role of a barbarian priest, and is not paying attention to the responsibilities of his position.

Weapon proficiencies: In addition to the weapons appropriate for a cleric or druid, the tribal priest is required to select one of the following weapons: knife, dagger, short bow, spear, or sling. These are the weapons of the nomadic tribes.

Nonweapon proficiencies: Bonus: Survival (in the terrain favored by the tribe), Water Find, Heat Protection. Recommended: Animal Lore, Direction Sense, Weather Sense, Fire-building, Hunting, Tracking, Herbalism.

Equipment: Tribal priests come from societies that are forced to make do with the most basic of materials. They may not purchase any metallic weapons when they begin play, but are unrestricted after that.

Special abilities: Tribal priests can always find shelter, food, water, and assistance with their protected tribe, no matter what the circumstances. The tribal priest can also arrange for up to one guest per level to receive similar aid. Note that while a tribe can always accommodate the priest himself, a large number of guests may severely strain the tribe's resources, and the tribal priest should never bring more guests than the tribe can support.

Tribal priests are recognized throughout the wastes of Athas as important people. When dealing with any nomad, raider, slave tribe, or herdsman, the tribal priest gains a +3 on his reaction check. This can be a disadvantage, as an outside tribe desperately in need of a new priest may be inclined to seize the PC tribal priest for their own if he impresses them too much.

Special hindrances: The tribal priest is tied to his tribe. Although it is assumed that he can occasionally leave the tribe to go adventuring, there are times when he is needed by his people. There is a 30% chance that the priest is required by his tribe anytime he considers undertaking an adventure that would take him away for a long time. The DM should enforce this rigidly for a character who tends to neglect his background, and be more generous with players who are role-playing their characters well.

Another hindrance lies in the fact that the tribe's enemies are the character's enemies as well. The character must select three distinct groups (for example, gith of the Black Spine Mountains, the Jura-dai elven tribe, and the slave tribe Werrik's Stalkers) to become his tribe's enemies. Whenever the character encounters these enemies, he suffers a -4 penalty on his reaction check with them, since his tribal markings and attitudes clearly mark him as a potential foe.

Wealth options: Tribal priests are impoverished, beginning play with only a

DUNGEONWORKS™

few hand-crafted items. They receive only 3d6 × 10 cp instead of the normal starting money of 3d6 × 30 cp.

Rogue kits

Caravaneer

Description: The caravans of the great merchant houses are the lifeblood of Athas, carrying goods, news, messages, and slaves from one city to another. The caravaneer is a character who makes a living in these roving islands of civilization amid the desert wastes. He is a skilled guide and trader, and in many cases a smuggler and a fence. Each new village or town, each new oasis or desert tribe holds the promise of wealth and fortune. Caravaneers are infamous rogues who appear again and again in the legends of Athas as untrustworthy, avaricious characters who think nothing of cheating on a deal. This is only part of the truth about these wanderers.

Characters of any race may be caravaneers, but dwarven caravaneers find that a life of simple thievery does not make up a focus. Thieves and traders may take the caravaneer kit; if the optional thief ability rules of the *Dragon Kings* volume are used, the thief caravaneer has the abilities of Forge Document, Bribe Official, Pick Pockets, Open Locks, Move Silently, Hide in Shadows, Detect Noise, and Read Languages. Caravaneers may be of any alignment and have no special ability prerequisites.

Role: The caravaneer is an arranger. If he is a thief, then he is a thief who relies on cons, swindles, short-dealing, and smuggling. He rarely resorts to actual acts of theft like burglary or brigandage. In short, he is a very traderlike thief. If the character is a trader, then he is a dirty trader who prefers to avoid declaring all of his imports and who seems forgetful of bargains he makes—in other words, a very thieflike trader.

The caravaneer is a character with his ears and eyes open for opportunity. He is at the heart of the action, on the front lines of the mercantile wars of Athas. The caravaneer can prove to be an excellent plot vehicle for a Dungeon Master, as he constantly hears interesting rumors and seeks out new ways to get rich quickly.

Weapon proficiencies: Since he is often called upon to defend the caravan against raiders, the caravaneer is required to be proficient in at least one weapon that can be used in mounted combat and one weapon that can be used in missile combat.

Nonweapon proficiencies: Bonus: Appraising, Land-based Riding, Bargaining. Recommended: Animal Handling, Cooking, Direction Sense, Etiquette, Firebuilding, Weather Sense, Disguise, Local History, Reading Lips, Alertness, Information Gathering, Looting, Observation.

Equipment: No special requirements.

Special benefits: Caravaneers may "sign on" with a caravan of their choice, receiving an appropriate wage to accompany the caravan in some capacity—scout, guard, purchasing agent, officer, etc. Generally, the wage and the position is commensurate with the character's level. A wage of about 1 cp per week per character level is appropriate, but as the character reaches higher levels the DM should increase the character's financial share in the venture by appointing him as an officer or senior agent in charge of the caravan. (Caravaneers of the trader class actually own some amount of goods and rent space on a caravan to transport their wares.)

The character is always guaranteed to receive shelter, food, water, and transportation to any common crossroads, trading stop, or city-state in addition to his wages. The character can also arrange for the hiring of one companion per two levels, although the companion may have to settle for a guard's or laborer's position.

Caravaneers are master smugglers and can conceal caravan goods of up to 50 lbs. per level so that they will not be discovered in the caravan during routine searches. Intensive searches require the rogue to make a roll against his Intelligence, with a modifier applied for the amount of preparation the character makes. Smuggling a small pouch of gems in an armored wagon is nearly foolproof; smuggling an escaped slave in the packs of a kank is much more difficult.

Caravaneers understand the life of trade and the people who can be found interacting with caravans. When dealing with merchants, other caravan persons, or innkeepers and stablemasters who deal with caravans, the caravaneer gains a +3 on his reaction checks.

Special hindrances: Known as scoundrels and gossips, caravaneers are often perceived as untrustworthy and avaricious. The character suffers a -3 penalty on his reaction check when placed in a situation where he is trying to win the trust of an NPC other than those with whom he receives a positive reaction check. For example, an elven chieftain may be perfectly willing to buy and sell goods with a caravaneer, but he would never give the caravaneer a secret message or package to carry.

Wealth options: Caravaneers begin play with the normal amount of money for their class. The accumulation of wealth is of great importance to the caravaneer character and he rarely, if ever, abandons riches or gives away money he has no use for.

Sycophant

Description: All cultures and societies seem to have their share of flatterers and yes-men who gravitate towards wealth and power. The sycophant is a character who constantly schemes to advance his own position through his association with the right people. His life is a constant climb through the social ranks as he seeks more influence and wealth than he currently enjoys. In some cases, the boldest and most daring of sycophants hope to win a rich inheritance, a marriage into wealth, or even a noble title in the court of a sorcerer-king. It is a dangerous game, and even the slightest misstep can spell ostracism or even death.

Of all the PC races, only humans, elves, and half-elves possess the wit and charm necessary for this kit. Sycophants are usually bards, but clever and personable thieves can survive as sycophants. Sycophants are generally self-centered individuals and may not choose to be of good alignment. In addition to all other requirements, sycophants must have Intelligence and Charisma scores of 14 or better.

Role: The sycophant begins his career as a gossip and wit. He is a slave to fashion and makes a point of appearing with the correct escort at the proper time. Above all, he must be entertaining; a sycophant whose company is not enjoyable is a sycophant who will soon be forgotten.

Very few sycophants rise out of the lowest classes or come from slave stock, although it is conceivable that a slave could take this kit as a recently freed concubine or artist. In the adventuring party, the sycophant functions as an excellent information gatherer, spokesperson, and spy. Most importantly, the sycophant knows people in high places, and he can often pull strings through his current contacts to free people from prison, finance risky mercantile ventures, or make introductions. A clever and unscrupulous sycophant with a weak-willed contact can completely dominate his benefactor—and, in some cases, even replace him.

Weapon proficiencies: Sycophants are not noted for carrying heavy armament. If there is a weapon fashionable to nobility (for example, the rapier of the Renaissance), the sycophant is required to be proficient in its use. The noble weapons of the Seven Cities are: short sword (Balic), javelin (Draj), bow (Gulg), club (Nibenay), flail (Raam), steel long sword (Tyr), and lance (Urik.) All other weapon proficiencies must be selected from small, easily concealable weapons such as the knife, dagger, or sling.

Nonweapon proficiencies: Bonus: Dancing, Etiquette, Heraldry, Observation. Recommended: Artistic Ability, Land-based Riding, Singing, Appraising, Disguise, Gaming, Musical Instrument, Reading Lips, Reading/Writing.

Equipment: The sycophant must possess one outfit of noble quality to move among the elite of his city. This can cost 10-30 cp, depending on the city. The sycophant may wear armor and carry weapons when journeying or adventuring, but generally goes unarmored and carries only a dagger or other small weapon as he makes his rounds of the nobility. If he attends a party in full armor or visits a high lady while armed to the teeth, he suffers a -2 to -4 reaction penalty based on the DM's assessment of the situation.

Special benefits: The sycophant manages to infatuate a few powerful patrons for a time. The character has a number of contacts equal to his level. Each of these contacts is perfectly willing and able to put the sycophant up for 10 days plus three days per level of the character. He lives in the lap of luxury during this time. After visiting, the sycophant cannot visit again until 100 days pass. The sycophant may subtract twice his level in days from this figure. As he increases in level, the sycophant is eventually able to live his entire life in one palace or another, since he is in so much demand. The sycophant always leaves on good terms when his time expires, since he avoids offending people by staying too long or not long enough.

Sycophants can also call upon favors from their patrons. Obviously, the patron must be in a position to help. Asking a merchant to free someone from the templar prisons is useless, and asking a sorcerer-king to protect a preserver is equally futile. Each time the sycophant calls for a favor, roll a reaction check. The sycophant gains a +1 bonus per three levels on the favor check. If he asks for more than one favor per 100 days, each subsequent favor check suffers a -2 cumulative penalty.

The sycophant's patrons are very important to the campaign, and the DM should go out of his way to develop the social ladder of the city-state. A clever sycophant uses his influence with one patron to win an introduction to an even more important and influential patron, slowly climbing the social ladder. The most daring (and foolhardy) of sycophants stand by the sorcerer-king himself.

Special hindrances: As noted under "Equipment," sycophants are usually unarmored and lightly armed (weapons of size S only.) The sycophant wears armor only in the most obvious of circumstances—accompanying a patron to war, duelling, or carrying a message through a dangerous area. Even in adventuring, the sycophant rarely brings his armor unless a fight is very likely, and even then he waits until the last minute to put it on. DMs should feel free to impose reaction penalties on sycophants who insist on a martial display.

Because he is unused to the weight and tactics of wearing armor, a given armor type protects the sycophant as if it were one place worse than it actually was; thus, plain leather armor (normally base AC 8) is actually base AC 9 for the sycophant. This hindrance applies to magical armor but does not apply to magical items like a *ring of protection* or *bracers of defense*, so long as they are the only protective devices worn.

Wealth options: Sycophants begin play with 2d6 × 60 cp. At least half of their treasure and earnings must be spent on clothes, luxuries, exclusive memberships, and other such fineries.

Psionicist kits

Noble

Description: Almost all humans and demihumans have some potential with the Way, but very few people are fortunate enough to find a tutor for their mental powers. These untutored potentials are fated to go through life as wild talents, possessing only a fraction of the powers they would if they had studied. On Athas, learning and study for its own sake is often a luxury only the wealthy and the noble can afford.

The noble psionicist is a character who was enrolled in a rigorous training regime by her family when she was young. Like children of our own world who take piano lessons, most find the study of their own minds to be unpleasant work, but others stay with their tutors and develop into formidable psionicists. These nobles enjoy a powerful edge over their rivals and are some of the most clever and cunning of opponents.

Noble psionicists may be humans, elves, half-elves, or dwarves. They may choose to be of any alignment open to the psionicist. There are no special ability requirements.

Preferred disciplines: Telepaths and clairsentients are greatly preferred for their information-gathering abilities.

Role: The noble psionicist is virtually a pariah among Athas's degenerate nobility. Her clear mind and self-discipline are virtues seldom found among the elite of the Seven Cities. Despite her distance from the social scene, she is still well-treated and respected by both her allies and her enemies. To her family, she is a valuable asset, a steel-bladed sword to be wielded against their rivals. In time, as the head of the family, she possesses the wisdom and the clarity of thought to bring the house even greater power and influence.

As an adventurer, the noble psionicist often has a challenging agenda mapped out for her by her family. Whether or not she follows that agenda is her own business. Until she actually assumes the mantle of leadership and the noble title, she is often free to pursue her own studies.

Weapon proficiencies: Nobles enjoy access to excellent weapons training. Many are taught the basics of self-defense at an early age. The noble psionicist receives a bonus weapon proficiency that can be used to learn martial arts or to specialize in punching or wrestling (see the

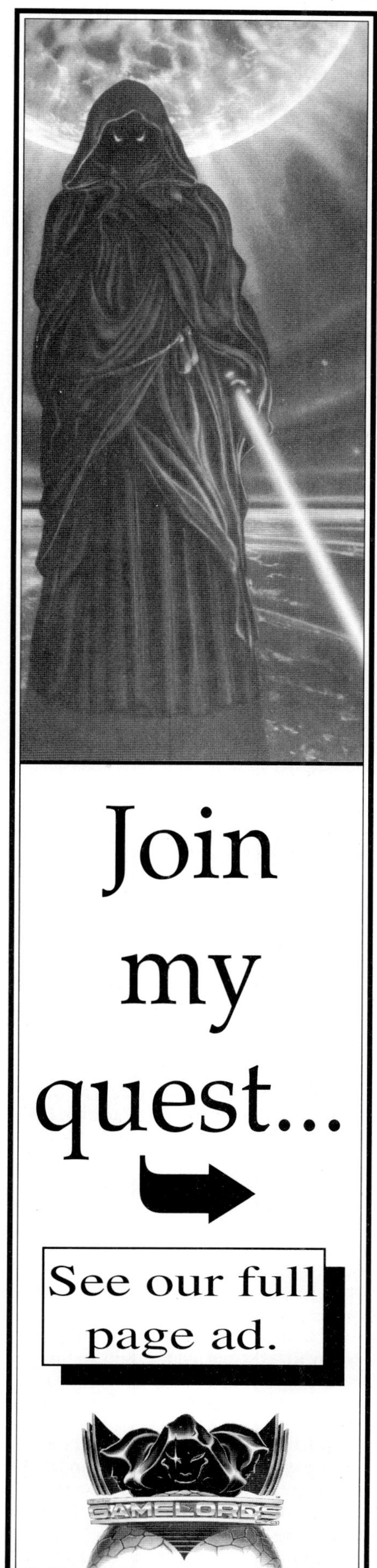

Complete Fighter's Handbook).

Recommended weapon proficiencies include any weapon generally associated with the nobility of the character's home.

Nonweapon proficiencies: Etiquette, Heraldry. Recommended: Meditative Focus, Rejuvenation, Harness Subconscious, Dancing, Land-based Riding, Reading/Writing.

Equipment: While a noble psionicist does not particularly enjoy the display of wealth, she also understands that appearances must be maintained. The psionicist must pay 150-200% (d6+14 ×10%) the normal cost of any clothing or equipment she purchases in order to make it clear that she is a person of privilege. If the noble psionicist cannot look the part, she will have a difficult time convincing NPCs that she is a noble.

Special benefits: The noble psionicist begins play with more money than a psionicist without a kit. She also has a family, clan, or estate to support her. If she wishes, the noble psionicist can live with her relations indefinitely, enjoying a life of ease and luxury. However, a noble psionicist who lives off her family's fortune will find that the family expects her full loyalty.

The noble psionicist receives a +3 bonus on reaction checks with any member of her culture or society who recognizes her as a noble. Many of Athas's lower classes have no love for nobility, but every citizen of a city-state has learned to respect it. A noble character in common clothes will not be recognized as a noble, no matter how many people she tells.

Special hindrances: As noted above, the noble psionicist must maintain appearances. She must always purchase the finest version of any clothing or gear she needs. This effectively raises the cost of any piece of equipment to 150%-200% of its listed cost.

The second hindrance of a noble psionicist applies only if she is living off her family and using their estate as her home base. Her relations are glad to have her around, and will often ask her for favors or support. At least once a week, the character will have to fulfill a family obligation; she may need to use her mental abilities against the house's enemies, she may be asked to spy on another rival house, or she might even be "invited" to attend to the sorcerer-king as the house's representative. The DM should use this as a tool to reinforce good role-playing; a wealthy PC who asks her family to buy steel weapons for all her friends had better be prepared to pay for it with her time and effort!

Wealth options: The noble psionicist begins play with 3d4 × 90 cp. At the DM's option, the character can also receive a stipend from her family equal to 10 cp per month per character level.

Untutored one

Description: The powerful manifestations of psionics in Athasian peoples often run in strange courses. Sometimes students with access to the most understanding and powerful of teachers barely master the basics of the Way; sometimes rogue talents of unbelievable strength arise in the most savage of tribes. The untutored one is a psionicist who has learned from no one but himself. He is often found living as an escaped slave or a savage raider of the desert. Most are brilliant blazes that flare and die beyond the sight of civilization, but others have shaken the world with their power.

Psionicists of any race or alignment may be untutored ones. There are no special ability requirements.

Role: The untutored one is often a hunted character. Templars and psionicists loyal to the sorcerer-king often pursue the PC under orders to capture him and learn the secrets of his power. At very high levels, the untutored one often runs afoul of the Order, a secret group of high-level psionicists. Despite this concentration of enemies, the untutored one often escapes their grasp—his abilities are often unknowable and uncontrollable. He is a true wild card who represents a threat to the established powers of Athas.

By necessity, untutored ones are loners. Other psionicists scorn them, and the nonpsionic savages or slaves that raised them fear their great power. The untutored character is often forced into a wanderer's life, and few ever call a place or people home.

Preferred disciplines: Unusual gifts can affect any discipline, but the most famous and powerful untutored ones are psychokineticists or telepaths.

Weapon proficiencies: Required: spear or knife. Recommended: short bow, short sword, hand axe, sling, or club.

Nonweapon proficiencies: Bonus: Rejuvenation, Endurance. Recommended: Heat Protection, Water Find, Survival, Hunting, Fire Building, Direction Sense, Land-based Riding, Running, Harness Subconscious, Meditative Focus.

Equipment: No special requirements.

Special benefits: The untutored one is completely free to develop his own potential, without the guidance of the established methods of learning the Way. After the untutored one chooses his disciplines, sciences, and devotions, he gains a random wild talent, just like a nonpsionicist character. This wild talent does not count against the allowable devotions and sciences he may know when he creates his character, and it does not matter if the talent is in a discipline he does not yet have access to. The normal rules for wild talent PSPs are used, and the total added directly to the psionicist's normal PSP pool.

The character cannot gain more than three devotions or sciences in this way. If the player rolls high enough to gain two or more wild talents, any combination of prerequisite powers and wild talents that would add up to more than three is simply discarded. If the wild talent (or any bonus prerequisites) duplicates a devotion that the character had already selected, he gains a special enhancement of that power but no new talents.

Enhanced powers that are successfully initiated (i.e., a power check is made) automatically have the effect listed under the "Power Score" entry in the power description. The only exception is a roll of 1 or 2 on the power check, in which case the power takes effect as normal. A psionicist with an enhanced power never suffers the ill effects of rolling a 1 on his power check.

Special hindrances: The untutored one is unfamiliar with many of the common teachings of psionics, including psionic defenses. Unlike most psionicists, the untutored one does not automatically gain psionic defenses and so must use new devotions or sciences to acquire them. The defenses are all telepathic powers, and the normal restrictions for choosing devotions and sciences applies when a character selects a psionic defense.

Secondly, the untutored one suffers a -3 penalty to reaction checks with normal psionicists who recognize him for what he is, and a -1 penalty with all other characters except those of his tribe or family. The character is markedly unusual and carries himself awkwardly; the burden of his unasked-for powers and his lack of self-knowledge erodes his social grace.

Wealth options: The untutored one rarely owns more than the clothes on his back. He begins play with only 3d4 ×15 cp.

Other kit ideas

The DM is not limited to the above character kits; many other DARK SUN characters exist on Athas, and many would make fine character kits. For example, a good one might be an elven runner, a multiclassed fighter/thief. Halfling shamans, dwarven sappers, or thri-kreen stalkers all would be good nonhuman kits. Other ideas for human kits might include an outrider (a fighter or trader who specializes in guarding caravans), a dilettante (a bard or thief born of the nobility), or a hidden priest (a character who maintains a shrine and practices elemental magic beneath the noses of the sorcerer-kings.)

The Dungeon Master shouldn't be the only one coming up with new kits. If you are a player and you have a great character concept, talk to your DM about customizing a kit just for that character. Be creative and have fun; after all, isn't that what it's all about? Ω

Castle Falkenstein

A world that could have existed.
A time that might have been.
A battle to save a Good and Golden Age
from a Revolution of
Steam & Steel.
Humanity's last and best Hope.

CASTLE FALKENSTEIN™

A new Roleplaying Experience.
Coming this Summer from R.Talsorian Games

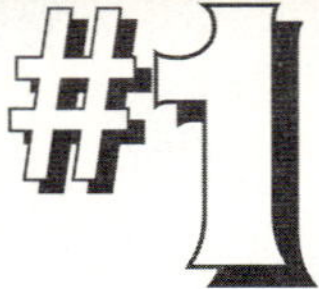

#1

Not just another bug hunt: TSR's BUGHUNTERS™ game

by Lester Smith

If you haven't heard it before, here's some news: TSR has been working on an entirely new line of role-playing games, all part of the AMAZING ENGINE™ system.

Even as you read this, the first two products in the line—the BUGHUNTERS™ and FOR FAERIE, QUEEN, AND COUNTRY games—are winging their ways to hobby

stores, each with a copy of the 32-page *System Guide* that serves as the core rules for all games in the AMAZING ENGINE line-up. Later this year, the MAGITECH™ and GALACTOS BARRIER games will join those products, and work has begun on next year's offerings as well.

As the designer of the BUGHUNTERS game, I'm taking this opportunity to tell you something about the thoughts that went into that game's creation—the whys and wherefores of its final shape. In order to do so, I'll first need to explain a bit about the AMAZING ENGINE system in general, so this article will also serve as a quick introduction to the AMAZING ENGINE line.

An amazing idea

The title of the AMAZING ENGINE system gives a hint as to the line's purpose. Just as AMAZING® Stories magazine covers a wealth of short fiction, the AMAZING ENGINE roleplaying system covers a wealth of role-playing milieux. For starters, there's the Victorian fantasy world of the FOR FAERIE, QUEEN, AND COUNTRY game, the horrific science-fiction setting of the BUGHUNTERS game, the modern magic-as-technology environment of the MAGITECH game, and the far-future universe of the GALACTOS BARRIER game, with lots more to come. Just as a short story is constructed differently from a novel, with an eye toward getting you into the action quickly, the AMAZING ENGINE system is designed to do the same. All of its member games are based upon the same core rules systems, and everything else you need for any particular milieu is packed within a single 128-page book.

When I joined the TSR staff last October, Zeb Cook had pretty much finished the core rules for the system, and he was working on the FOR FAERIE, QUEEN, AND COUNTRY game. Being the nice guy that he is, and wanting to make the "newbie"

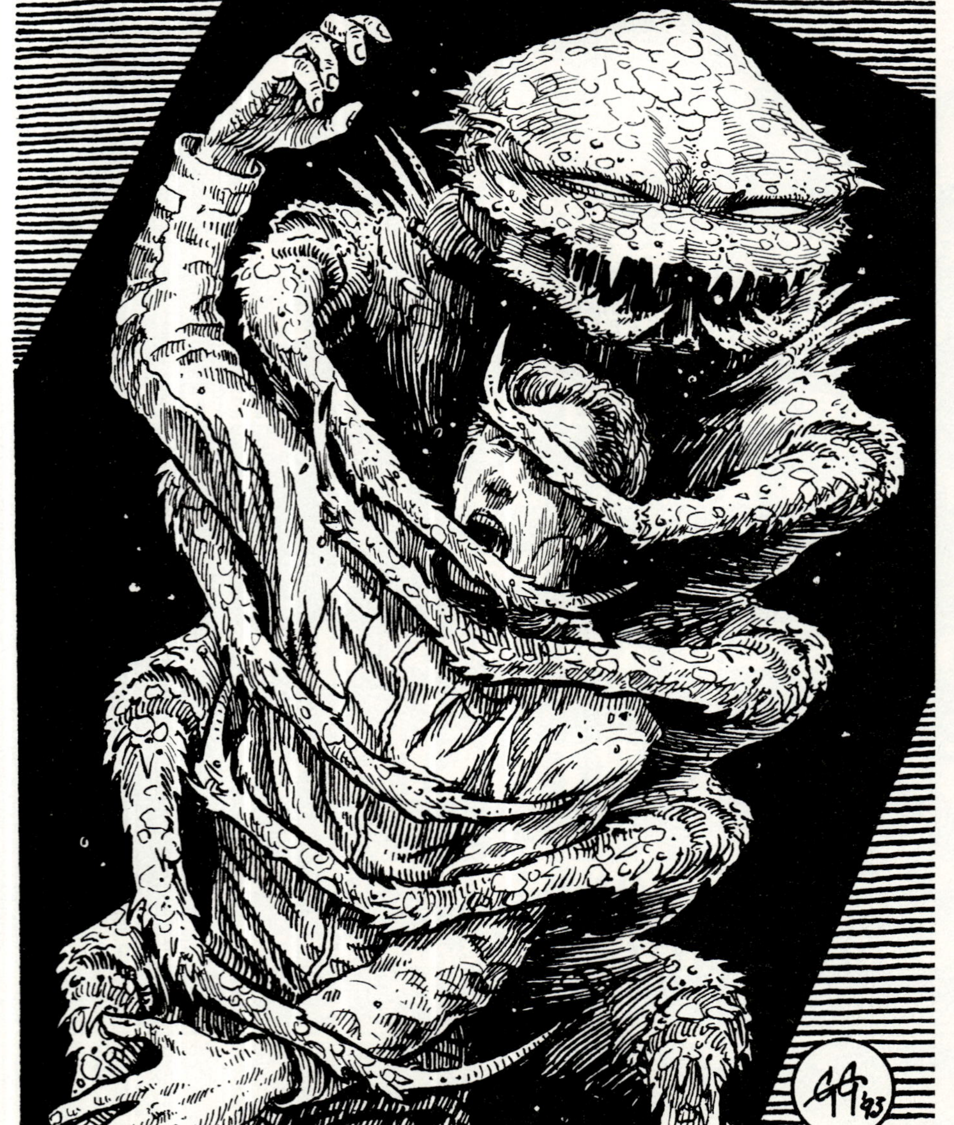

feel welcome, Zeb invited me to join his playtest group for that game. I was immediately excited by the milieu he was creating. For one thing, the genteel vs. bawdy tensions of Victorian England are quite entertaining, particularly when a goodly portion of the citizenry is possessed of at least a bit of fairie blood. For another, Zeb's take on the magic system is fascinating. Casting a spell is basically like constructing a sentence: You designate a subject (the "victim"), decide upon a verb phrase (the "action" of the spell), then load the spell up with modifiers to reduce the power cost (such as speaking it in rhyme while dressed in green and standing on one foot). I'll leave it to Zeb to reveal further details of the game at a more appropriate time in the future.

The bughunt begins

I felt great excitement over the shape the AMAZING ENGINE system was taking. So, when I was asked if I'd like to design the BUGHUNTERS game—a game of personal combat versus deadly alien creatures in the not-too-distant future—I jumped at the chance, despite the fact that there was something of a time crunch involved. It had been decided that the best way to launch the brand-new system was to release the FOR FAERIE, QUEEN, AND COUNTRY and BUGHUNTERS games simultaneously, thereby showing off the AMAZING ENGINE system's range of possibilities, from unusual fantasy to gritty sci-fi. This plan called for delaying release of the first game a bit while pushing the BUGHUNTERS game ahead in the schedule. Fortunately for me, a number of people volunteered to help out with the BUGHUNTERS game project (you can find them listed by chapter in the game's credits). It isn't an easy thing to write to match someone else's peculiar vision of a new game, especially when that writer is a brand-new member of the staff. These peoples' willingness to help out and to ease my initiation into the company made all the difference, and I bless them for it, and their children, and their children's children . . .

The mechanics

When I started working on the BUGHUNTERS game, there were a few "givens" I had to take into account. First, of course, whatever I did had to match up with the core rules in the *System Guide*. Not only did that apply to the specifics of the dice mechanics, character attributes, etc., it also directed the feel of any new rules I was to come up with. As a prime example, the fact that each skill in the AMAZING ENGINE system defaults to a related character attribute, rather than having a separate number value to keep track of, served as a constant reminder to keep my attention on fast and easy play. There were times when I chafed at this;

it's easy for a designer to keep adding levels of complexity like new layers of snowfall, losing track of just how deep the drifts are growing. However, as the whole took shape, I became increasingly won over by Zeb's vision of how easy the game play of an AMAZING ENGINE session should be. Of course, the fact that I had to fit an entire milieu within 128 pages served as another pointer to the age-old K.I.S.S. maxim ("Keep it simple, stupid").

Another "given" was that the BUGHUNTERS game would have a more detailed combat system than most other AMAZING ENGINE projects. The *System Guide* itself makes reference to that fact. I opted for a tactical design that limits the actions available to a character by how far the character moves in a turn, with individual actions defined in fair detail. For instance, in fire combat, aimed shots can only be performed by a stationary figure, while snapfire can be conducted by a walking figure, and burst and autofire even by a running figure. This results in appropriately tactical personal combat situations for the milieu. My thanks to Tim Brown for the work he contributed to this section of the rules, and to Colin McComb, Karen Boomgarden, and Newton Ewell for related work on the equipment chapter.

In my opinion, the starship chapter is another high point of the BUGHUNTERS game's design. Tim Beach took my desire for a modular approach to ship creation and turned out an impressively designed set of statistics, floor plans, and matching text. Together, we worked out a simple but wide-ranging system of how ship speed relates to mass and drive power. Thus, within a very few pages, the reader is provided with a system for quickly creating many different starships at widely ranging sizes and speeds. Working with Tim on this chapter was a distinct pleasure.

Character creation is the third leg of the tripod skeleton of the BUGHUNTERS game. I'll have more to say about PCs later, but for the moment I'll point out that the character-creation chapter provides not only stats and beginning equipment for characters, but also a sense of history and future goals.

The milieu

Having spoken about the skeleton, let me now tell you something about the flesh of the BUGHUNTERS game.

From the project's inception, a year or more before I joined the crew here at TSR, the game was intended to cover the sorts of gritty human-versus-alien conflict portrayed in such films as *Aliens, Enemy Mine, The Deep,* and *Predator,* as well as in a host of novels and lesser-known B-movie thrillers. This suited me perfectly. As a GM, I like to draw adventures from lots of different sources, and I frequently find myself finishing a movie, TV program, or

book with the thought, "I wonder how my players would respond in this situation?"

At the same time, both as a gamer and a game designer, I've noticed how important it is for people to be able to convey the essence of a game succinctly to their friends. New players are much more likely to join a game whose premise is readily grasped than one whose premise is not. The second sort of game may be loads of fun to play once a player is familiar with it, but new players are going to feel uncomfortable and unsure of their roles until then. Given that the AMAZING ENGINE system is designed to get you quickly and easily from milieu to milieu, it would be especially counterproductive to expect players to founder for a while before becoming familiar with each new game in the line. Taking such things into account, I like to set things up so that there is a clear central premise, but one specifically designed to accomodate a wide range of adventure types.

How does this all reflect on the BUGHUNTERS game? Well, the central

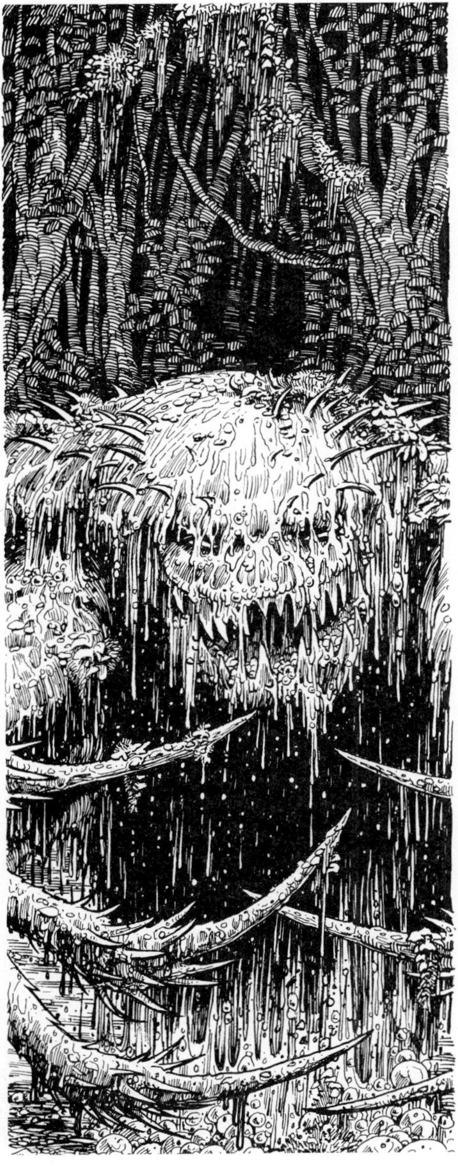

premise I settled upon is that Humanity has begun its first efforts to colonize the stars. However, the race is discovering that the galaxy is a much deadlier, nastier place than could have been expected, full of bloodthirsty creatures of all sorts, including savagely evolved animals, murderous intelligences, and even mechanical assassins. (There is a very good reason for the existence of these things—a simple secret that is revealed to GMs and empowers them to adapt nearly any sort of science-fiction adventure plot to a BUGHUNTERS campaign. It is intended that players discover that secret only through the course of play.)

A united Terra has responded to this threat by creating a special aerospace and marine force consisting of physically and mentally enhanced humans, each cloned from normal human volunteers. The PCs, then, are larger-than-life warriors, with their donors' memories, personalities, and dreams—but bound to serve as soldiers for the duration of Humanity's need (in other words, indefinitely). Of course, because they are bigger and tougher than normal people, these synthetic humans (typically called "synths" or "synners") are mistrusted and feared, though often secretly envied.

The PCs may not get respect, but they do get big guns, high explosives, and plen-tiful targets. The problem is, of course, that those targets tend to be quite tough in their own right. The result is a game that combines combat and fear, horror and heroism.

Establishing the right imagery for hardware in this game was a bit tricky. I think people have come to expect spaceships in this genre to travel faster-than-light but still have dim corridors lined with oil-stained pipes and bundles of grimy wiring. Although the ships do move faster than light, they still take quite a while to get anywhere, so the isolation during voyages contributes to the sense of horror when something goes wrong. What's more, in this genre people expect to see the stars drift by outside the portholes. To account for all this, I decided upon a FTL drive that skips in and out of hyperspace like a stone skipping across the surface of a pond, powered by a fusion engine which drives turbines to generate electricity.

There are other presuppositions for this genre, of course. For example, weightlessness is never a problem in films of this genre—there's an unspoken assumption that artificial gravity exists. Suspended animation is common, too. That's all pretty high-tech stuff. Still, the weapons tend to be very similar to today's slug-throwers, with visible smoke and recoil, and the typical combat uniform is highly reminiscent of Vietnam-era fatigues and web gear. That's all rather low-tech stuff.

My solution to this high-tech/low-tech dichotomy was to posit a future in which the United Nations (now United Terra) has become the predominant government, and national wars are pretty much a thing of the past. Consequently, technology has pursued space travel rather than the production of more advanced guns. What's more, a ballooning global population stretches world resources ever thinner, in the process creating rising pressures for colonization of other worlds.

Conclusion

One of the most fascinating things about working on this game was creating a logical rationale that would take all of the "givens" and presuppositions into account. I had a great good time working on the BUGHUNTERS game, and from the response of playtesters, I suspect that a great many people will have much fun playing it, as well.   Ω

Here it comes!

Wondering what TSR is about to do next? Turn to "TSR Previews" in this issue and find out!

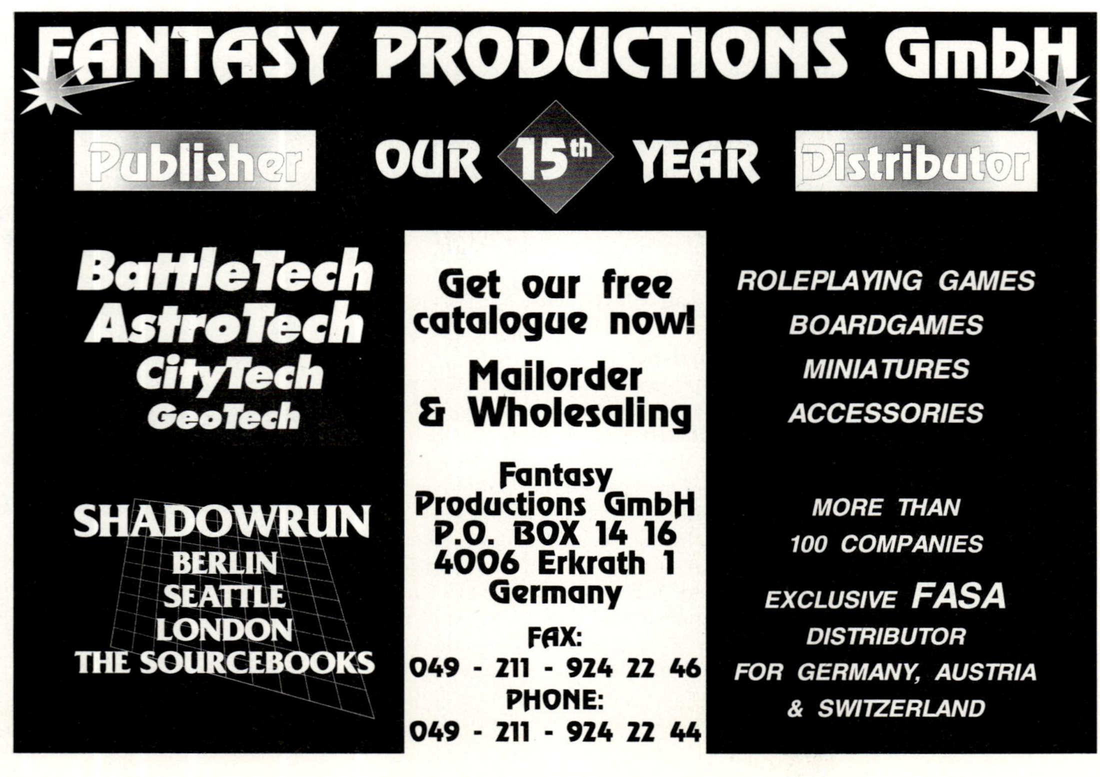

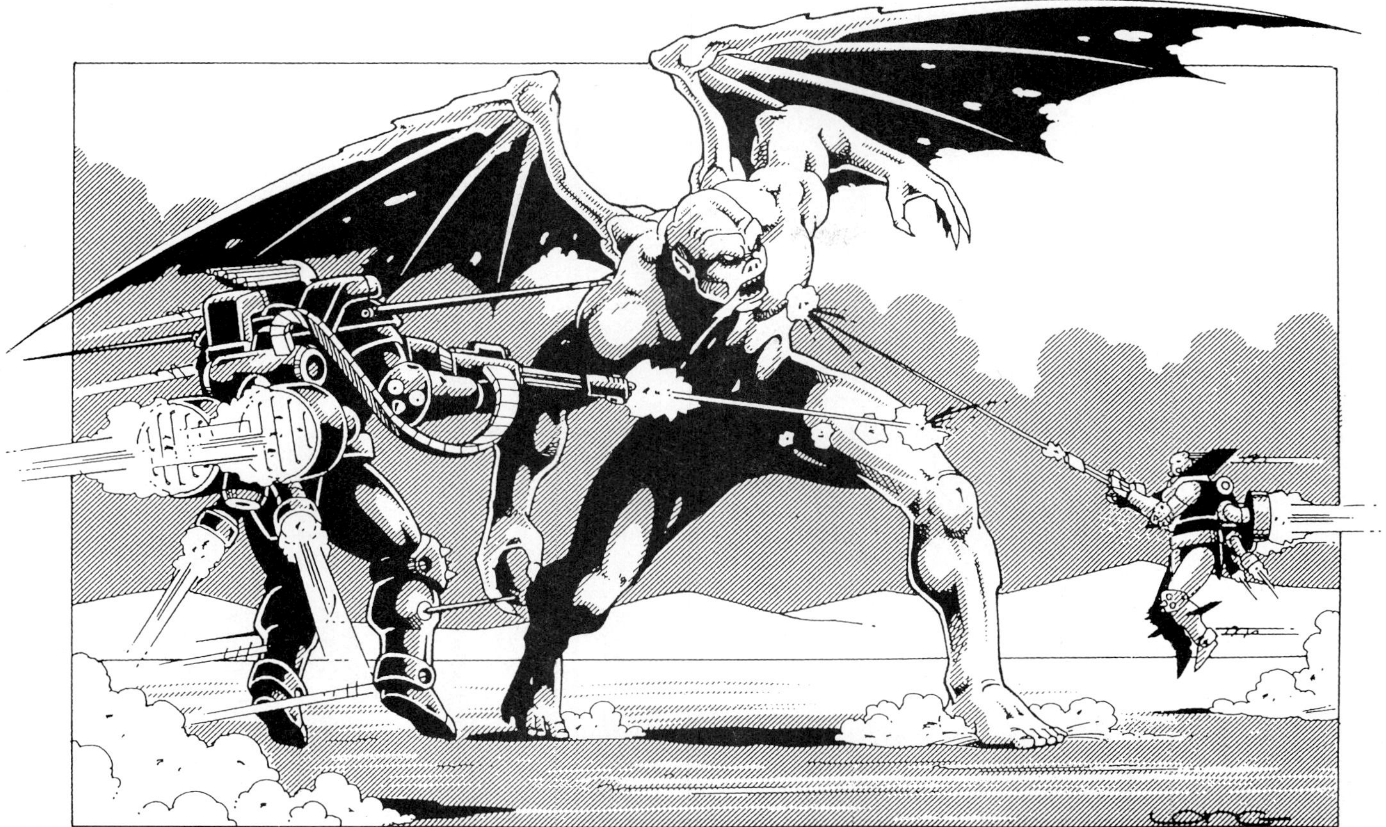

The endless adventure of Rifts®

The Rifts® RPG

**Nearly 70,000 copies have sold
and it continues to sell like crazy!**

That's right! Nearly 70,000 copies of just the RPG book alone have been sold! When we include all our **Rifts RPG products,** including supplements and sourcebooks, it adds up to well over a quarter of a million copies! Isn't it time you discovered the adventure of **Rifts**?

The Rifts RPG provides all the rules and world information players need to launch a campaign. The many sourcebooks only add to the rich, multi-dimensional worlds of **Rifts**.

Earth has been transformed into a doorway to a thousand different worlds and dimensions. A place of challenge and endless adventure where humans explore strange new worlds and struggle against a menagerie of supernatural and alien invaders.

Rifts Earth is a place of dramatic contrast where magic and super-science coexist in a hostile environment. Mystic energy flows in lines of power known as ley lines, empowering humans and monsters alike. High technology enables humans to augment their frail bodies with cybernetic implants, bionic reconstruction, power armor and giant robots.

Nearly 30 character classes, including dragons, cyborgs, robots, psi-stalkers, cyber-knights and glitter boys. Psionics, magic and super-science, plus 16 pages of full color paintings by Long, Parkinson and Siembieda, presented in a 256 page masterpiece. **$24.95 plus $2.00 for postage and handling.**

Palladium Books®	**12455 Universal Drive**
Dept. D	**Taylor, Mi. 48180**

Rifts Metal Miniatures! At last, your favorite **Rifts** characters are available as safe, non-lead, metal miniatures. The Glitter Boys, Ulti-Max, Dog Pack, Line Walker, Coalition soldiers, Cyborgs and SAMAS are among the first to be released. Watch for 'em late this summer.

The Entire Rifts® Megaverse®

Rifts Sourcebook One™. More details on the Coalition States, their soldiers, war machines, skelebots, and plans for conquest. More robots, power armor, body armor, weapons, monsters, new villains, and world information. Plus adventures introducing A.R.C.H.I.E. 3, Hagan Lonovich and their mechanized minions. **$11.95 plus $1.50 for postage and nandling.**

Rifts Sourcebook Two: The Mechanoids®. A.R.C.H.I.E. Three and Hagan are back with more insidious schemes. Only this time they may have bit off more than even they can chew — The Mechanoids! More mechanical creations from A.R.C.H.I.E. Three & Hagan. The Mechanoids — old and new; complete stats. Adventures, adventure ideas and other good stuff. Cover by Long, interior art by Long, Ewell and Siembieda. **112 pages — $11.95 plus $1.50 postage and handling.**

Rifts World Book One: Vampire Kingdoms™. This book offers more than just info about the hordes of wild vampires that ravage the American southwest, vampire intelligences, or the even the powerful vampire kingdoms of Mexico. It introduces new techno-wizard devices, methods of fighting vampires, Reid's Rangers and other vampire hunters, the mysterious and deadly Yucatan Peninsula which straddles at least two dimensions, werepeople, new monsters, traveling shows and carnivals (which are far more than they seem), world data and more! **$14.95 plus $1.50 for postage and handling.**

Rifts World Book Two: Atlantis™. Atlantis is a multi-dimensional wonderland. Ley lines crisscross the land and their energy is tapped by giant, mystic pyramids. At the Dimensional Market in the city of Splynn it is said one can purchase anything or travel anywhere. Scores of alien creatures lay claim to the land and hundreds more are sold at the trans-dimensional slave markets. 30 optional player characters, including Tattooed Men, Stone Masters, Atlanteans, Undead Slayers, Sunaj Assassins, & others. The secrets of rune magic, bio-wizardry, stone magic, pyramid technology, tattoo magic and more. Written by Siembieda, cover by Parkinson, interior art by Long and Ewell. **160 pages — $14.95 plus $1.50 for postage and handling.**

Rifts Conversion Book™. Over 100 different monsters, 40 optional player races, adult dragons, super-heroes, warlock, witch and diabolist character classes. Specific rules and general guidelines are provided for converting characters, super powers, robots, magic, weapons and vehicles from all of Palladium's role-playing games to **Rifts**. Plus more magic and world information. Written by Siembieda, art by Long and Gustovich. **$19.95 plus $2.00 for postage and handling.**

BAZAAR of the BIZARRE

Tenser's Bottling Co., Inc.

by Spike Y. Jones

Artwork by L.A. Williams

The most useful and yet potentially the most dangerous class of magical items are the potions and other magical fluids that store magical energies in fragile glass bottles. While a flask of *oil of fiery burning* is obviously useful, it is also obviously dangerous to have one in a back pocket when you fall into a pit! Even relatively harmless potions can still cause problems if their bottles break, such as the embarrassment (and reduced effectiveness) caused by scrabbling across the ground on your hands and knees looking for uncontaminated drops of *healing potion* to drink. Here is one solution to the problem of fragile potion bottles (along with a number of new potions and other fragile magical items), *Tenser's tantalus*, also known as *Tenser's potion caddy*.

Tenser's tantalus (Wizard)

A tantalus is a nonmagical piece of furniture, a liquor-stand that uses wooden or metal rods to keep the bottles and glasses in the stand from moving about. *Tenser's tantalus* is a mobile, magical version of the same sort of device, designed to transport magical potions or other fragile items, keeping them safe and within easy reach for the mage's use.

Although there is no evidence that this magical item was created (or even used) by Tenser, the famed wizard of the WORLD OF GREYHAWK® setting, the reasons its origin was erroneously attributed to him are obvious; *Tenser's tantalus* is a flat metal disc, 3' in diameter, which floats at a constant 3' above the surface of the ground (under most circumstances) and at the same 3' distance from its user unless specifically commanded otherwise. But while it shares much in common with the *Tenser's floating disc* spell, it also has a number of significant differences, the primary one being that *Tenser's tantalus* is a permanent magical item, not a temporary magical spell.

The disc's upper surface emits a soft glow extending for about a foot above the metal. Any objects placed entirely within this field are subject to a powerful quasi-magnetic force that holds any nonliving matter (including once-living materials such as paper, leather, or a small dead body, as well as completely inanimate matter like glass, metal, or crystal) firmly to the surface of the disc, but that has no effect on living flesh, even creatures small enough to fit within the field's confines. No matter what pressures are exerted against it, the tantalus will protect objects within its field from the effects of violent motions and other external shocks unless those shocks are powerful enough to destroy the metal disc. For this purpose, treat the disc as a metal shield, using the Item Saving Throws table on page 39 of the *Dungeon Master's Guide*.

Since the quasi-magnetic force doesn't affect objects only partially within its area of effect, bottles taller than the 1'-tall field will not be held by a *Tenser's tantalus* unless laid on their sides. Bottles can be stacked, but that is difficult. Reaching through the glowing field and grabbing an object on the disc frees the object—when an object is grabbed, the field reacts as if the object is physically connected to the arm and thus as if it extends beyond the edge of the field.

Because objects only partially within the field aren't affected, a thrown spear can wreak havoc on the disc's load—a spear is long enough that part of it is always outside of the field. On the other hand, a sling bullet hurled at the bottles cannot break them because the field affects it as soon as the bullet is fully within its boundaries, leaving the bullet suspended in mid-air just inside the edge of the field. For maximum protection, potions should be placed as close to the center of the *Tenser's tantalus* as possible, protecting them from weapons shorter than the 1.5' radius of the disc. If the disc is fully loaded, items close to the edge can be easily affected by short weapons such as hand axes or daggers.

A *Tenser's tantalus* can hold up to 20 lbs. of bottles and contents (the average potion in a glass bottle weighs about half a pound), and will smoothly accelerate and decelerate to safely follow its owner at any speed up to 18, including following him as he climbs stairs. If the user moves beyond the 50' effective range of command, the tantalus ceases all movement and hovers in place until either its user returns or another wizard takes control of it.

A *Tenser's tantalus* will follow its owner if he falls into a pit, but because of the owner's rapid acceleration, he will soon out-strip the disc's power to follow. In a pit 75' deep or less, the disc will gently descend to the bottom a few seconds after its owner, but if the pit is any deeper the owner will eventually accelerate out of the 50' range, meaning that the disc will stop in mid-air some 20' down from the upper end of the pit, waiting for someone to come within range and take command.

Because such an obvious display of treasures increases the possibility of theft, many *Tenser's tantaluses* are equipped with a permanent *alarm* spell with a volume loud enough to be heard from 50' away but not farther. The alarm sounds when anything enters the field without speaking the *alarm*-deactivating command word. Semi-solid manipulators, such as *unseen servants*, *telekinesis* or *Bigby's hand* spells, air elementals, or *gusts of wind* are all too tenuous to reach into the field and take or destroy items, but all of these will activate the *alarm*.

A thief could attempt to steal the entire disc away from its owner. This requires a Strength check on 4d6 to break the disc's attraction to its owner. If the thief takes the disc more than 50' from its owner (and remember, the *alarm* will sound unless the thief manages to touch only the bottom and rim of the disc), it is free to be commanded by another wizard.
XP Value: 3,000 (3,500 with *alarm*)

Bottle of preservation

While they look like normal glass bottles from the outside, these common magical devices are invaluable to wizards or other collectors who use them for storing odds and ends. The bottles come in a variety of sizes and shapes, but all share one property; their interior walls project a spell designed to preserve indefinitely the freshness of anything placed within them, including spell components or ingredients for the manufacture of potions and other magical items. A more mundane use for a large *bottle of preservation* would be the storage of perishable food items, but the use of even a common magical item to preserve inexpensive food seems a little wasteful.
XP Value: 200

Bottle of trapping (Wizard)

These magical bottles look absolutely normal when empty except for their large, flaring mouths, and the elaborate, hinged stoppers that close them. The bottle's magic is activated when it is pointed at an object or person of less than 120 cubic feet volume (which includes most humanoids 12' or less in height) and the

lid is opened. When this happens, a beam of multicolored light lances out from the bottle's mouth to strike the target. If the target fails a saving throw vs. spells, it shrinks (as if affected by a *reduce* spell cast by a 12th-level wizard; a 12' tall creature would shrink to 3" tall) to a size that lets it fit within the bottle. Then the target is sucked toward the bottle's mouth.

At that point most inanimate objects are irresistibly sucked into the bottle, but living creatures can attempt to grab the lip of the mouth and hold on against the force of suction. To cling to the edge of the mouth, they must succeed at a Strength check on 1d20 each round that they wait for rescue. The bottle can only hold one shrunken object at a time, so if the target does end up in the bottle, it is entirely empty of previously-affected objects. While the bottle's walls are as fragile as normal glass from the outside, they are stronger than steel from the inside, foiling most attempts to escape.

There are two ways to exit the bottle. At the command of the holder, the bottle can expel its contents the same way that it trapped them, shooting them outward and subjecting them to an *enlarge* spell so that they return to normal size within seconds of escape. Less commonly, someone may escape a *bottle of trapping* when the bottle is destroyed, an easy task from the outside. Unfortunately, destroying the bottle also prevents it from *enlarging* its contents, so that anyone escaping from a shattered *bottle of trapping* will still stand just a few inches tall until a *dispel magic* or *enlarge* spell is cast on him.
XP Value: 3,500

Nerve tonic

This potion allows the imbiber to take control of his own emotions, remaining calm, cool, and collected no matter what the situation around him. All outside influences on his emotions are either eliminated or minimized. If used by an NPC, his morale rolls are made at +3.

No *scare*, *charm*, *fear*, or other emotion-

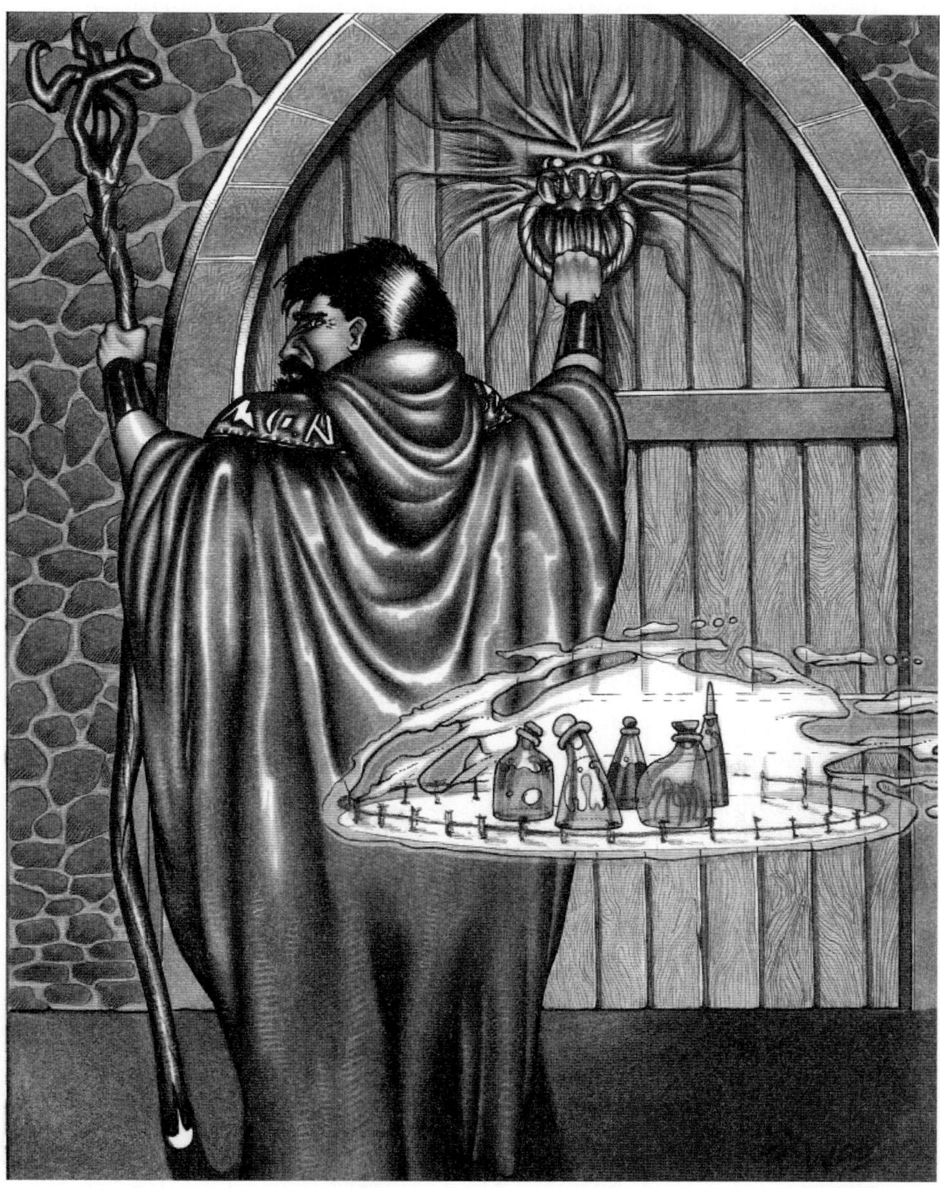

altering spell has any effect on the user of this potion, and the user also gains a +3 bonus to saving throws vs. spells that affect the victim's emotions indirectly, such as *spook* or *phantasmal killer*. The potion has no effect on mind-controlling spells without an emotional component such as *hypnotism* or *domination*. All of these effects last for 2-5 turns. Each bottle contains a single dose.

XP Value: 150

Oil of monster repulsion

Like many other oils, this liquid meant to be applied to a single person's clothing and skin rather than taken internally. It quickly soaks in and works continuously for 12 hours (unless removed by a strong solvent). Once applied, this oil releases a scent that is odorless to all creatures except the one type of animal or monster (lion, tiger, troll, blue dragon, goblin, etc. at the discretion of the maker) that it was formulated to affect. That type of creature smells an odor so disgusting that it will not willingly approach within 80' of the offending person. An intelligent creature can overcome its revulsion and force itself forward, but as it gets closer the odor increases so that each halving of the 80' distance gives the affected monster a cumulative –1 on all combat rolls (such as attack, damage and saving throw rolls); –1 at 40', –2 at 20', –3 at 10', and –4 at 5' or closer.

This oil can also be painted on inanimate objects such as fence posts to create a large zone of exclusion that no member of the target species can enter. One dose of oil can coat up to ten objects this way.

XP Value: 250

Oil of neutral scent

This magical oil's volume and duration resemble the *oil of monster repulsion*, but unlike that oil it doesn't make the user emit a special scent. Rather, it neutralizes all scents that the wearer and his coated equipment emit, making him effectively odorless. While this could have some bad effects (for instance, the user's pet dog may not recognize him), it is generally helpful, preventing the wearer from being sniffed out by giant ants, carrion crawlers, griffons, minotaurs, rust monsters, wolves, snakes, and other creatures dependant on scent to hunt or track. Even if such a monster blunders upon the wearer accidentally, the lack of a scent is likely to make it hesitate in combat (–2 on initiative rolls).

Unless the user can bathe a monster's entire body in *oil of neutral scent*, this oil is useless against the crippling scent attack of troglodytes and other smell-emitting monsters.

When the effects wear off, the wearer is instantly assailed with his own normal scent. It takes 1-4 turns before he is again so used to his scent as to be unaware of it.

XP Value: 300

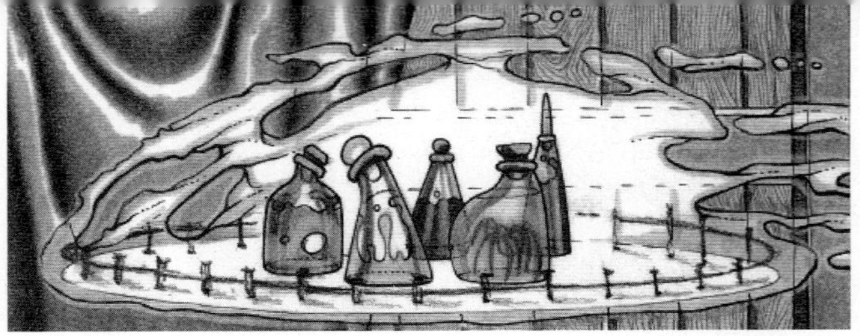

Pox potion

Although this potion is often the result of a failed attempt at creating some beneficial potion, it is sometimes intentionally manufactured or substituted for some other potion (for reasons ranging from con games to assassination attempts). When first swallowed, the potion has no apparent effects. After about an hour, boils, rashes, warts, and sores appear on the user's body. These grow in number and size until they cover the victim completely, but while they resemble the symptoms of many contagious diseases, the effects of a *pox potion* are not catching. For every hour after the elixir's ill effects first manifest themselves (up to a maximum of seven hours) the pox increases in stages, with the victim's Strength, Dexterity, and Charisma dropping by one point and his hit points by two points each hour (a maximum loss of 7 and 14 points, respectively).

The only known cures for this poison are a full dose of *sweet water*, a *dispel magic* spell (the poison resists as if created by a 12th-level wizard), or a *cure disease* spell cast by a priest of 12th or higher level. There is rarely more than one dose of *pox potion* found in a single place.

XP Value: 50 if created deliberately

Ship-in-a-bottle

To all appearances, this seems to be just another example of the sailor's hobby of building miniature vessels and sealing them into large glass bottles. As with most of its kind, this magical model is a highly detailed replica, so much so that one could almost believe that it was a real vessel shrunken by way of powerful magics. In fact, the magical ship-in-a-bottle is actually constructed in the same way as any other such model, but with expensive enchanted construction materials. The impression that it is a ship that has really been shrunken is only strengthened when the item is used. At the moment it is smashed against a pier or seashore rock, the model expands to form a full-size version of the same ship in a single round; this can be anything from a two-man row-boat to a trireme war-galley or beyond.

Although the enlarged vessel radiates a mild aura of magic, it has no magical powers and behaves exactly as a normal ship. The ship is permanent, barring accidents of fate and the depredations of time, tide and barnacles. It is equipped as the builder depicted it in miniature, with the exception of a crew. Any sculpted crew members in the miniature become man-

sized sculptures on the decks of the full-size ship, forcing the user to provide living crew members to replace them. Although a normal model ship would probably be destroyed if thrown against a rock, the magic of this item protects the bottle's contents until the *ship-in-a-bottle* is fully enlarged. Thus, the boat will be as sea-worthy in fact as it was in appearance in the bottle.

Lest anyone think this an easy way to create a fleet, the cost of the special materials involved in the creation of this item are the same as those required to make the full-size ships (see *Player's Handbook*, page 67), and the mage must perform all stages of the construction himself, meaning that he will have to study the art of bottled ship building before he can craft his magical models (Bottled Ship Building nonweapon proficiency: General, 1 slot, check vs. Dexterity at –2). Making a simple raft-in-a-bottle can take the wizard as much as a month, while a multi-deck galleon would certainly involve almost a year's effort; time enough for a shipyard to produce a small fleet.

XP Value: Half cost in gp to produce

Skunk water

This potion is not meant to be drunk, as it's not appetizing (although nonpoisonous on its own) to the human or demi-human palate. When added to other liquids it transforms them into impure, foul-smelling, undrinkable sludge. It has no effect on poisons, and *skunk water* automatically converts magical potions to poison. A single bottle of *skunk water* can foul 100,000 cubic feet of fresh water or turn 10 magical potions into poison (type G, H, or I, with full effects felt only if a complete dose is ingested; see *DMG*, page 73). While the effects of *skunk water* are permanent, an equal volume of *sweet water* can restore foul water to fresh. *Sweet water* has no effect on potions made poisonous.

XP Value: 100

Smoke of fire quenching

This small and fragile glass globe releases clouds of thick white smoke that extinguish all normal fires within 60' when shattered. Magical fires are entitled to a saving throw, requiring a roll of 15 or better, with a +1 bonus per level of the spell (so a *fireball* cast into an area protected by *smoke of fire quenching* would only ignite if a saving throw of 12 or better is made).

The spell has no effect on fires created by a creature's body (such as the breath of a red dragon) but secondary fires sparked by these flames are affected. The smoke dissipates in 3-6 rounds, and new fires can be lit in the area once every trace of the smoke is gone. The range of the thrown globe is 90' (see Grenade-Like Missiles, *DMG*, pages 62-63).

XP Value: 500 Ω

#2

The first game for all new gamers: the DRAGON STRIKE™ game

by Bruce Nesmith

Elation, frustration, hope, despair, relief, joy—no, these are not the emotional stages you pass through when you die. They are the emotional stages of game design. In particular, that's what I went through to design the DRAGON STRIKE™ game. It's new from TSR, Inc. and should be available in stores everywhere this month.

The DRAGON STRIKE game is a mass-market board game for young, novice gamers. It will be available in stores like Wal-Mart and Target as well as regular hobby shops. Experienced gamers will find that it makes a *great* gift for younger brothers, sisters, cousins, sons, daughters, kids down the street . . . sorry, got carried away there. Two to six people can play, ages 10 and up (lots of adults here at TSR have had fun playing it, too). Each player runs a character that is a fantasy hero, warrior, wizard, elf, or thief. One player is the Dungeon Master and sets up the adventures. The other players try to win the adventure before Darkfyre, the dragon, is placed on the board.

Of course, the game concept didn't start that way. Let me begin at the beginning. My boss, Jim Ward, gave me the choice assignment of rewriting the DUNGEONS & DRAGONS® game—you know, the black box with the red dragon exploding out of it. Boy, was I excited! Dare I say, I was even elated. It's not every day that a game designer gets to work on the world's premier fantasy role-playing game.

Everything went fine for the first month.

Then upper management had *the idea. The idea* was to produce a board game for kids that included a 30-minute, action-packed video tape. It would be a great way to introduce young people to fantasy role-

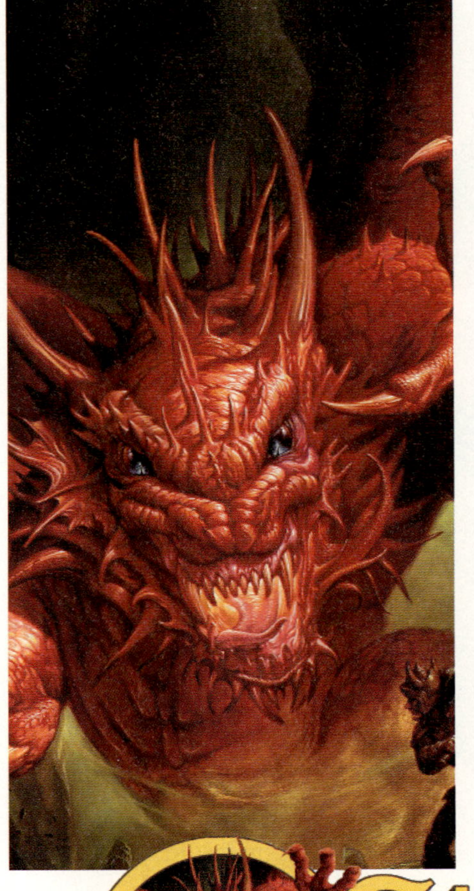

playing without wrestling with the complexities of the D&D® and AD&D® games. Once kids played this game, they'd be excited about getting into role-playing.

My rewrite of the DUNGEONS & DRAGONS boxed set was dropped faster than last year's DRAGONLANCE® calendar. Suddenly, I was making a mass-market board game that included a mini-movie. I was *definitely* elated. (By the way, *mass market* means that the game is supposed to appeal to everyone, not just role-players. A broad audience appeal means more sales, which means more gamers, which benefits everyone.)

Quicker than an editor's red pen, the plans for the game that was to become the DRAGON STRIKE system grew and grew. It got plastic pieces—24 of them, to be exact. It got two game boards. Then the game boards became double sided. It soon included 16 adventures, 110 cards, card sheets, counters, bases, and a screen. To cap it off, my boss was transferred to Marketing and I got a new boss. Over half my time at TSR was spent in meetings about the DRAGON STRIKE game. It became a monster out of control—and it was barely written down.

Then I heard those dreaded words: "Your deadline hasn't changed." I had only three months to design a game with all that stuff in it, and I was starting from scratch.

In no time, I had a game design and a prototype prepared. I was then ready for the most terrifying experience a game

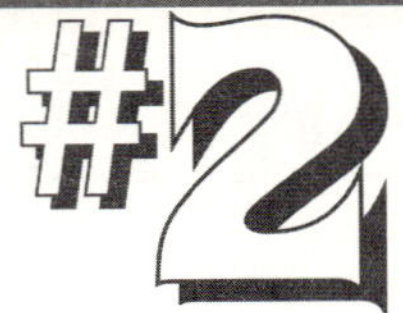

designer can have: a playtest by other game designers. I thought about wearing a bulletproof vest, but decided it would get in the way of my lunging across the table to strangle critical co-workers. Like all initial playtests, it ended disastrously and in frustration. I swept up the remains of my shattered ego, extracted the game board from the claws of my former friends and colleagues, and slunk back to my office. A warning to all aspiring game designers out there: Sell your egos and buy thick skins. If you can't stand the heat of the playtesting, don't bother applying for the job.

I set up several more playtests for those heartless people I work with. With their advice and suggestions, the game actually became playable. Then it became good. Finally, it became fun (far more important than being good!). There was hope yet.

Now I had to write down the rules. As you might guess, I had used up a lot of my three months getting to the point where I could begin to write. Fortunately, I had an editor. An editor is every game designer's best friend and worst nightmare, all rolled into one. I had the best of both in Andria Hayday. She was there for all the playtests, all the endless meetings, all the swift changes in direction. Andria pulled my fat out of the fire. All she asked in return was tireless devotion.

Although I can lay some claim to the game design, much of the actual writing is Andria's. She worked endless late nights and even cracked the whip to get me to work a few myself. Despair set in as the deadline quickly approached.

Just before Christmas, I became a father for the third time, and my DRAGON STRIKE game deadline arrived. I did my best to match Andria's pace while attending more and more important but lengthy meetings. Finally, after what seemed to be an eternity, the project was finished. What a relief! (Famous last words.)

Once a good editor gets hold of a manuscript, the manuscript won't be let go until it's perfect. Andria had more changes for me to make, more things to review, and more things to do. For over a month I worked on my regular project and did whatever she needed to have done. At last, even that was finished. What a relief! (Haven't I heard that somewhere before?)

During all this chaos, we received the results of our outside playtesting. The playtesters liked the game! After the shock wore off, I was even more relieved. But if you thought I would be overjoyed at this point, you were wrong. As a game designer, you pour your heart and soul into a game, giving it your best shot. All your co-workers can tell you that the game is great, but until real, live kids play it and say they like it, you really don't know for sure. Now I knew.

As I write this, the game is still in production. I am still waiting for that last emotional surge: joy. That will come only when everyone reading this goes out and buys a copy of the DRAGON STRIKE game. Joy comes when the game is a commercial success. Oh, it's nice to be a critical success, too, but I find it much more satisfying to know that regular people, not just critics, enjoy my games. What are you waiting for? Go out and make me happy! Buy the DRAGON STRIKE game. Ω

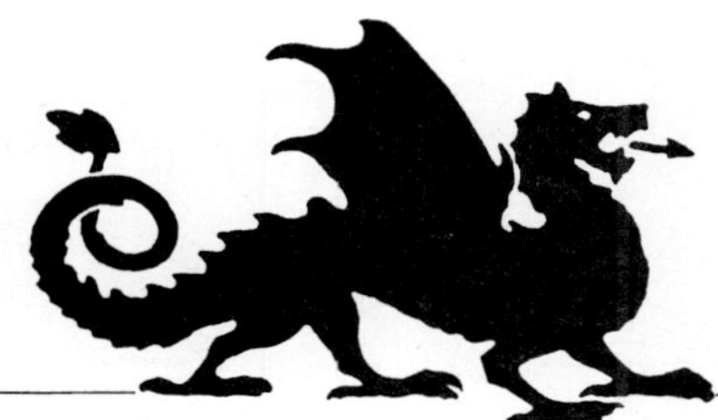

Give us the word!

What do you think of this magazine? What do you like best or want to see changed most? What do you want to see next? Turn to "Letters" and see what others think, then write to us, too!

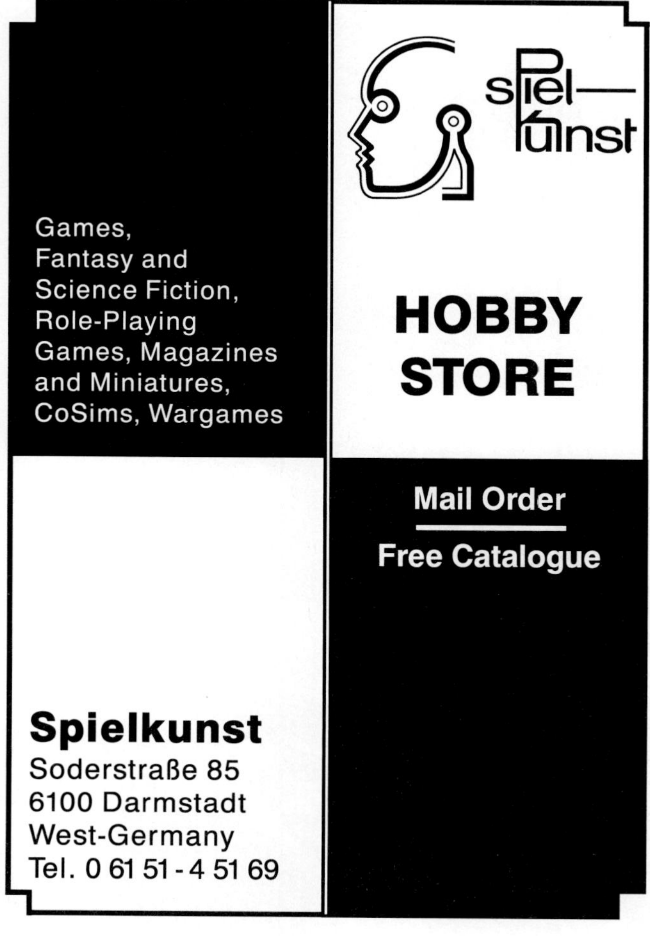

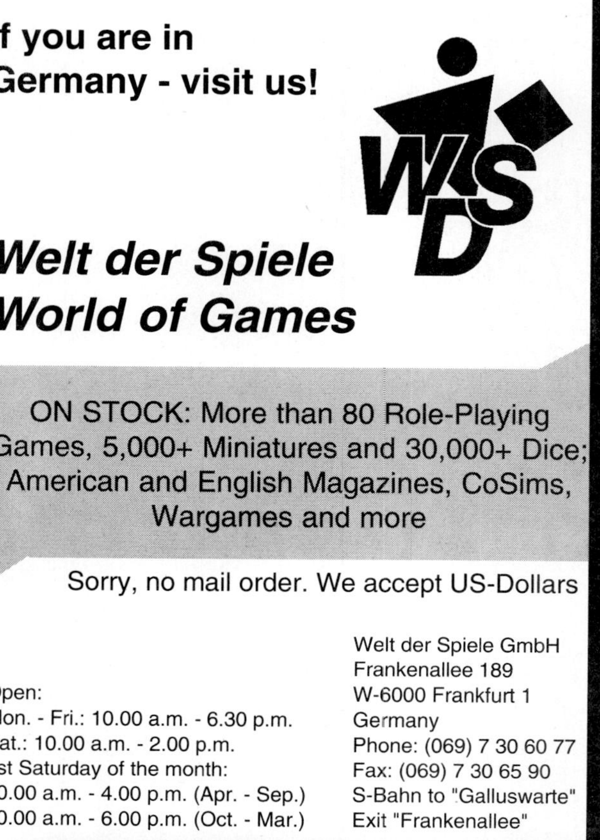

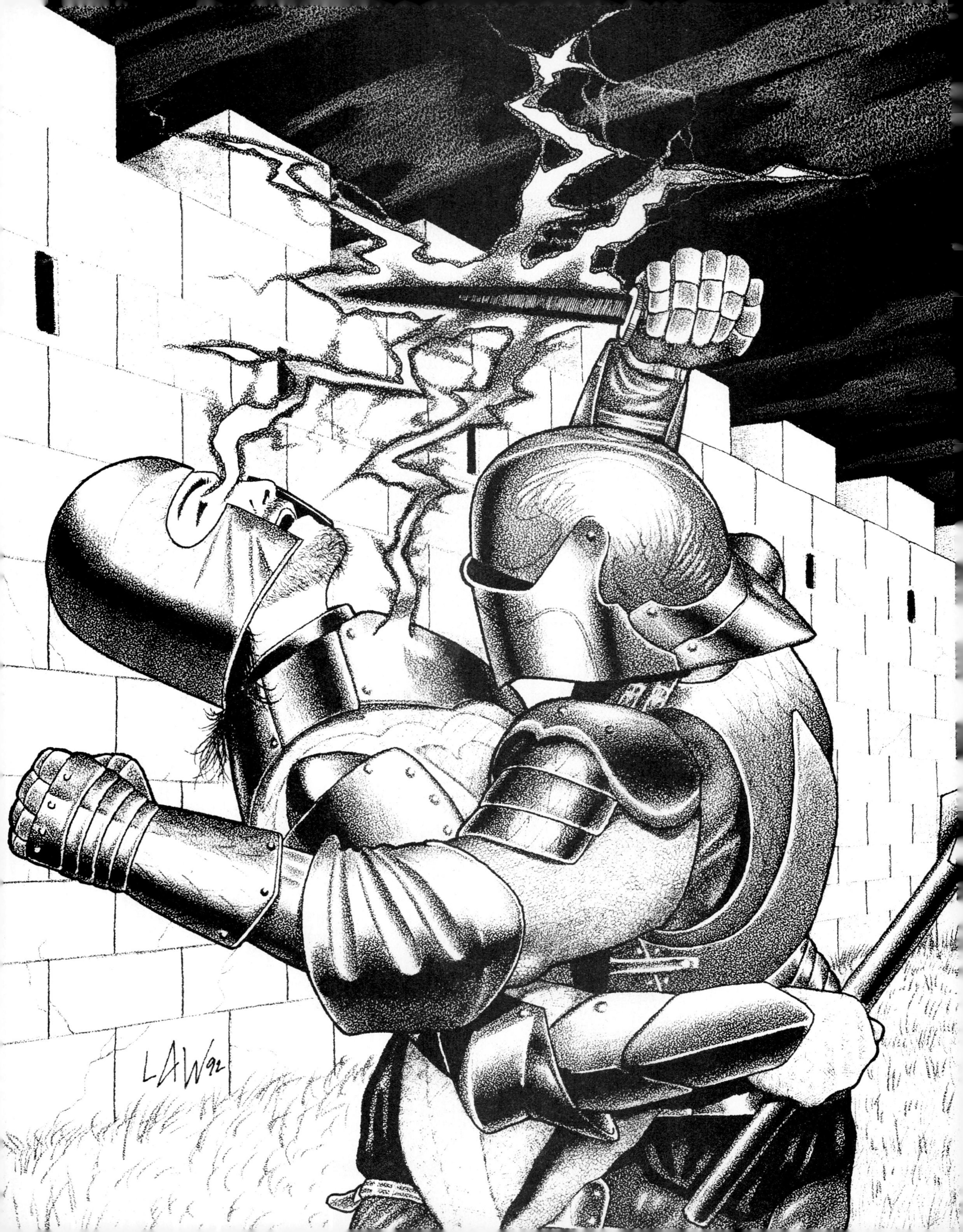

by Gregory W. Detwiler

Artwork by L. A. Williams

With a Bond of Magic!

This article describes a new type of magical weapon for the AD&D® game: the bonded weapon. What makes a bonded weapon different from a standard magical weapon is the fact that it is not an ordinary weapon with a dweomer of some sort placed on it. Instead, it is an element, material, or essence bonded together in the shape of a melee weapon. Thus, there can be a *fire axe* made of the element of flame, or a *fear sword* made of the essence of terror.

Players with spell-caster characters must already be wondering how to create such magical weapons. My reply is brief: You can't. These weapons can only be created by the gods themselves (who else has access to the essence of things like "fear" or "pain"?), and thus are relatively scarce. Not only that, but two-thirds of these weapons do not have a permanent dweomer. These temporary weapons have a limited number of charges; when they are used up, the weapons themselves simply dissolve into nothingness.

The basics

Bonded weapons come in four distinct classes: Minor Bond 1, Minor Bond 2, Major Bond 1, and Major Bond 2. A Minor Bond 1 weapon expends a charge anytime it scores a hit in battle, even when its special power would be useless or even counterproductive, such as stabbing a shambling mound with a sword made of bonded lightning (which will make the beast grow in power, as per its description in the *Monstrous Compendium*). This also means that even when the special power

works, it might be wasted on weak opponents that don't need that kind of power to kill them, causing the weapon to run out of charges rapidly. A Minor Bond 2 weapon lacks this fault, being magically attuned to its owner (a process that takes 24 uninterrupted hours). It expends charges only when its wielder actively wills it to do so. No more than one charge can ever be expended at a time.

Major Bond weapons 1 and 2 are like their Minor counterparts of the same numbers, but they are powered by permanent dweomers, with no charges to run out. Thus, the only problem with a Major Bond 1 weapon using its power against the wielder's wishes will come if the attack is counterproductive, as in the case of the *lightning sword* used against a shambling mound. Major Bond 2 weapons are the very best, being equivalent to the best "conventional" magical weapons.

Even when its special power is useless or unused during an encounter, the bonded weapon is still a great improvement over mundane weaponry. The material or essence, once bonded together, is held in place by a magical energy field shaped like the weapon the creator desired to make. This field interacts with the magical protection of creatures that cannot be harmed by ordinary weapons, enabling the wielder to hit and harm even monsters unaffected by +4 weapons.

One caveat: All that the weapon's energy field does is to nullify the special protection of supernatural creatures, enabling the wielder to hit them as he would ordi-

nary creatures. It does *not* bestow any attack or damage bonuses beyond what the weapon's special power may inflict. (Strength bonuses on attack and damage rolls still apply, of course.) If a hero is armed with the aforementioned *lightning sword,* and he runs into a gargoyle that has somehow been made immune to lightning, the hero will do only normal sword damage to it. If he meets up with a shambling mound, he should run!

As stated earlier, roughly two-thirds of these already scarce weapons are temporary (Minor bonds), while half of those remaining will not respond to an owner's will. Of all bonded weapons, Minor Bonds 1 and 2 each make up one-third of the total, while Major Bonds 1 and 2 each make up one-sixth. (Roll 1d6: 1-2, Minor Bond 1; 3-4, Minor Bond 2; 5, Major Bond 1; 6, Major Bond 2.) Reducing the number of permanent items helps reduce the dangers of game imbalance, the more so since half of both the Minor and Major Bond weapons will use their powers with every successful hit on an opponent, no matter how inappropriate that power use may be.

A freshly created Minor Bond weapon has 16 charges, which are gone for good (as is the weapon) when they are used up. For a weapon found in a dungeon or the like, roll 2d8 to determine the number of charges remaining. Remember that a weapon owned by an intelligent monster with manipulative organs will almost certainly be used in combat against the adventurers, further reducing the total number of charges or even discharging it, so that the party's prize vanishes before their eyes during the course of the fight.

Bonded weapons are never intelligent and never possess any other characteristics, such as the ability to detect items or communicate with a wielder. They have no alignment and may be used by anyone who picks them up, though severe religious restrictions may apply if a weapon falls into the wrong hands, as noted later.

The special powers of bonded weapons, unless otherwise stated (as in the case of bonded-rust weapons), always work against normal living creatures, although many normal foes may not need this type of power to be used against them. If a weapon's special power duplicates a spell or substance, its effect is no more versatile than that spell or substance. Thus, if Shanara the thief sneaks into a necromancer's lair, her *holy water sword* works perfectly well against the undead monsters guarding the place. If she returns to camp in time to see her partner Reland lovingly carrying a kelpie into the local lake, the short sword inflicts only normal damage because the kelpie, though evil, is not affected by holy water.

The reverse is true, too, of course. Special powers *will* inflict extra damage on creatures particularly vulnerable to that type of attack (see "The weapons"). A *holy water sword* inflicts extra damage on creatures such as the undead, and a bonded weapon of ice greatly harms fire-based beings such as salamanders. The special power descriptions state what, if any, creatures receive extra damage from the special powers, as well as what sort of creatures are immune to them.

Creating bonded weapons

As mentioned earlier, the gods themselves are the only ones who can create bonded weapons. Needless to say, they do not do this all the time, nor is each deity able to create every type listed herein. Aside from keeping the campaign world from being flooded with such weapons, this also means that the weapons that *are* created are quite typical of items in general that the deity in question would create. *Air* weapons are created by deities governing the air or atmosphere. *Fire* weapons are created by gods of heat and flame, *water* weapons by gods of water or the sea, and *earth* weapons by earth-based deities. *Lightning* weapons would be a specialty of gods governing thunderstorms, lightning, or electricity in general, and so on. Gods residing on the various elemental, para-elemental, or quasi-elemental planes can also make bonded weapons of the appropriate type; many weapons using fear are thought to come from the domains of the RAVENLOFT® setting. Other types of bonded weapons besides those detailed here are possible, subject only to the Dungeon Master's research and imagination (see details on the various inner planes in the AD&D 1st Edition *Manual of the Planes* or DRAGON® issue #73, pages 10-13, then consider the details on weapons of magma, steam, vacuum, shadow, and so forth). Those listed here are the most common.

In general, when a deity gives a bonded weapon to a character or temple of that god's faith, it is as a reward for some extremely beneficial service that was performed on behalf of the god's faith. Merely killing a few unbelievers or defiling a temple or two of the opposition won't do the trick; we're talking major quests here. The only exception to this rule would be if that deity or a high priest funding the quest gave a worthy character such a weapon before the quest was begun to ensure the quest was accomplished. This is particularly appropriate for those bonded weapons of a temporary nature; the thing would have just enough charges to defeat the main enemy (thus accomplishing the deity's goals) before vanishing entirely (thus preventing a super-powered character from conquering everything in sight by virtue of his nifty magical weapon). If this is the case, the PC who has been given the weapon might well be expected to safeguard it from all combat until the main goal of the quest has been reached, carefully husbanding the handful of charges until they are *really* needed. When fighting his way through a monster-infested wilderness to reach his goal, or cutting a path through the main foe's minions, the hero could use only mundane weaponry and such magical items as he had gained prior to the quest.

Improper use of a bonded weapon is grounds for serious divine reprisals. This should be spelled out very clearly by the DM in his role-playing of a high priest or deity. If the PC ignores a warning, show no mercy! Letting characters of inappropriate alignment or faith touch, much less use, the weapon is sacrilege, and vengeance might fall on the defiler as well. If a bonded weapon is captured by foes of another alignment or religion, this is reason for yet another quest, to "rescue" the weapon from its captors. The quest would be particularly vital if the weapon was a Major Bond 2 weapon.

Should your party of PCs discover a bonded weapon in a dungeon, don't forget the possibility of the deity or clerics of the appropriate faith sending someone or something after the device once it has resurfaced. This is an especially good plot device if more than one magical item was recovered from the dungeon; the PCs know everyone's after them because of something they took from the dungeon, but which item is causing all the fuss?

The weapons

Remember that in each case below, a bonded weapon does double normal damage against creatures that are especially vulnerable to that attack form or possess innate qualities opposed to that attack form. For example, a white dragon would take double damage from a *fire spear*'s hit. Also, creatures that are invulnerable to the attack form given still take normal damage from the weapon. Thus, a fire elemental still takes normal damage from that *fire spear*. DMs should carefully check the information on each monster encountered and make an appropriate ruling. For instance, an *ice axe* will probably do great harm to salamanders, red dragons, and fire elementals. It is possible for *water* and *holy/unholy water* weapons to doubly harm fire-based beings, too, though only a *holy water* weapon will do extra damage to an undead being.

Air weapons harm any creatures that can be harmed by air-based attacks, including such spells as *gust of wind* or an air elemental's whirlwind attack. They inflict an extra 1-4 hp of wind-burn damage against "normal" foes. Air elementals and vampires in gaseous form, among other monsters, take no extra damage. *Air* weapons seem very light and easy to use.

Earth weapons are effective against any creature vulnerable to earth-based attacks, such as *spike stones*. Normal foes take 1-4 hp scraping damage from each attack, in addition to any normal damage the weapon inflicts. These weapons seem unusually heavy.

Fire weapons do 1-4 extra hp fiery damage to ordinary creatures that can be harmed by fire but are not especially vulnerable to it. Note that though this type of weapon will be warm to the touch, it will not set material alight.

Water weapons inflict double damage on fiery creatures but do only an extra 1-4 hp watery (drowning or watery blast) damage against ordinary foes.

Lightning weapons do double damage against creatures particularly vulnerable to electrical attacks, including any humanoid opponent clad in metal armor. Again, 1-4 hp extra shocking damage is inflicted against mundane foes. The power is useless against electrical beasts such as blue dragons, and downright counterproductive against creatures such as shambling mounds. Holding this type of weapon usually causes the wielder's hair to stand on end from the static electricity around it.

Ice weapons, like *water* weapons, inflict double damage against fiery opponents, and 1-4 hp extra cold damage against most foes. However, their special power is useless against foes immune to cold-based attacks, such as white dragons. This type of weapon is cool to the touch.

Time weapons do no extra physical damage beyond the norm, but they age victims by five years per hit if a save vs. spells is failed. This can be a source of quick victory against most animals, which have relatively short lives, and may also be useful against human and humanoid opponents, but it is of little or no value against long-lived dwarves, elves, and dragons, or ageless golems and undead.

Rust weapons attack the foe's armor and (if parrying is used) weaponry, in addition to the foe himself. Any metallic item struck by this sort of bonded weapon is subjected to the same sort of rusting attack that a rust monster would inflict, or what the AD&D 1st Edition *Oriental Adventures* sixth-level wu jen spell *metal to rust* would accomplish if they fail their save (see the *Monstrous Compendium* entry on rust monsters for details). It thus does extra damage only indirectly against most foes, by depriving them of armor protection, though it can be decisive against iron golems and similar opponents. *Rust* weapons are produced, in general, by deities who have the defense of instantly crumbling any weapon that touches them.

Salt weapons, whenever they hit a foe, throw off a shower of salt grains that can blind the target for 1-4 rounds (assuming the foe has eyes and fails a save vs. spells) and inflict 1-4 extra hp damage due to dehydration, as the weapon absorbs the enemy's bodily fluids. Because of this, it does double damage against watery creatures such as water weirds, as well as semisolid opponents such as oozes, jellies, slimes, and puddings (giant slugs also take double damage). Sea deities produce such bonded weapons.

Ash weapons, created of the leavings around the forges of blacksmith gods or from the quasi-elemental plane of Ash, behave similarly to *salt* weapons in their blinding effects, though ashes are thrown off instead of salt. The foe takes 1-4 extra hp burning damage; since these are ashes instead of flames, there is no doubled damage against opponents specially vulnerable to fire-based attacks. Fire-immune foes take no physical damage, though they are still blinded if they fail a save vs. spells.

Holy/Unholy water weapons are two separate types of weapons, lumped together here because their effects are so similar. Any good or evil deity can make the appropriate weapon out of holy or unholy water. They do double damage against strongly (and innately) evil or good beings such as undead, paladins, devas, baatezu, tanar'ri, or lammasu, as appropriate to the weapon type. They are generally constructed for characters such as paladins or clerics and are not meant for use against humanoids and dragons, doing no extra damage to these plain opponents.

Musk weapons do all the damage that the special attack of a giant skunk would. That is to say, the foe will be blinded for 1-8 hours, losing 50% of his Strength and Dexterity for the next 2-8 turns if the victim fails a save vs. spells, and any cloth item hit by the weapon will rot away. Magical items are allowed a save vs. acid. If the victim survives, the foul stench will still linger until he has thoroughly washed and aired all his gear for several days. Nature deities make these weapons, often for druids (rangers prefer weapons that do not stink and thus give away their positions).

Positive energy weapons, often created by good-aligned gods, do 1-4 hp extra damage due to burns from positive-plane energy, or double damage against evil creatures of darkness, such as undead and shadow dragons, as well as all evil creatures from the Outer Planes. Undead cannot touch these weapons without sustaining the extra damage; even vampires may be permanently destroyed by them. Using such a weapon to attack good-aligned beings from the outer planes or highly good beings such as paladins will cause the

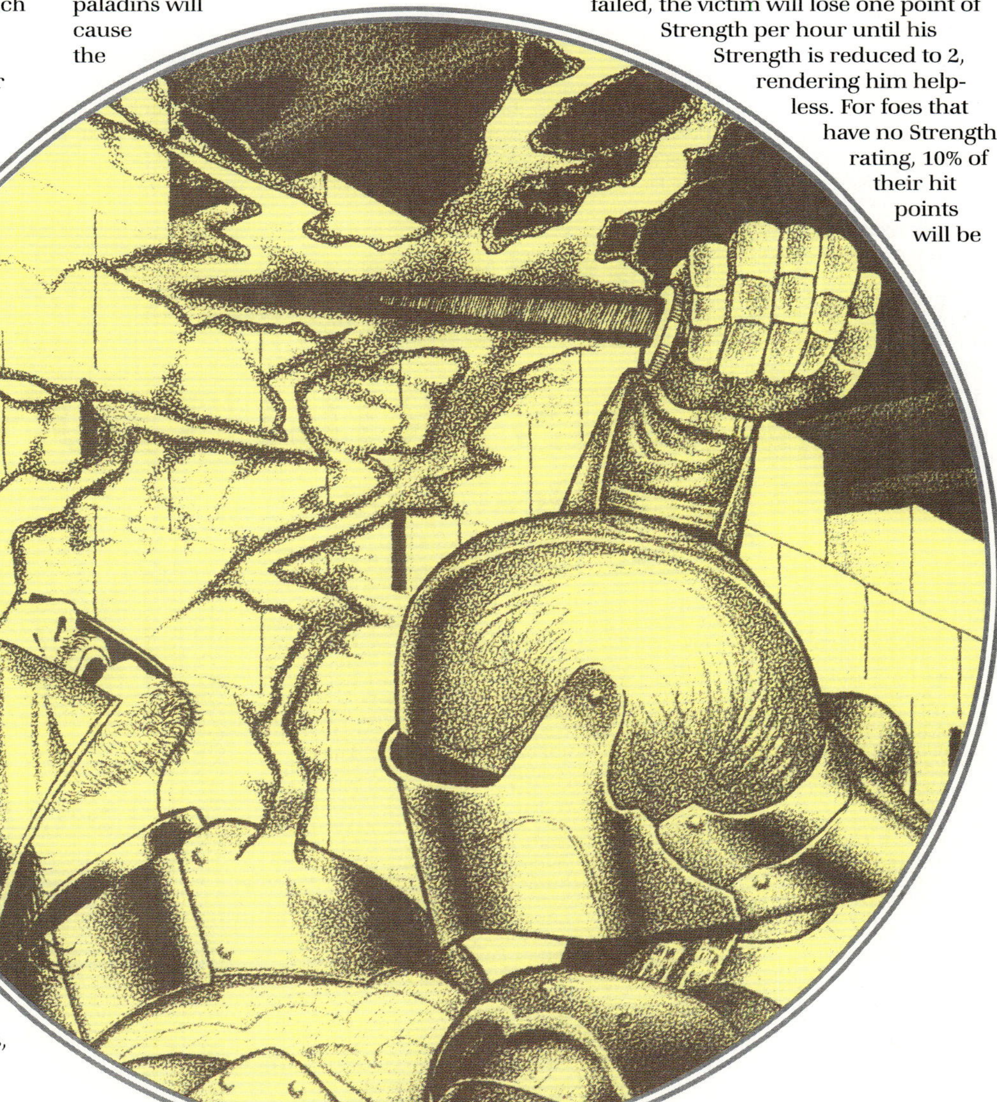

wielder to sustain the burn damage himself; the opponent will take normal weapon damage.

Negative energy weapons, made by death- or evil-oriented deities, drain 1-4 extra hp from the foes they strike, an effect similar to that of the spell *energy drain* or the attack of undead such as spectres (this damage can be healed, however). Humans or humanoids slain by *negative energy* weapons can be animated as juju zombies, but unless the spell-caster is also the one who wielded the killing weapon, they will be free-willed. If a *negative energy* weapon is used against energy-draining undead, the wielder loses 1-4 of his own hit points, as the weapon's dweomer interacts with the "energy vacuum" inside wights, wraiths, etc. A character who uses this weapon against undead can turn himself into an undead monster, even if the monster doesn't fight back!

Disease weapons, created by gods of disease and plague, infect victims as the spell *cause disease* if a save vs. spells is failed. From one to six turns after the save is failed, the victim will lose one point of Strength per hour until his Strength is reduced to 2, rendering him helpless. For foes that have no Strength rating, 10% of their hit points will be drained per "Strength point" loss, down to 10% of their original hit points. Without a *cure disease* spell, full recovery takes 1-3 weeks, assuming the victim survives the battle. Beings immune to disease or able to cure it by their innate powers (such as paladins) are immune to this effect, but not to normal damage.

Slow weapons cause the victim to make all movements (including combat) at one-half normal rates for the next four rounds if a save vs. spells is failed. Repeated blows do not make for a cumulative effect; the effects of the first blow must wear off or be dispelled before the victim can be *slowed* again. Copper dragons, stone golems, and other creatures with an innate *slow* ability are immune to this effect. Speed- and travel-oriented gods favor this sort of weapon.

Wood weapons, favored by forest deities, let off a shower of wooden splinters every time they strike a foe, doing 1-4 extra hp damage to any creature that can be harmed by normal weapons.

Bone weapons, built by gods of death, act the same as *wood* weapons, but the tougher bone splinters do 1-6 extra hp damage.

Fear weapons induce magical *fear* in foes for the first four rounds after being struck, unless they save vs. spells. Undead and other *fear*-immune enemies are not affected. Gods of terror (and the Dark Powers of the RAVENLOFT setting) are thought to make these items.

Sleep weapons, made by sleep- and dream-oriented gods, cause victims to instantly fall asleep for four rounds unless they make successful saves vs. spells. Undead, golems, and similar unsleeping monsters are not affected.

Paralyzation weapons paralyze victims for four rounds after a blow is struck, unless a successful saving throw vs. paralysis is made (the effects are noncumulative). Undead and similar beings, as well as any creatures with an innate power of *paralyzation,* are not affected. Violence-hating and speed-oriented deities prefer such weapons as these.

Silence weapons affect those they hit as though the priest spell *silence, 15' radius* were cast on them, although only the struck enemy will be silenced. The foe cannot call for help or cast any spells requiring verbal components, and monsters such as harpies, androsphinxes, and dragonnes cannot use their special attacks. Music-loving gods make these weapons.

Pain weapons, crafted by pain-loving deities, affect the victim as per the *Oriental Adventures* sixth-level wu jen spell *pain.* A fantastic pain is felt upon being struck, which passes swiftly. However, for the next four rounds, the foe's Strength and Dexterity will be reduced to 3, making him −3 on attack rolls, −1 on damage, −3 on reaction attacking adjustments, and −4 on defensive adjustments if a save vs. spells is failed.

Magnetism weapons are unusual in that they *do* provide an attack bonus, but nothing else. Against metallic opponents such as iron golems, as well as human or humanoid foes in metallic armor (even as little as that in studded leather armor), the weapon is +3 on attack rolls though it does normal damage. The wielder also gains a +3 bonus in any attempt to parry metallic weapons. Metalsmithing gods are the main producers of weapons of *magnetism* weapons.

Radiance weapons (also called *light* weapons) are produced by light- or sun-related gods. They give off a flash of light that effectively blinds enemies they strike for 1-4 rounds if the target fails a save vs. spells. No extra physical damage is inflicted beyond the norm. Only the struck foe is blinded; even nearby enemies are not affected. Eyeless or blind enemies are immune to this power. Furthermore, these weapons do double damage against evil creatures from the plane of Shadow, as well as any darkness-related evil beings such as the undead shadows and shadow dragons. Undead who are vulnerable to sunlight, such as vampires, also take double damage and may be permanently slain by these weapons.   Ω

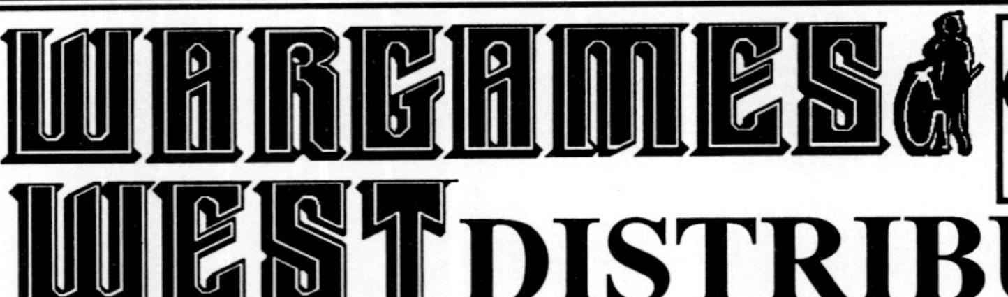
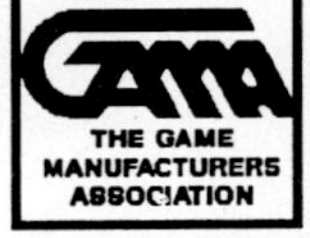
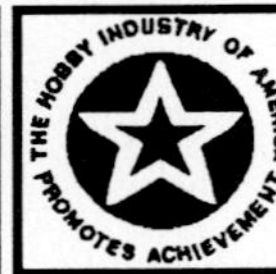
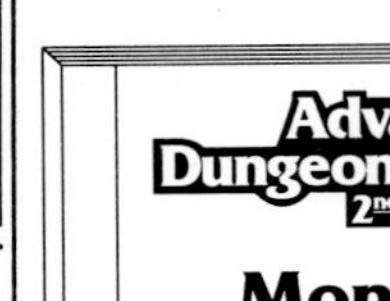
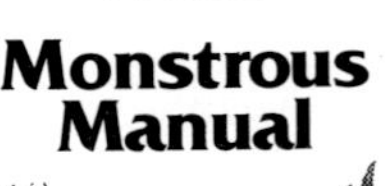
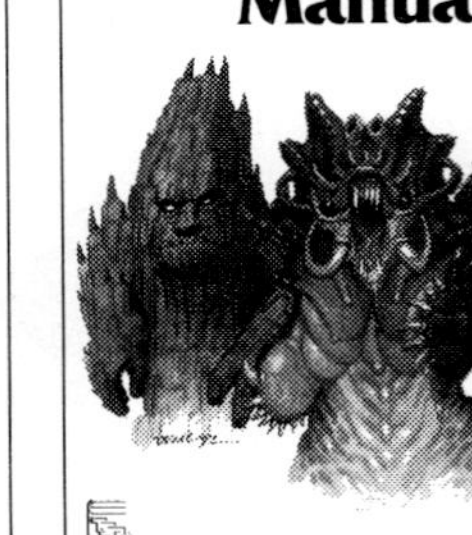

® designate trademarks owned by TSR, Inc.

I am Jodar...

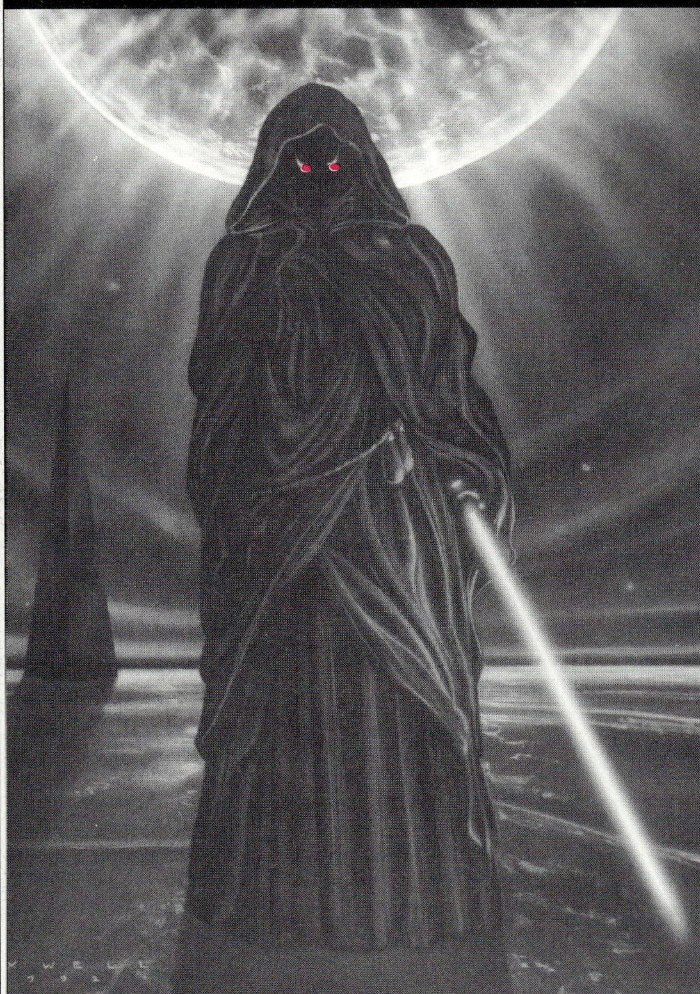

...an alien from a distant, besieged reality. I have returned to this reality by the power of The Sorce, seeking those few who dream to fight for truth, freedom and justice. I call upon the bravest and strongest to embark upon a quest to save my universe. I can provide few rewards, but I can reveal the secrets of Scaping™, and unlock the ultimate power within!

The keystone is delivered through the portal. Go beyond imagination.

As I speak, the MetaScape™, game system is being distributed throughout this world. It contains all the tools necessary to tap into the power of Scaping, open a portal between realities and begin the battle to save my universe.

Now I must return to my own domain... and wait... and hope that the brave and strong will come and aid me on this ultimate quest!

The MetaScape™ Game:

A new and innovative roleplaying system, featuring:
* Unique die mechanics - any outcome from a single roll;
* A fast, flexible system designed for ease of play;
* The new 16-sided die, never seen in any other system;
* Full rules for miniature play;
* The first 1,000 games numbered for collectibility;
* An international ranking system, with membership benefits.

The Guild Space™ Setting:

An exciting science fiction setting, featuring:
* Six powerful player-character races;
* An exciting setting, developed over years of playtesting;
* Dozens of skills, weapons, and equipment items;
* The secrets of super-technology, cybernetics and biotech;
* Mysterious powers: psionics, psychosomatics, and The Sorce;
* *The adventure: Shakna — Assault on the Hive*;
* Six highly detailed metal miniatures;
* Aliens, NPCs, starships, vehicles, and a galaxy of adventure!

Order Today! Call 1-800-880-8880

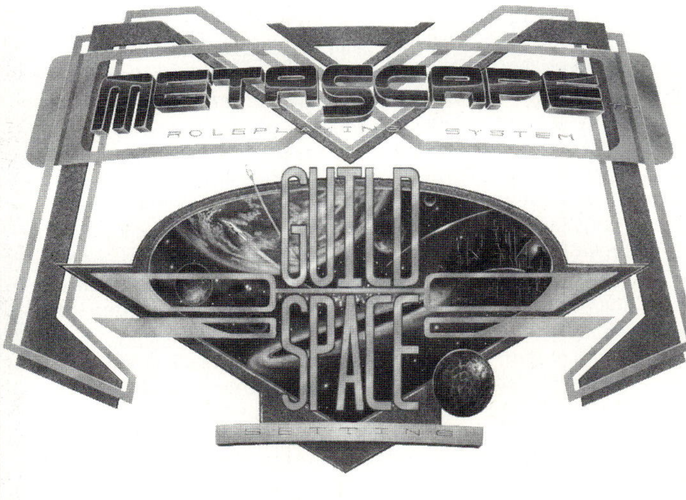

YES! I want a copy of the MetaScape™ roleplaying system!
Price: $29.95 + $3.50 shipping. (Shipping is **FREE** during June, '93.)

(Please Print)

Name:______________________________________

Address:____________________________________

City/ST/Zip:________________________________

Phone: (_____)______________________________

Form of Payment (check one):

❑ Check (Make payable to The Game Lords, Ltd.):

❑ Visa/MC/Discover/AMEX

ACCT.#:_____________________________________

EXP. Date:____/____ Signature_______________

The Game Lords   1-800-880-8880 (Orders only)
P.O.Box PP   1-303-878-4042 (FAX orders)
Meeker, Co 81641   1-303-878-4048 (Questions)

Collaborators: an interview with Michael and Teri Williams

by Will Larson

DRAGON® Magazine wishes to thank Carla Vaananen of Louisville, Kentucky, for her interview and indispensable help in the preparation of this article.

The reasons why authors collaborate are nearly as many as the collaborations themselves. A skilled ghostwriter helps a celebrity tell his or her story. A commercially successful author lends his name (for a fee, of course) to a project largely handled by a relative unknown in an effort to boost sales. A writer simply has too many projects in the fire, and a second author is sought to insure adherence to the schedule. Two writers with considerably different strengths are paired together in an effort to showcase both of them at their best. One author is a terrific idea person, while the other has strong writing skills. And—let's be perfectly honest here—every once in a while, a writer simply screws up and needs to be bailed out.

From an editor's perspective, one can hardly help but be curious about which contributor created what. There are no physical clues in the neatly numbered and labeled pages of the manuscript as to authorship. The clues are more subtle and generally stylistic in nature, but they are inevitably there for an editor familiar with the work of the authors in question.

Thus, when a highly stylized writer with several impressive efforts to his credit announces that his latest effort is a collaboration, the collaborator is none other than his wife, and the resulting collaboration proves to be absolutely seamless, with no hint whatsoever of where one left off and the other took over—that, my friends, makes an editor sit up and take notice.

Michael and Teri Williams's *Before the Mask*, the first volume in the DRAGONLANCE® Villains series, is the book that caught this editor's attention for the aforementioned reasons, and a dandy book it is. It tells the tale of how Verminaard, the notoriously villainous Dragon Highlord of DRAGONLANCE Chronicles and Legends fame, became so despicable. The book came out just this April.

To discover how Teri and Michael came to work so flawlessly and apparently

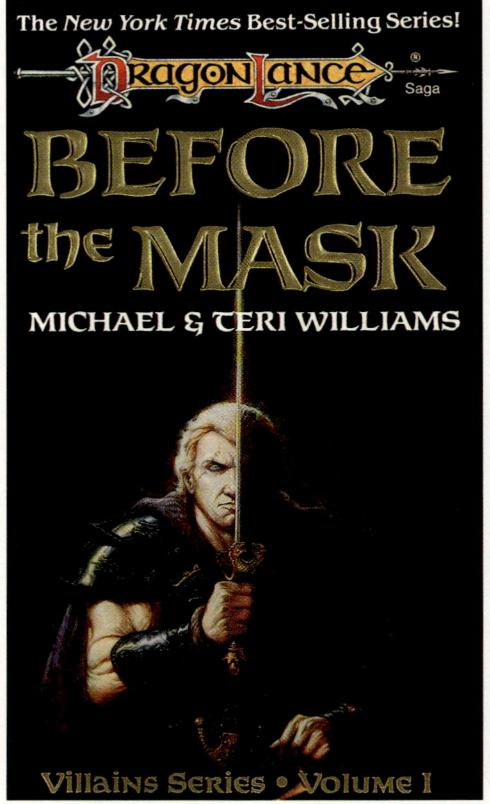

effortlessly together, we (the TSR Book department and DRAGON Magazine) decided to interview them.

In one way or another, Michael and Teri Williams have been partners for years. Almost six years of marriage have led them through all sorts of collaboration: teaching together at the University of Louisville, raising dachshunds and daylilies, and running Teri's busy pottery studio in the Louisville suburbs. Recently the couple joined their talents in writing fantasy fiction with a story, "Mark of the Flame, Mark of the Word," in 1992's *DRAGONLANCE Tales: The Cataclysm*. Then came their novel, *Before the Mask*.

Opposites often attract in romance and marriage, but rarely make for a successful writing partnership. Michael and Teri abound in differences. He's a big-city boy, and she's from a wide place along a Florida road. She wears bright colors, likes Jimmy Buffett, and never knows or cares what time it is. He prefers tan, Russ-

ian Orthodox chants, and gets himself and Teri where they should be—way before it's time. He orders char-broiled steak and french fries. She eats half a salad and saves the rest for later. Somehow, somewhere between the salad and the steak, between purple and khaki, between Margaritaville and Moscow, the partnership thrives.

At their dachshund-infested house in Louisville, Kentucky, Michael and Teri talked with our interviewer about how they make their collaboration work.

TSR: What method do you take to collaborate? Do you sit down and write together as you talk through the ideas, or do you each write a part, then exchange them for the other to read? And how do you decide who gets what part?

Teri: We both invent the characters, unless we're working on something like DRAGONLANCE [stories], where some of the characters are already created. In all cases, we work from plot outlines, which we put together over long walks and conversations. Once we have an outline talked through, Michael generally writes the first draft, scene by scene and chapter by chapter. Then I take the hard copy and make additions, cuts, and revisions, generally late at night when Michael and the dachshunds are asleep. Most of my writing is done in longhand, on the backs and margins of pages. The manuscript passes back and forth between us several times—in the case of one short story, sixteen times! In later drafts, I try to eliminate any narrative confusions and check for things like chronology, plausibility, and small character consistencies—so that everyone's eye color and name spelling stays the same. But the work decides what is needed, and who does what. It's never really a case of the same person always focusing on the same aspect. We talk it over and see who has the best idea for every particular part of the story.

Michael: Usually I knock down the first draft, as Teri said, after a lot of consultation over what goes on. I do it early in the morning, before sunrise, because there's something right about working in the dark hours as you wander into the dark of a blank page. Teri and the dachshunds are usually still asleep at this time—as you can see, the dachshunds have the easy part in the process. Then the text passes between us, taking shape and rhythm and direction, kind of as I imagine improvisation would be in a jazz piece. When the story's path is still dark ahead of you, outlines and character sketches are a good point of departure, but they can guide you only so far. Then you proceed on instinct and on the unique pressures that rise up in the story as it begins to tell itself. Generally both of us work on every part of the book, but sometimes, after we've agreed on a particular idea for a scene, the responsibility for working on it falls to the one of us who really wants the scene more. It's as simple as that: Enthusiasm in the writing makes for a good read.

TSR: What do you do when you hit a disagreement over characterization or plot? And how do you handle it if one of you wants to put something in the story that the other person really doesn't like? Is it hard to get to a point in collaborating where you don't fear being honest about something you don't like?

Teri: When we come across disagreement, each of us makes a case for how we think the story should go, then we come to a consensus. It's not hard to be honest. It's not about us, or primarily *for* us. It's about a story and a reader, and we have to get out of the way. If you keep that in mind, the really weak or inappropriate things become surprisingly obvious. Something that one of us wouldn't like gets stopped long before the manuscript gets to a final stage. Occasionally one of us might get attached to a detail—maybe even one word—that we think the story may turn on, and we tend to get more particular about things like that as we get closer to the final stage. Hemingway calls it the "*mot juste*," the precise word. Early on, we try not to get attached to particulars, but once we've agreed on everything, we don't like for it to be changed. We work to balance idea, story, and style, and last-minute tinkering often destroys that balance.

Michael: When we disagree, I usually buckle under to Teri. But seriously, folks, we always talk out the disagreements and follow the direction of whoever provides the most convincing argument. Although we're very different from one another, we've spent a good deal of time writing, and simple experience and technique tell when a scene, a plot turn, or a bit of dialogue just won't work. So the disagreements are relatively minor and easy to resolve. Each of us trusts how hard the other presses a point, and each of us listens especially closely if the scene is more important to our partner than it is to us. Disagreements are usually no more than detail, but even something as apparently minor as a word choice can be momentous at times. We work very hard to make all parts of the story connect and resonate, and that means we have to be honest to the story and to each other. If you

aren't honest, the story shows it. I'm honest with my suggestions to Teri as well, but she takes criticism marvelously. I admit my ego gets in the way at times, but for the most part, I take criticism well—at least from her.

TSR: What do you do when one of you is inspired to write, but not the other?

Teri: Generally I find my great ideas late in the day and want to discuss them *right then*. Michael's more of a morning person. We have learned to talk about work in the middle of the day, when both of us are awake enough. Michael is great at applying intuition to the direction of the story when he's working past the point we've outlined. I enjoy discovering where he's taken it, and most of the time, it's the same place I would have gone, too.

Michael: We have a little time friction here. Teri's late hours and my early ones mean that she's bleary if I want to talk early, and that I'm nodding off if she wants to start an hour-long discussion just a little before midnight. As she said, midday is the best discussion time. If the ideas we come up with in the wee hours—late or early—are any good, they'll hold until noon when both of us are clear-eyed and awake.

TSR: Do you feel any lack of individual identity because of collaborating?

Teri: No. I'm not defined by my work. I would have an identity if I wrote with twelve people, or if I didn't write another word.

Michael: I don't feel a lack there, either. Collaborating is a different process than writing individually. And in fact, Teri's had a part in my work increasingly since *Galen Beknighted*, so much of late that in the new book, *Before the Mask*, we've acknowledged what I think has been the case for a while now—that she is indeed coauthor. I still have individual irons in the fire, but remember that even the "individual" work a reader takes off a shelf is the product of many collaborators. It's not only the writer's judgment and insight, but that of the friends who first read the manuscript, of the editors and copy editors, and of the artists, whose illustrations give a shade and feel to the world of the book. Still, there's a peculiarly solitary pleasure in the single-author book for me. My natural tendency is that I write to learn, and there are lots of things you need to learn on your own. I wouldn't want to give up either individual or collaborative work, since both satisfy me in different ways.

TSR: Do you feel it's easier to come up with ideas or inspirations with another person, or do you ever feel that you have to compromise a lot in order to collaborate?

Teri: Compromise? You grow, building on one another's ideas. It's like being at an idea bazaar with thousands and thousands of available choices that haven't come from your own experience. And you don't have to use them all at once; many

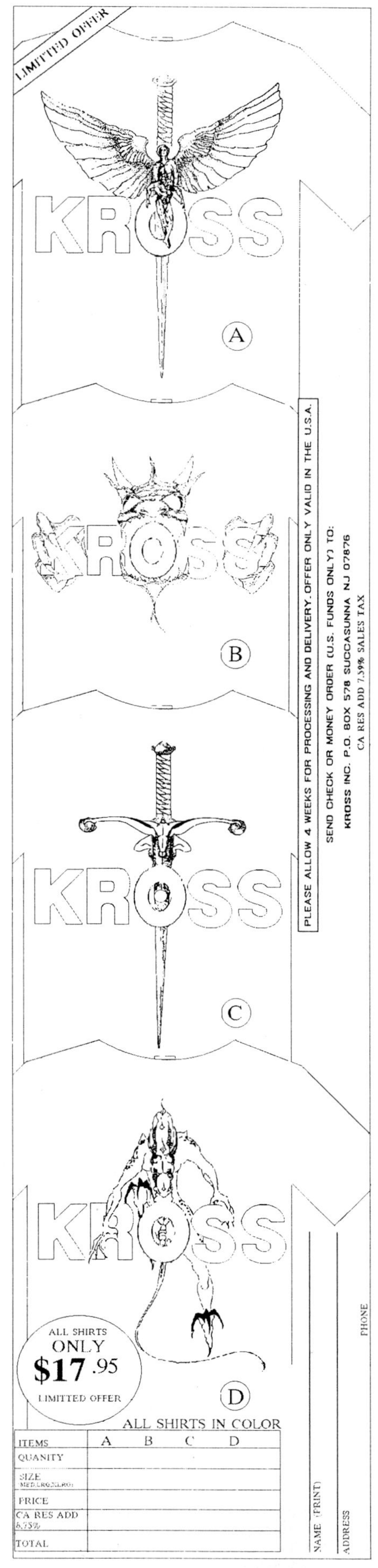

ITEMS	A	B	C	D
QUANITY				
SIZE (MED, LRG, XLRG)				
PRICE				
CA RES ADD 6.75%				
TOTAL				

of them will wait for your next book and the one after that.

Michael: You probably get more ideas in collaboration, because something is always happening in the exchange. Collaboration is strangely competitive, as though you try to top one another in a way. If you've ever seen a basketball team with two superb athletes—the Chicago Bulls, say, with Scottie Pippen and Michael Jordan—you know that in the game, those guys play for the good of the team, but they're inspired to outdo one another in the process. I think that kind of striving makes for better work.

TSR: As collaborators who live together, what do you do to separate work from time off? How do you deal with stress together as the deadline looms?

Teri: First of all, it's not a "deadline" to us. We call it a "due date," because reference words are important as well, and "due date" is more peaceful and less ominous. We look at how long we have to complete something, then we arrange the tasks to get it done on time. It's really a matter of considering the work, not the stress and worry. At any point in the project, our schedule is roughly the same: We discuss ideas and editing six days a week, but we rest and renew on Sundays. Basically we keep a traditional Sabbath. Every work idea I've ever had on a Sunday showed great promise and no delivery.

Michael: There are also some boundaries during the other days. I have to be vocal and say, "It's too late to discuss that. I'm shutting down for the night." When we go out, we often insist on "no book talk." I handle stress by working constantly and gradually, so that there isn't a blinding, breakneck rush in the last weeks before a due date; even so, the last week is almost nonstop work. I tend to worry more than Teri, and I'm probably more difficult to live with when the stress begins to build up.

TSR: Now that you've been collaborating, would it be hard to say "I want to do this one on my own"?

Teri: I have always approached writing in a collaborative way. I even teach it that way. Michael will always be my first reader, and even if only my name is on the cover, he will be a large part of the creation of the work. But I don't think I would ever need to say, "I want to do it on my own." However, if Michael had no time for a project that I wanted to do, I would just forge ahead.

Michael: No, I wouldn't have a problem saying that. I still want to do individual work. There's a certain sense of daring and exploration on a solo flight.

TSR: Why do you think your collaboration works so well?

Teri: Actually, given our differences, I see no reason it *should* work well. I truly believe that only grace helps us communicate so well.

Michael: I think Teri's answer to that is excellent.

The dachshunds were loudly proclaiming their opinion that suppertime was long since due, and with considerable reluctance, we took our leave of the Williamses, the dachshunds, and Louisville, Ky., with fervent wishes that their writing partnership continues to flourish.

Two months from now in this same space, watch for Jim Lowder's enlightening explanation of the intricacies of the FORGOTTEN REALMS™ time line. In the meantime, check out Michael and Teri's *Before the Mask*. You'll be glad you did! Ω

What's *your* opinion?

What is the future direction of role-playing games? What problems do you have with your role-playing campaign? Turn to this issue's "Forum" and see what others think—then tell us what *you* think!

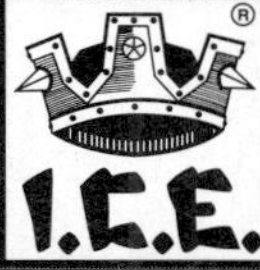

NEW FOR CHAMPIONS

DARK CHAMPIONS™
HEROES OF VENGEANCE

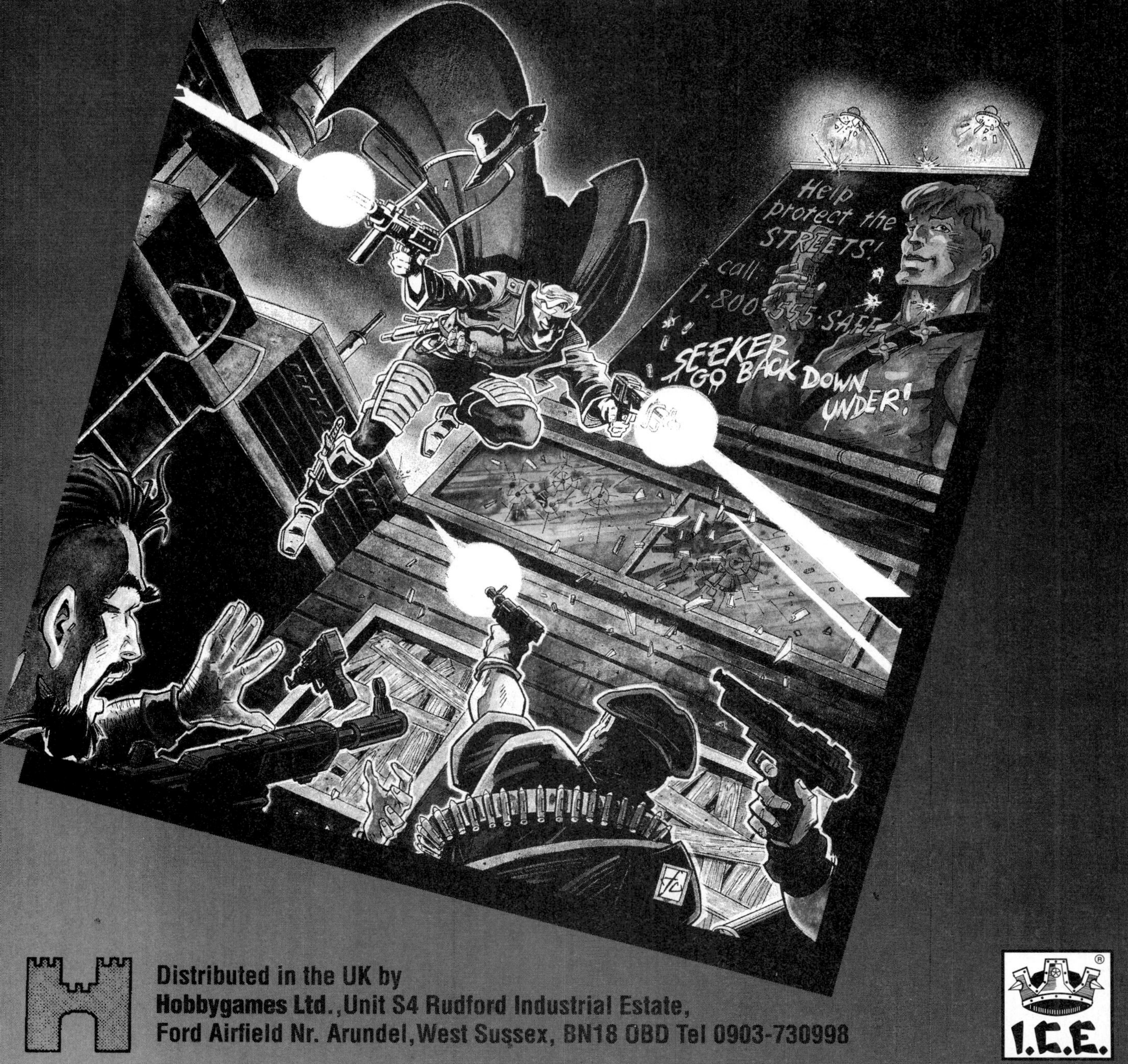

DRAGONMIRTH

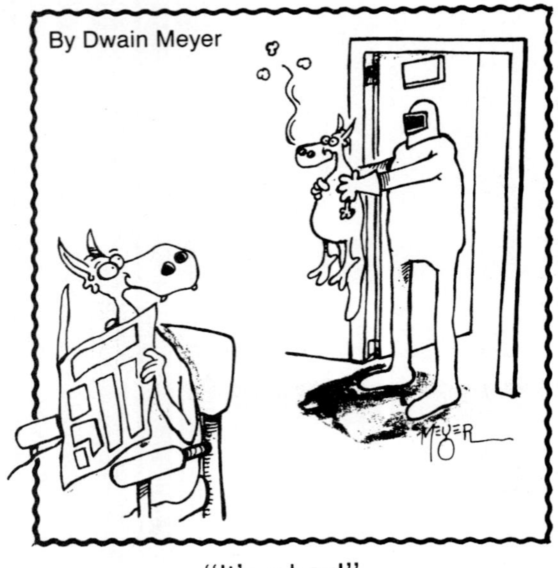

By Dwain Meyer

"It's a boy!"

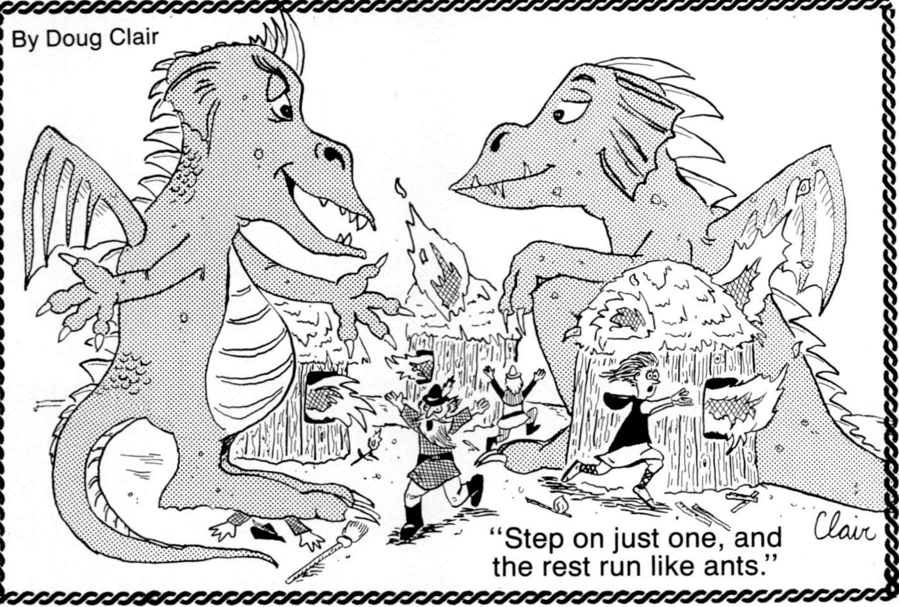

By Doug Clair

"Step on just one, and the rest run like ants."

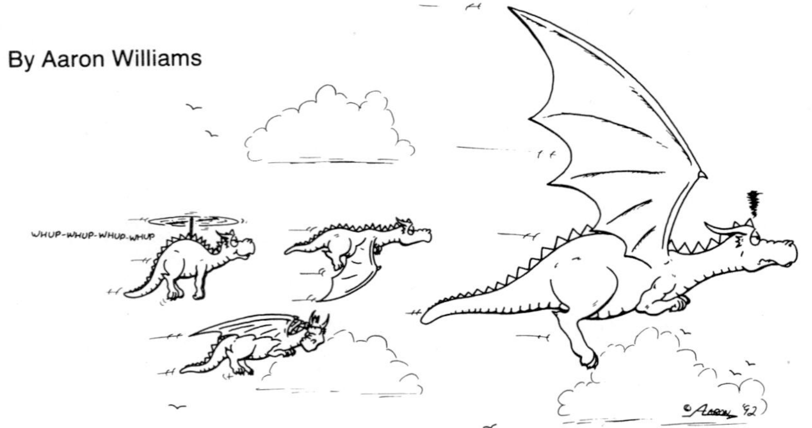

By Aaron Williams

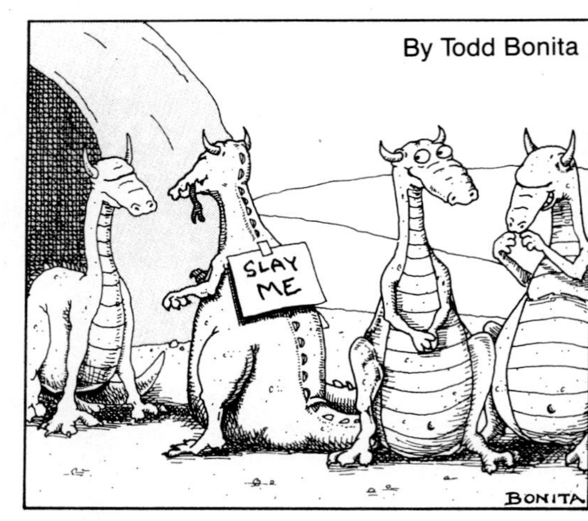

By Todd Bonita

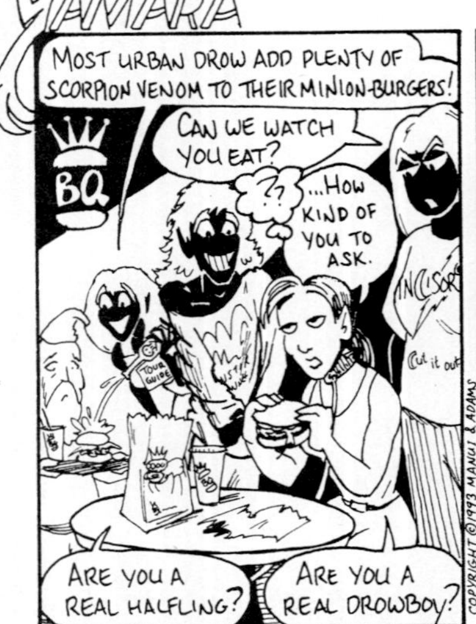

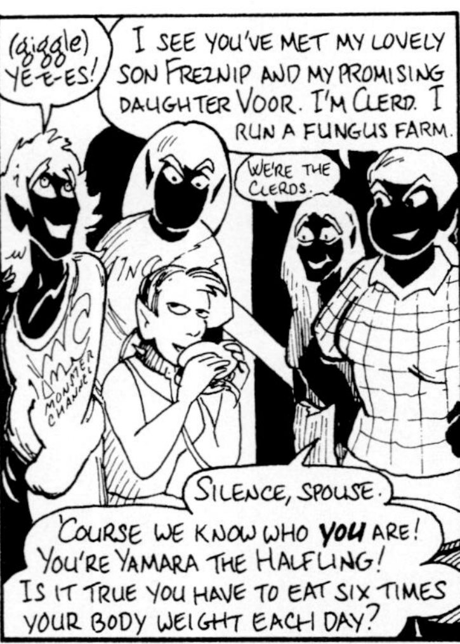

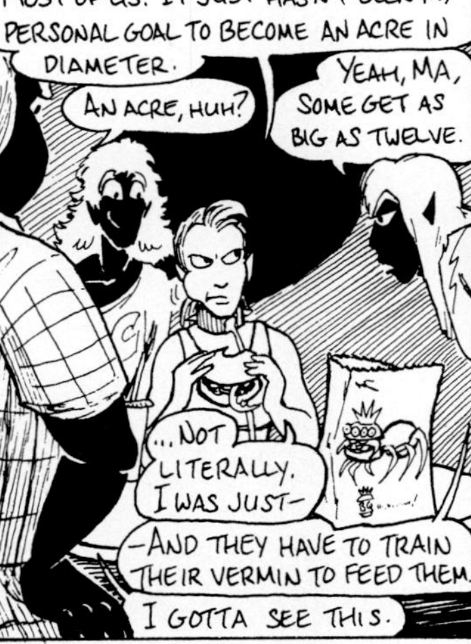

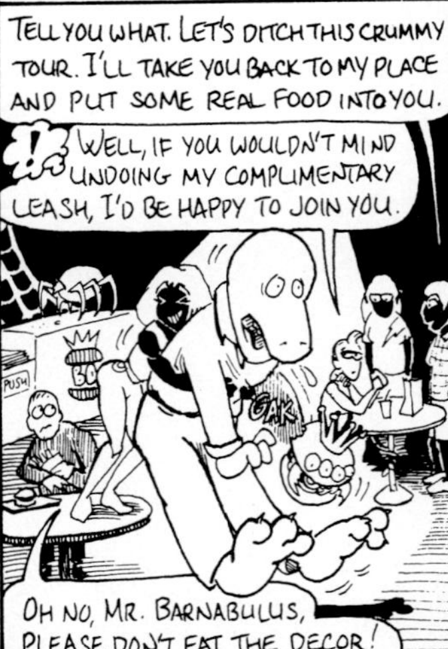

By Barbara Manui and Chris Adams

By Jim Martin, Jr.

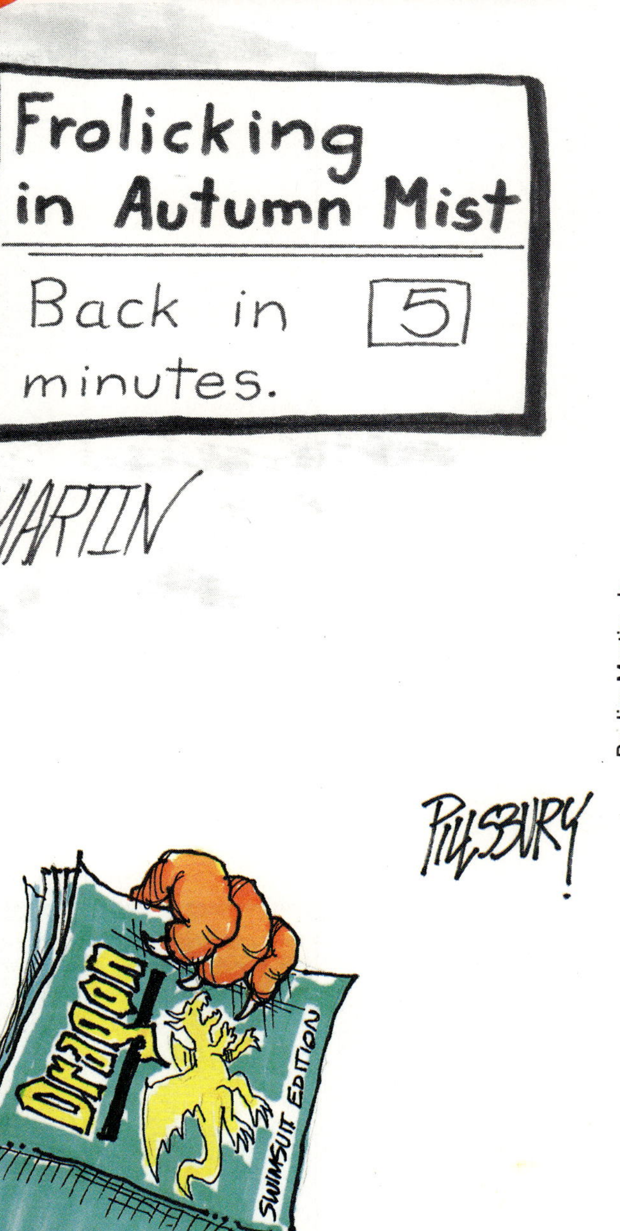

By Joseph Pillsbury

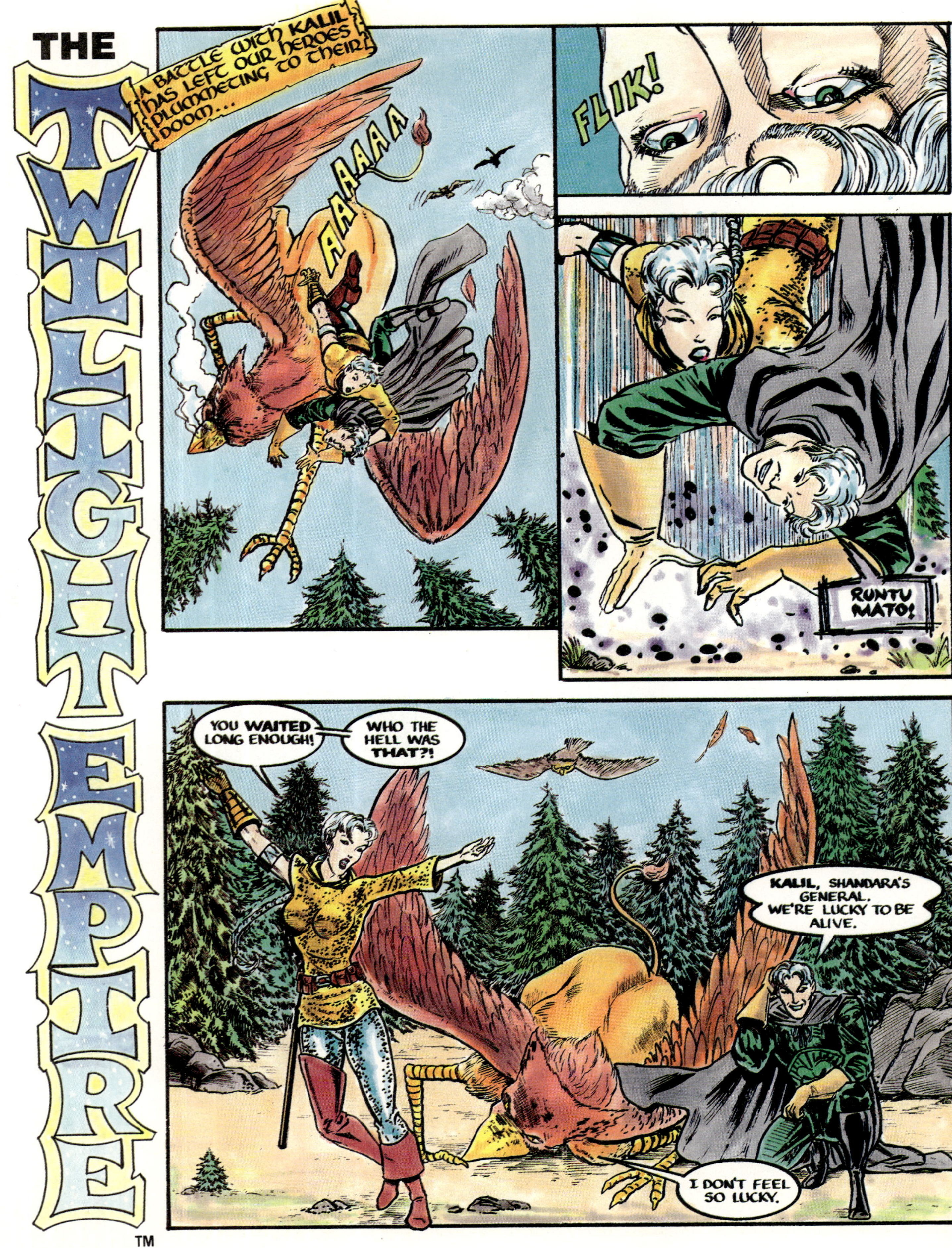
THE TWILIGHT EMPIRE
™
A BATTLE WITH KALIL HAS LEFT OUR HEROES PLUMMETING TO THEIR DOOM...
AAAAAA
FLIK!
RUNTU MATO!
YOU WAITED LONG ENOUGH!
WHO THE HELL WAS THAT?!
KALIL, SHANDARA'S GENERAL. WE'RE LUCKY TO BE ALIVE.
I DON'T FEEL SO LUCKY.

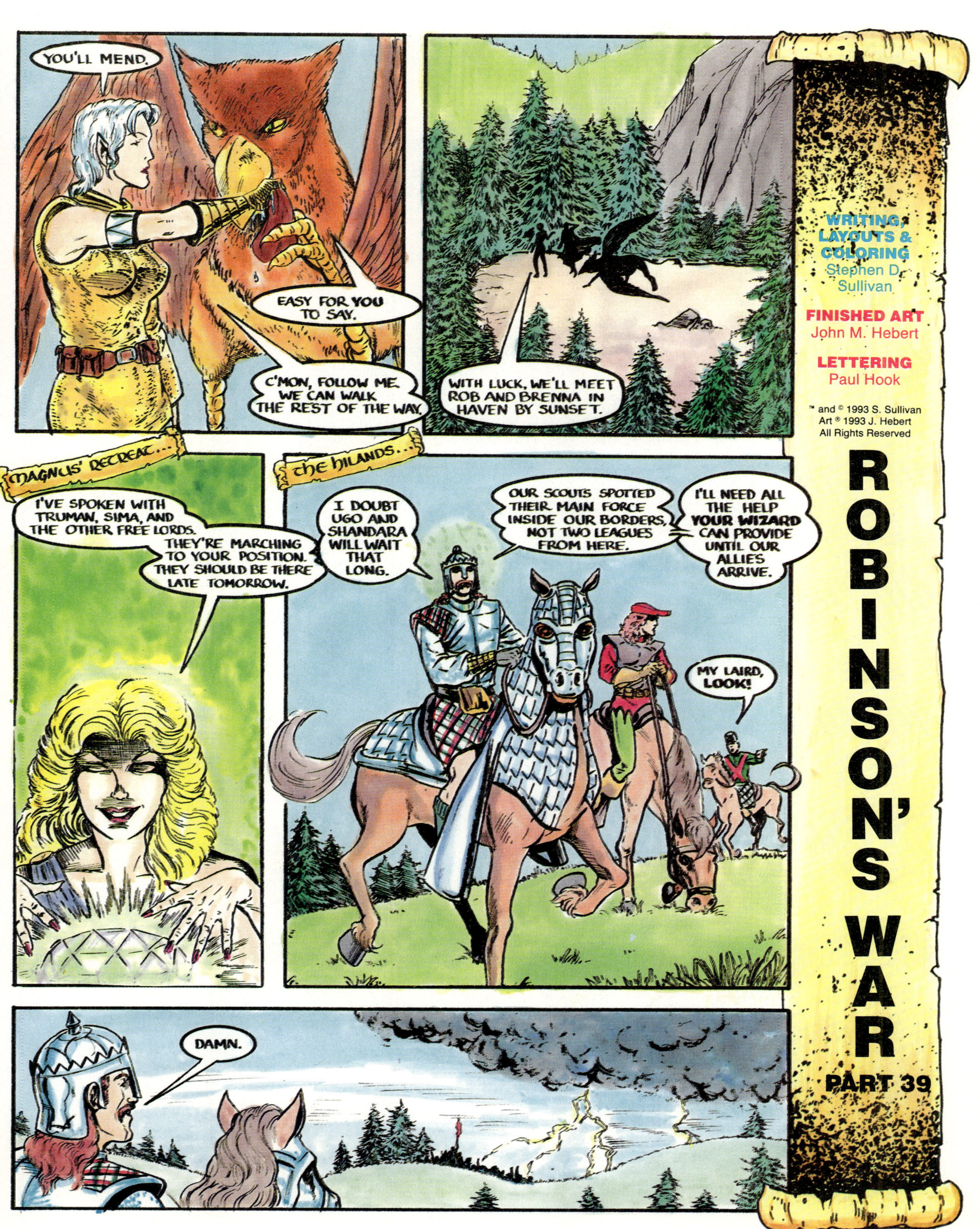

YOU'LL MEND.
EASY FOR YOU TO SAY.
C'MON, FOLLOW ME. WE CAN WALK THE REST OF THE WAY.
WITH LUCK, WE'LL MEET ROB AND BRENNA IN HAVEN BY SUNSET.
MAGNUS' RETREAT...
THE HILANDS...
I'VE SPOKEN WITH TRUMAN, SIMA, AND THE OTHER FREE LORDS. THEY'RE MARCHING TO YOUR POSITION. THEY SHOULD BE THERE LATE TOMORROW.
I DOUBT UGO AND SHANDARA WILL WAIT THAT LONG.
OUR SCOUTS SPOTTED THEIR MAIN FORCE INSIDE OUR BORDERS, NOT TWO LEAGUES FROM HERE.
I'LL NEED ALL THE HELP YOUR WIZARD CAN PROVIDE UNTIL OUR ALLIES ARRIVE.
MY LAIRD, LOOK!
DAMN.
WRITING, LAYOUTS & COLORING
Stephen D. Sullivan
FINISHED ART
John M. Hebert
LETTERING
Paul Hook
™ and © 1993 S. Sullivan
Art ® 1993 J. Hebert
All Rights Reserved
ROBINSON'S WAR
PART 39

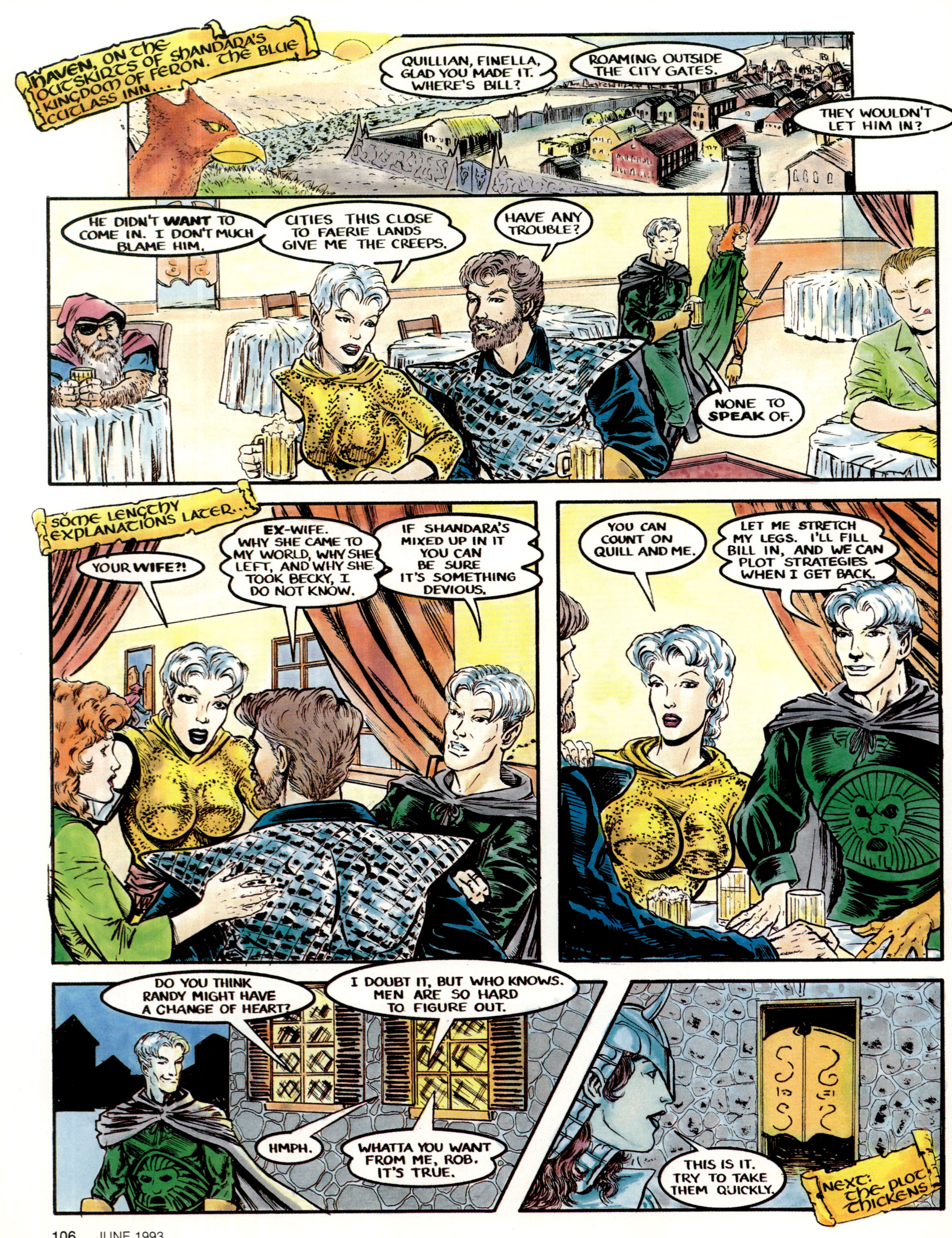

HAVEN, ON THE OUTSKIRTS OF SHANDARA'S KINGDOM OF FERON. THE BLUE CUTLASS INN...
QUILLIAN, FINELLA, GLAD YOU MADE IT. WHERE'S BILL?
ROAMING OUTSIDE THE CITY GATES.
THEY WOULDN'T LET HIM IN?
HE DIDN'T WANT TO COME IN. I DON'T MUCH BLAME HIM.
CITIES THIS CLOSE TO FAERIE LANDS GIVE ME THE CREEPS.
HAVE ANY TROUBLE?
NONE TO SPEAK OF.
SOME LENGTHY EXPLANATIONS LATER...
YOUR WIFE?!
EX-WIFE. WHY SHE CAME TO MY WORLD, WHY SHE LEFT, AND WHY SHE TOOK BECKY, I DO NOT KNOW.
IF SHANDARA'S MIXED UP IN IT YOU CAN BE SURE IT'S SOMETHING DEVIOUS.
YOU CAN COUNT ON QUILL AND ME.
LET ME STRETCH MY LEGS. I'LL FILL BILL IN, AND WE CAN PLOT STRATEGIES WHEN I GET BACK.
DO YOU THINK RANDY MIGHT HAVE A CHANGE OF HEART?
I DOUBT IT, BUT WHO KNOWS. MEN ARE SO HARD TO FIGURE OUT.
HMPH.
WHATTA YOU WANT FROM ME, ROB. IT'S TRUE.
THIS IS IT. TRY TO TAKE THEM QUICKLY.
NEXT: THE PLOT THICKENS

The Rifts® Megaverse®

Rifts World Book Three: England™

Rifts England is a sourcebook packed with idea after idea: new occupational character classes, mystical beings, strange races, monsters, herbs, plants, philosophies of magic and new magic powers.

England is a place of magic and magic creatures. It seethes with mystic energy from hundreds of ley lines and nexus points, transforming the British Isles into a land of enchantment. An alien environment that attracts a host of creatures and characters unlike any place else in the world!

Highlights include:

- **The return of Erin Tarn.**
- **21 New O.C.C.s/R.C.C.s, including the super-human Earth and Star Child, Chiang-Ku Dragon, temporal wizard, Nexus Knight, herbalist, druids, sectles, and many others.**
- **Temporal magic, including 25 unique new spells.**
- **Herb magic with its many magic teas, potions, wands, staves, leaves, sprigs, poisons and more!**
- **The majestic and magical 1000 foot tall Millennium Tree and its Millennium Druid O.C.C.**
- **Monsters like the Fomorians, Cernun serpent men, flash beetles, cobra vine, brain tree, ghost knights, alien intelligences, Celtic gods & supernatural menaces.**
- **New Camelot, with lots of surprises!**
- **Places of magic and other locales mapped and described.**
- **Written by Kevin Siembieda.**
- **Illustrated by Long, Ewell, Breaux, and Siembieda**
- **Cover by Parkinson.**
- **152 pages — $15.95 plus $1.50 for postage and handling.**
- **In stores everywhere right now!!!**

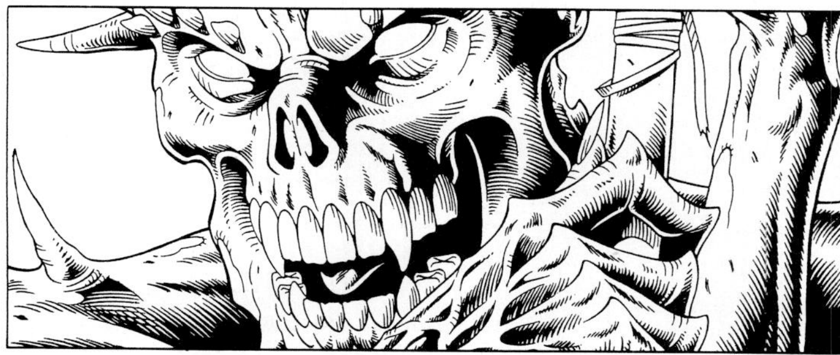

Rifts World Book Four: Africa™
The Four Horsemen of the Apocalypse

The Four Horsemen of the Apocalypse are unbelievably powerful supernatural forces bent on the destruction of the Earth. Once all life has been obliterated on Earth, they will use its thousands of dimensional rifts to carry their destruction throughout the Megaverse!

If they are going to be stopped, it must be now! The four were separated when they rifted to Earth. They seek to find each other, unite and become one unstoppable force. If they can be defeated one at a time, the Earth and the entire Megaverse may be spared. Failure means almost certain oblivion.

Highlights Include:

- **Four of the most unique and powerful monsters ever presented by Palladium! But that's not all!!**
- **The Phoenix Empire (Egypt), the enslaver of humans, inhabited by monsters and ruled by the Lord of Death, Pharaoh Rama-Set, an evil Chiang-ku dragon.**
- **The return of Egyptian Gods and their minions, but are these gods on the side of mankind or do they work toward its destruction?**
- **The gathering of heroes (including some surprises).**
- **Mind Bleeder R.C.C. (finally, and you won't be disappointed).**
- **The Necromancer O.C.C. and his dark, deadly magic.**
- **Additional O.C.C.s, villains, adventure and more.**
- **Written by Kevin Siembieda**
- **Cover and interior art by Kevin Long. Additional art by Siembieda and Ewell.**
- **152 pages — $15.95 plus $1.50 for postage and handling.**
- **Available Now!**

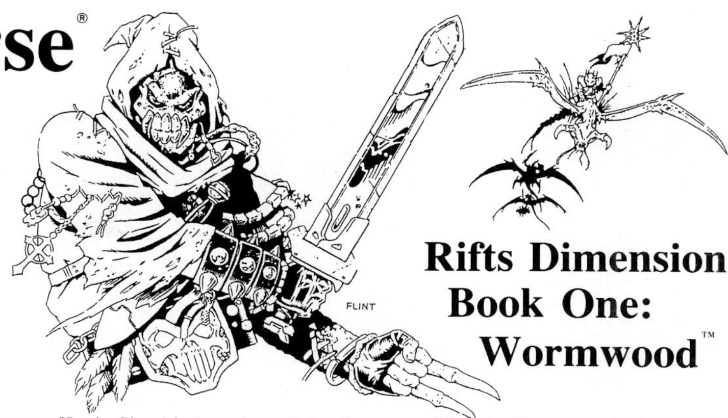

Rifts Dimension Book One: Wormwood™

Kevin Siembieda and comic book creators *Timothy Truman* and *Flint Henry* join forces to take **Rifts** fans into the fantastic alien world of **Wormwood**. A filthy, decadent, violent and deadly environment ruled by maniacal dictators and clergy who control powerful cults. These political powers are so blatantly manipulative and consumed with the acquisition of power that the Coalition States pale by comparison!

Wormwood is the first of many dimension books to be presented by Palladium; alien worlds linked to **Rifts Earth** by the many dimension spanning ley line nexus junctions.

Highlights Include:

- **A brand new 20 page comic strip by Truman & Henry!**
- **New Occupational Character Classes and heroes.**
- **Many new and horrific monsters, villains, and characters.**
- **Magic weapons, technology and dark secrets.**
- **The world mapped and key places described.**
- **Written by Siembieda. Based on concepts and characters created by Timothy Truman and Flint Henry. Additional text by Truman.**
- **Art by Truman, Henry, Long and Siembieda.**
- **152 pages; $15.95 plus $1.50 for postage & handling.**
- **Available in August.**

Rifts World Book Five: Triax™ & The NGR™

An in depth look at the government, structure, technology and creations of **Triax** and the **New German Republic (NGR)**.

The New German Republic is a refuge for humans amidst a turbulent Europe seething with inhuman invaders. Triax is the high-tech industrial giant of the world. It works hand-in-hand with the NGR government, supplying mankind's defenders with the super weapons to fight the supernatural invaders that threaten all of Europe. Triax is responsible for the creation of the Ulti-Max, Dyna-Max (new) and a huge variety of incredible power armor, cyborgs, robots and war machines (all presented in this book).

Highlights Include:

- **Page after page of new cyborgs, robots, weapons, vehicles and power armor created by Kevin Long, including the "Dyna-Max" and other mind boggling designs.**
- **New Occupational Character Classes.**
- **Juicers, Crazies, strange augmentation and dark secrets.**
- **The New German Republic, their allies and enemies.**
- **The Gargoyle Empire, adventure and more.**
- **Written by Kevin Siembieda and Kevin Long.**
- **Cover and artwork by Kevin Long, with additional art by Newton Ewell and Kevin Siembieda.**
- **180+ pages; $19.95 — available late October.**

32 page Summer Catalog

The Megaverse® of Palladium Books® includes **Rifts**®, Heroes Unlimited™, Villains Unlimited™, Robotech™, Beyond the Supernatural™, Mystic China™, TMNT®, Macross II™, Palladium Fantasy RPG®, RECON®, T-shirts, miniatures and more, all described in our latest 32 page catalog; only 75 cents (postage and handling included).

Palladium Books®   12455 Universal Drive
Dept. D   Taylor, Mi. 48180

Available at hobby shops and comic stores everywhere!

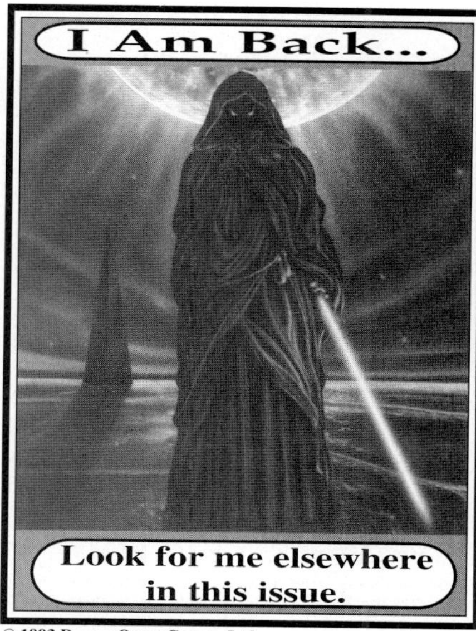

© 1993 Dream Quest Games, Ltd.

PLAY BY MAIL GAMING

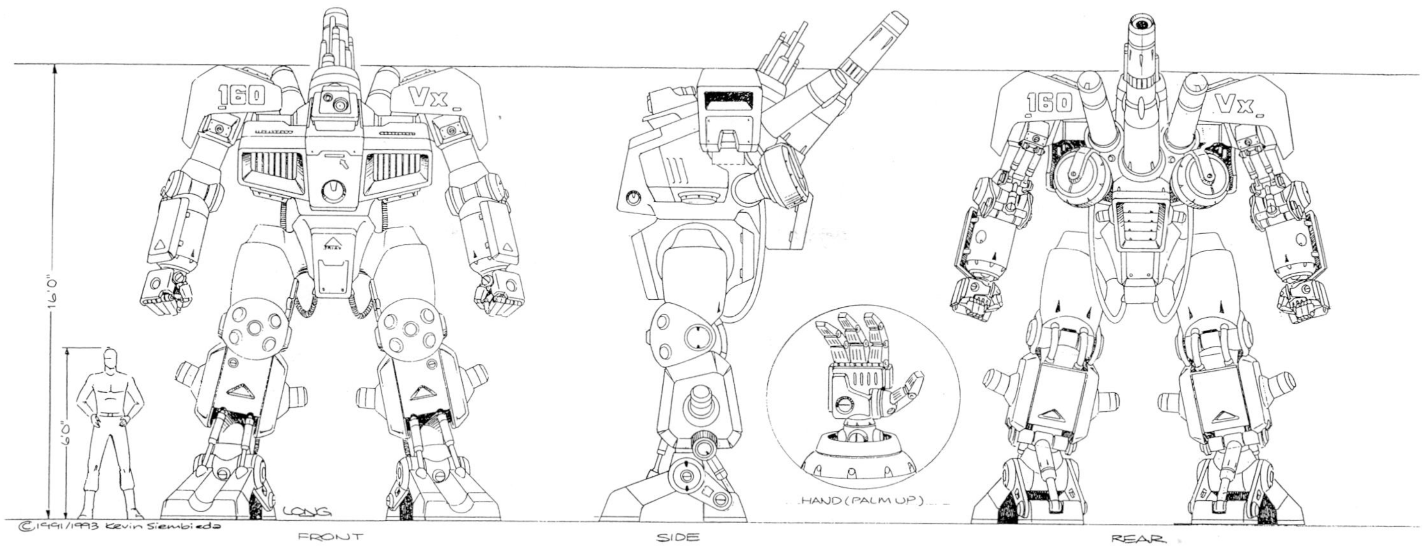

Palladium Books® Characters now available as Metal Miniatures

At last! **Palladium Books** presents its dynamic robots, cyborgs, dragons and characters in the three-dimensional splendor of metal miniatures!

Palladium has been quietly planning this for two years now and is finally ready to launch a complete line of non-lead, metal miniatures. All will be of the highest artistic and manufacturing quality we can muster.

Palladium Books will handle everything from the selection of characters to the assigning of sculptors, advertising, packaging, and marketing. **Rafm** has been selected as the manufacturer because of their quality and professionalism.

What you can expect

Unfortunately, we don't have any photographs available yet to show you what we have planned. The best we can do is show some of the front, side and back views created as reference guides for our sculptors.

Initial figures will be **Rifts** characters and, with time, will include just about every major player character, D-Bee, bot, cyborg, dragon, monster and villain in the series. **Other figures** will include characters and mecha from **Macross II** and we have several other plans up our sleeves, so keep an eye out for all our products.

Rifts® Miniatures
The First to be released

The following will be the items in the first series of releases, beginning in July or August of 1993.

- **The Glitter Boy and GB pilot:** Blister Pack: $7.95 (looks great).
- **Dog Pack:** Four different dog boys ready for action! $6.95
- **Xiticix & Black Faerie:** A dynamic xiticix warrior armed with a TK rifle, plus the maleficent black faerie. $6.95
- **Borgs Pack One:** Four different cyborgs, including the red borg. $7.95
- **Coalition Soldiers:** Four different soldiers, including grunts, and officer. Blister Pack: $6.95
- **CS SAMAS:** Two figures. $7.95
- **CS Sky-cycle and pilot:** Two figures (one seated & one standing) and cycle. $7.95
- **Skelebots:** Four different menacing CS robots. $6.95

Boxed Sets

- **Ulti-Max Boxed Set:** One of the most popular Triax power armor suits ever! Plus the Triax Terrain Hopper and Explorer body armor. Price and date of release not yet determined.
- **UAR-1 and CS troopers Boxed Set:** Price and date of release not yet determined.
- **Dragon Boxed Sets:** Specific dragons, price and date of release not yet determined (probably not before 1994).

Highlights Include:

- **No lead content! All of Palladium's miniatures are made of non-lead metal alloys.**
- **25 mm scale with figures ranging from one to seven inches tall for a real and consistent feeling of scale!**
- **Excellent quality and appearance.**
- **Produced, packaged and distributed by Palladium Books.**
- **Manufactured by Rafm.**
- **Average prices: $6.95 and $7.95 per blister pack.**
- **Available starting July or August 1993. Watch for them!**

NO LEAD! There has been a long, controversial debate regarding the potential dangers of lead and lead poisoning. The well being of our fans is too important to take chances with, so all of Palladium's miniatures are made of *non-lead* metal alloys. This may mean higher prices, but one can never put a price on health, safety or the preservation the environment. We hope to make up for the cost with quality, dynamic figures.

Warning: Metal miniatures should be kept out of the reach of small children. The figures are small items and/or may contain small parts that can be harmful if swallowed. Miniatures are recommended for people 10 years of age and older.

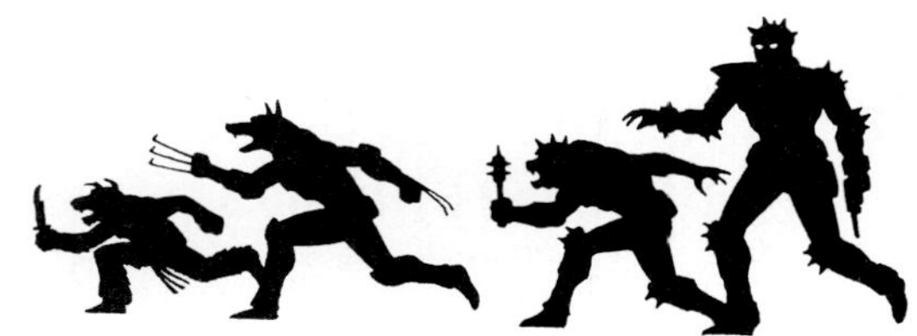

32 page Summer Catalog

The Megaverse® of Palladium Books® includes **Rifts**®, **Heroes Unlimited**™, **Villains Unlimited**™, **Robotech**™, **Beyond the Supernatural**™, **Mystic China**™, **TMNT**®, **Macross II**™, **The Lazlo Agency**™, **Compendium of Modern Weapons**™, **Palladium Fantasy RPG**®, **RECON**®, T-shirts, miniatures and more, all described in our latest 32 page catalog; only 75 cents (postage and handling included).

Palladium Books®   12455 Universal Drive
Dept. D   Taylor, Mi. 48180

Available at hobby shops and comic stores everywhere!

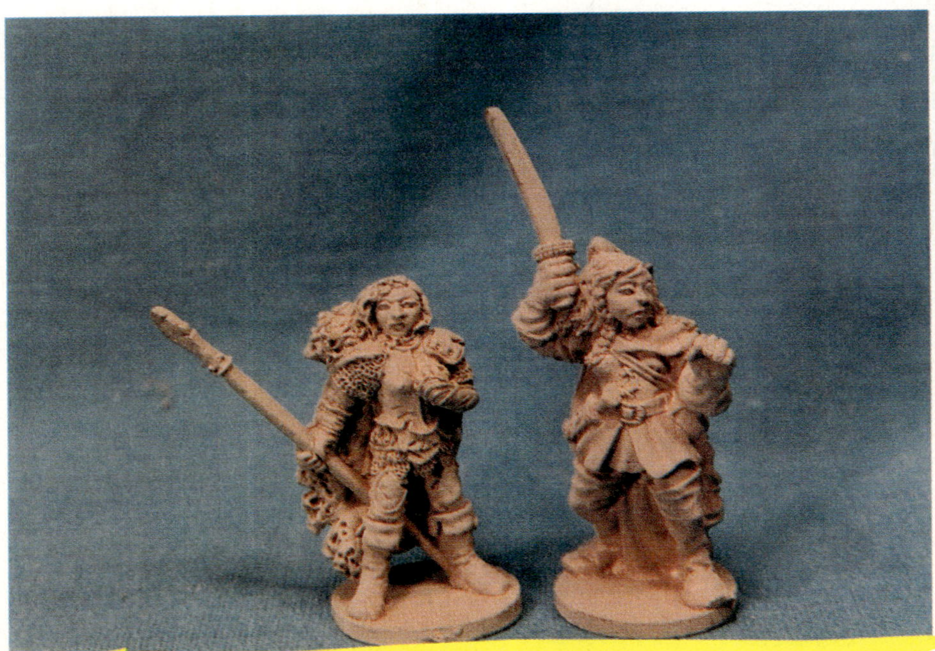
Female Fighters (Metal Magic)

Can lead be saved? It's all up to you!

©1993 by Robert Bigelow

Photographs by Mike Bethke

A small bright spot has appeared on the horizon for those of us who want inexpensive miniature armies. The courts found on close inspection that the research done by the New York Health Department, and the conclusions drawn from that research, were seriously flawed. This has led to the sidetracking from June to late fall of the New York bill prohibiting lead in miniatures. This also sidetracks similar bills in other states, since many of those bills were based on the information and studies passed on by New York. Most other states are now waiting for New York's final bill to be drafted before taking action.

This does not mean we can celebrate, however. Residents of New York should write polite and concise letters to their congressmen to explain that miniatures are collectibles and should be exempt from any lead-banning bills. Residents of other states should write to their congressmen as well, basing their concerns on the New York legislation, asking for a similar exemption for hobby materials. Point out that this ban affects not only our games but the model railroad and dollhouse hobbies as well, harming hobby shops and much of the rest of our industry. You must keep the pressure on; the outcry that reaches the legislators tells them how important the passage (or stopping) of a bill is to the people the congressmen represent.

Several people asked me to suggest ways to keep lead out of the environment if the owner of some lead figures decides to get out of gaming or if his parents (or spouse) decide to get rid of the figures. If you want or need to get rid of your figures, look for a nearby gamer or gaming club and donate your figures to that person or the club members. If you cannot find anyone to accept your figures, send your figures to me, using the address at the end of this article, and I will find a good home for them. We might be able to start a miniatures "pool" from which people can check out figures for gaming use.

I also want to thank the individuals who have responded to my requests for a player opponents' list and interconnecting-club set-up. The feedback has been very positive, and we are well on our way. If you have not sent in a note detailing your playing forces or gaming periods, please do so (this includes clubs as well as individuals). I want to assure everyone that this is going to be a noncommercial list that will be available to gamers and *not* to game companies for their mailing lists.

The bad news this month is that lead miniatures are undergoing a price increase, supposedly reflecting the growing cost of lead bought in bulk by these companies. I am not sure that this price increase is entirely due to bulk-lead prices, and I feel that most miniatures' companies should rethink their pricing structures. The hobby is getting too expensive, and the prices are scaring off prospective new gamers.

I apologize for the lack of dragon figures in this month's column. While at the GAMA show, I churned out more reviews than I had thought, and the overflow from May swamped this month's offerings. Now, on with the show.

Miniatures' product ratings	
*	Poor
**	Below average
***	Average
****	Above average
*****	Excellent

Metal Magic

c/o Wargames
P.O. Box 278, Rt. 40 East
Triadelphia WV 26059

Hobby Products

Postfach 10 10 20
4200 Oberhausen 1
GERMANY

C1006a Female Fighter with Spear *****

One of the most frequent complaints from my female customers is that all of the fighters must have been designed by men, as there seems to be few practical female fighters. Here, we present one from Metal Magic (we reviewed another last month; this issue has a picture of both last month's miniature and this one's).

This fighter is scaled to 25 mm and is a demure 23 mm tall to the eyes from the circular base. (The figure is made of lead, but the company has no plans to change the content until the laws have settled out.) Her pants are frayed and have holes in places, and a metal plate rides high on one thigh. A long-sleeved shirt is covered by a tattered chain-mail shirt. A leather jerkin covers a slight bust, and there is a protective plate on her left shoulder. Both hands and arms are covered by plates; her right hand grasps a long spear with a nicked point. Her upper body is covered by a tattered, fur-lined cloak. Her facial features are plain, and her lip is curled as if to protect it from the cold. Curly hair streams out in a breeze. This figure is highly recommended at $1.79.

RAFM Company, Inc.

20 Parkhill Rd. E.
Cambridge, Ontario
CANADA N1R IP2

3045 Dark Elves Spider Cavalry ****½

The possibilities of spider cavalry as "vertical assault troops" was mentioned when we reviewed the goblin spider cavalry from Grenadier. Unfortunately, morale and intelligence are not strong points for goblin soldiers. Now, RAFM has presented us with a perfect morale-enforcement unit, one with initiative and intelligence.

The package contains eight pieces that assemble into two spider-mounted troops. The figures are scaled to 25 mm and are made of lead, and are very flexible.

The four leg assemblies, each of which has four legs, fit into the slots on the side of each spider body. The spider has an armored head and body with a simple chair for the rider. The pincers are extended out and eyes are visible, although not faceted. The thorax is covered by well-done hair, with enough detail to withstand primer. The legs have some mild flash but are easy to clean. There was no flash, and mold lines needed only light

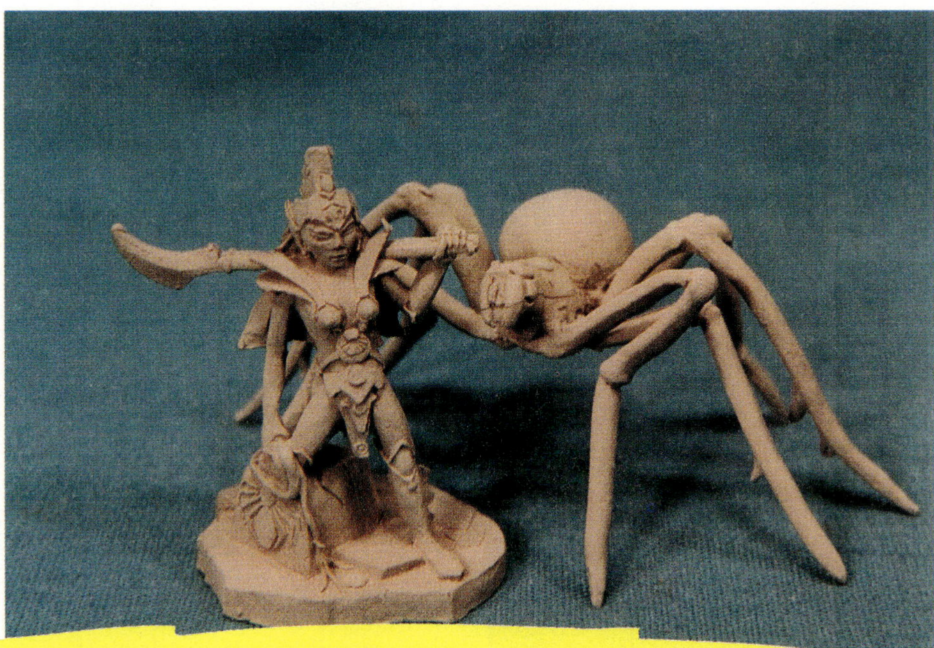

Dark Elf Queen Arachnia & Pet (RAFM Co.)

cleaning with a knife.

The rider's body consists of two parts. The lower part consists of knee-high boots in stirrups and pants. The body is divided at the wide belt. The body top fits into a depression in the lower body, but needed to be trimmed slightly as the holes looked like they had filled partially during casting. The warrior is dressed in chain mail covered by plate mail in front and a lighter armor in back. A neck decoration is the only ornate part of an otherwise functional outfit. The elf's high cheek-bones and stern face are topped by a Mohawk-style haircut that ends at the neck and frames the pointed ears. He is armed with a huge sword held at the ready, with only gloves softening the weight.

This is a well-done kit that requires patience to finish well. This kit is highly recommended, and I'll probably pick up about three more sets for my dark elves. The cost per pack is $4.50 (it may go higher after the metal changeover).

4001 Dark Elf Queen Arachnia & Pet ****

This 25-mm set consists of a nine-piece spider and a queen figure, made of lead. The spider is smooth skinned, with mouth, pincers, and even eyes well visible. The problem is that there are no instructions with this kit, and the eight separate legs will fit almost anywhere in the spider's body slots. The front legs have several bends, but also had cracks in each bend (the cracks were fixed by using drops of super glue). There was some flash, and care had to be taken to remove it and not the sensory organs on the legs. Mold lines are present but easily cleaned.

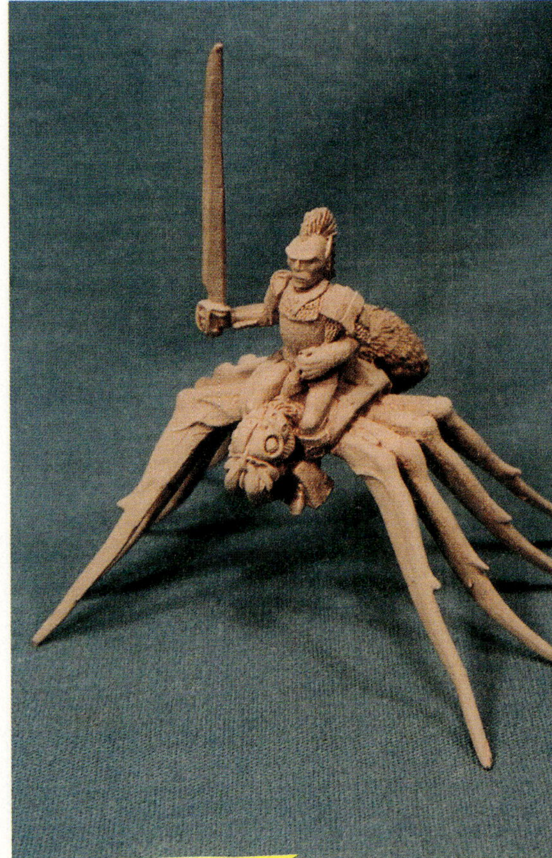

Dark Elves Spider Cavalry (RAFM Co.)

The queen is dressed in knee-high spiked boots, with the rest of her body being covered by a brassiere, an ornate loincloth, and shoulder plates, all linked together with a thin strand of chain. Her back is covered by a short cape that is

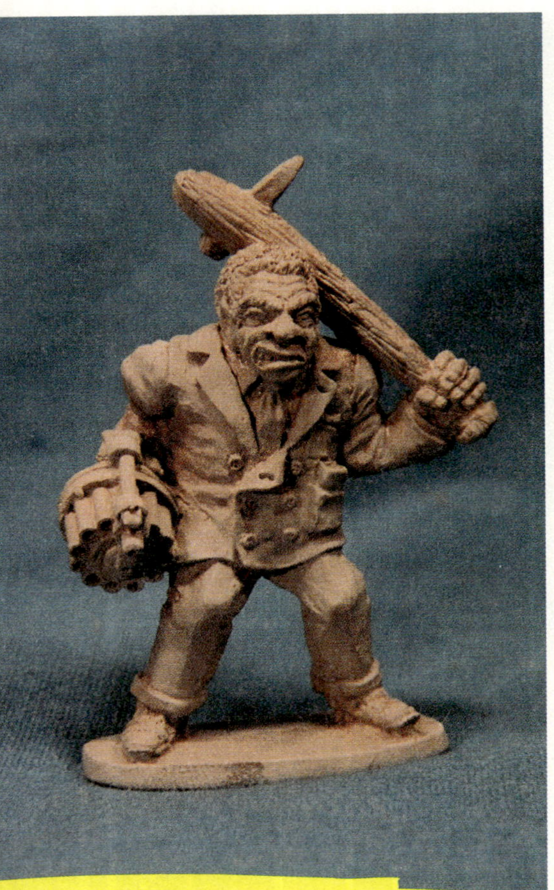

Giant Bruiser (Lance and Laser Models)

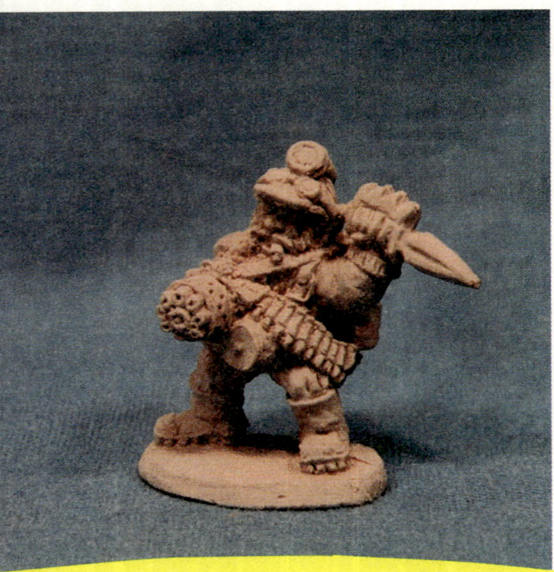

Dwarf Tunnel Fighter (Lance and Laser Models

realistically wrinkled. She is half-kneeling on a block with a bas-relief spider. Her straight, shoulder-length hair is capped by a headdress with a spider insignia and a high crest. Her face is cruel, and she is armed with a hooked bill and a whip. The limbs are slightly out of proportion, but not glaringly so. With no mold marks or flash, the queen lives up to her name. This kit is recommended, but you will probably need only one queen. The price is $5.

Lance and Laser Models Inc.

P.O. Box 14491
Columbus OH 43214

TORG 017 Giant Bruiser ★★★★

The giant bruiser is a modern-genre, 25-mm scale lead figure on an oval, flat base. The figure stands 34.5 mm high, which puts it at just under 9' tall. He is dressed is a double-breasted suit with slight leg cuffs, shirt, tie, and what look like cowboy boots. The suit buttons have holes, and a couple look like they are threaded. A rolled paper sticks out of the bottom left pocket. Buttons are on both sleeves, and the figure is molded so as to have creases in the pants. He is armed with a spiked, wooden club in his left hand and a grenade launcher with a long rotary magazine in his right. His hair is tightly curled, and his facial expression is a toothy sneer. The eyes are nicely done and the facial wrinkles are a nice touch, but the ears came out different sizes.

This is a very good figure for use with everything from West End Games's TORG* system to FASA's SHADOWRUN* game. The figure is menacing and makes a good enforcer. The only problem is that the detail seems to be superficial. Careful cleaning of the figure and a good paint job will fix this. It is recommended at $3.50 each.

TORG 014 Dwarf Tunnel Fighter ★★★½

This is a 25-mm scale lead figure on an undetailed oval base. The figure stands about 18 mm tall and is dressed like a miner with a serious attitude problem. He wears a jump suit with knee-high cleated boots. Most of his upper torso is covered by a huge minigun, complete with motor, that he holds in his right hand. Detail is fair, but the holes are more oblong than round on the barrels. His left hand is covered by a glove and a wrist device, but also grasps a combat knife complete with knuckle guards. On his head is a construction worker's hard hat with a mounted light and goggles; on his back is a large pack with an ammo belt that snakes its way around to the front of the figure to the gun.

The face is poorly executed. Basic details such as eyes are indistinct, and the left side of the face seems to be almost blurred. There is a cigar in his mouth, but teeth are not visible. Even the expected large dwarven nose is lost.

This is another figure that needs careful attention and can be redeemed by a careful paint job and a sharp, pointed blade. This type of figure is not available for the sci-fi genre anywhere else, and it would provide a unique addition to any SHADOWRUN*, TORG*, or CYBERPUNK 2020* world. The cost is $1.50 each.

Fortress Figures

P.O. Box 66
Jonesboro IN 46938

WW201 Infestor Pod ★★★★

The infestor pod is scaled for 25 mm and represents a possible horror for your dungeon stompers. The figure is 20 mm high by 17 mm with a sprawling base. The pod is horizontally ribbed with a group of interjoined sections. Tubular growths like plants or vines grow along the sides towards the opening on the top. The sack-like top emits large drops of a viscous solution that run down the sides of the pod to the sprawling base. It costs only $1.50.

XL26 Ooze Creature ★★★★

Scaled for 25 mm, this figure could be a real shock at underground pools, lava flows, or surface swamps. The figure is mounted on a 23-mm circular base that lends itself well to modeling fluid or substances. This figure is a simple mix of slimy, dripping substances that has formed a troll-like face with pointy teeth. It has runny, oozing hands and the consistency and appearance of an often-used candle.

The figure has the advantage of being almost universally useful in any game system as everything from mutated chemicals to elementals. It's worth the $2.50 price tag.

Ral Partha Enterprises

5938 Carthage Ct.
Cincinnati OH 45212-1197

Minifigs

1/5 Graham Rd., Southampton
UNITED KINGDOM S02 0AX

02-162 Dwarf Flamethrower ★★★★★

This 25-mm scale, lead weapon set contains 12 different parts that form a wheeled platform-mounted flamethrower. Its finished dimensions, not including crew, are 40 mm × 67 mm × 31 mm high. The wheels are molded to look like they are made from heavy planks trimmed by a wide metal band and secured by strip metal and nails. The axle on the outside appears to be secured by a spike and joins the wooden pegs easily, though the hole is a bit large. The bed is a box frame supported by three braces and a huge front spur with bolted spikes. A plank deck is nailed to the frame, as is a push handle frame. The front shield is made out of planks held together by metal strips and exhibiting a number of front pointing spikes. The fuel tank is glued to the second and third boards and consists of a metal drum with a handle-locking side door and a lock-down top. Bands with double rows of rivets join the planks. The flame dispenser is a metal pipe that extends from the tank through the shield, ending in a dragon head with a nicely done hole in the mouth and good teeth and board detail. The last part of the piece is an air pump, with plunger-type compression and a pipe going to the tank. Both pieces have female ends, so carefully secure the piece. This pump is part of a crew casting.

Two of the dwarven crew are assigned the unenviable task of pushing the cart. The two are identically cast, with hands set to push a bar. They wear loose, unarmored clothes and loin guards. They are armed with sheathed short swords. Facial expressions reveal looks of exertion; you can almost see sweat drip into their beards. Their heads are covered with hoods. There was some flash on the circular textured base, but this was easily cleaned. As a note, you might wish to trim the bases down, as both figures are only partially protected by a shield.

The pump operator wears an ankle-length great coat with a wide sash belt. His hands are gloved, and his upper back is protected by studded leather. A large fur cap and a short sword complete the adornments on this figure. His face is thin, with a long nose and gaunt cheeks, and he has his mouth open as if puffing from exertion.

The crew chief is holding a long pole with the flaming brand used to ignite the weapon. He wears a full set of chain mail covered by a great coat and cape, with gloves on his hands. A map pouch hangs from his belt. His face is thinner than expected, and he is squinting while staring ahead. His head is covered by a pill-box-type cap with a band and a skull on the front. All clothes and the brand are molded as though there is a wind.

This would be a perfect support weapon for the Iron Lords Orc Foes set, with the dragon totem held by their cleric/shaman. This is recommended at $9.95 per set.

54-473 Crossbowmen   ****½

This set of 25-mm scaled figures consists of three different castings for a total of six figures. The figures are all mounted on circular bases that are nontextured and come from the Conquistador line. The height is slightly shorter than for standard adventurers, but this is hardly noticeable.

The first set consists of two figures wearing slipper-type boots and tights known from conquistador times. Each wears a regular shirt with a drawstring closure and puffed shoulders and elbows, and a set of knee-length trousers with

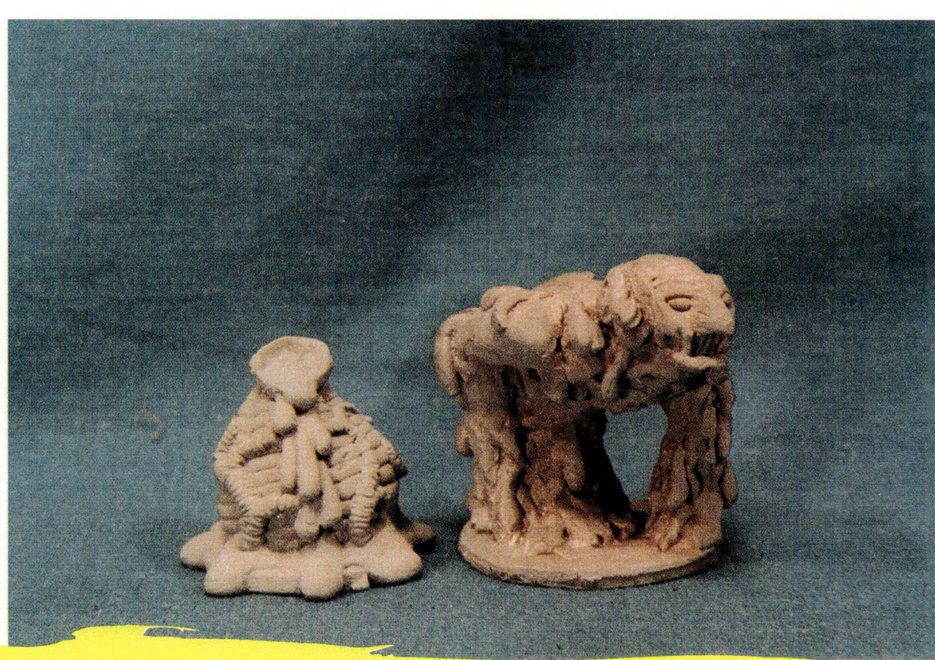

Infestor Pod and Ooze Creature (Fortress Figures)

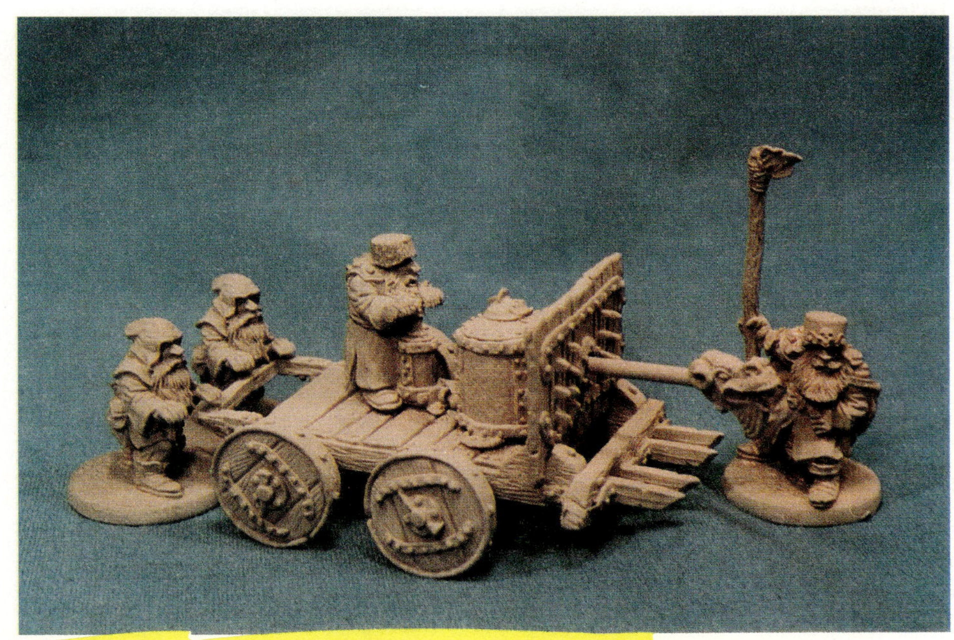

Dwarf Flamethrower (Ral Partha Enterprises)

puffed cuffs; this uniform has no armor value. Each wears a soft hat with a feather. The hands are uncovered; the left hand holds a crossbow and the right is drawing a bolt from a weapon pouch. A sword with hand guard hangs at the left hip. Each face is serious and has a neatly trimmed beard and moustache. These figures would make excellent merchant militiamen for a town, or a defensive unit for field marches. There was no flash on these figures, but the legs looked very

angular.

The second group consists of two figures with crossbows at the ready. They are dressed in knee-high boots with fold-over tops. The previously seen type of knee-length pants with puffed upper thighs and knees adorn their legs. Shirts with long sleeves and padded, sleeveless vests cover their upper torsos. A scarf is tied around their throats, and their heads are covered by a Spanish-type helmet. Curly hair is visible, and facial hair is

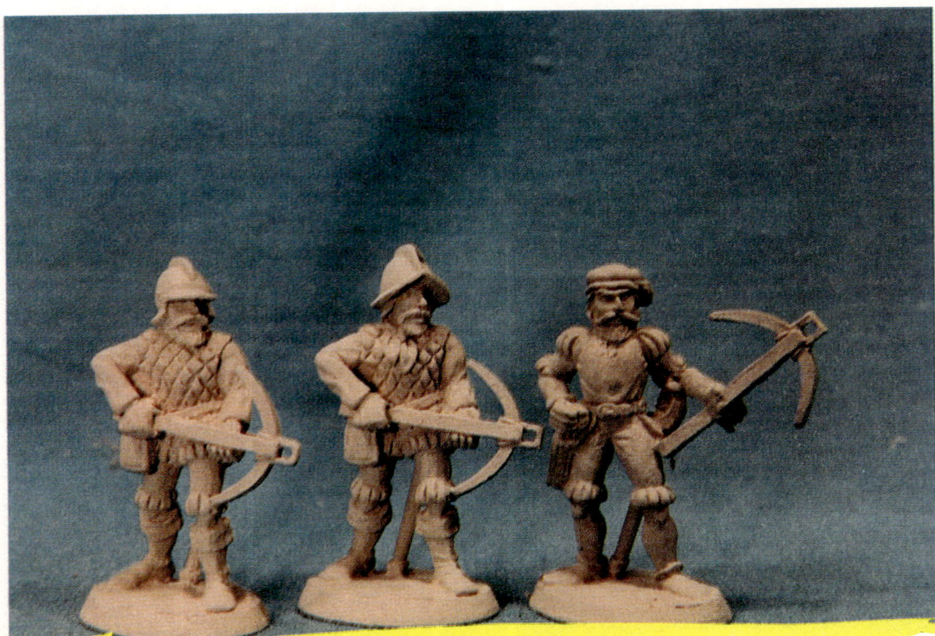

Crossbowmen (Ral Partha Enerprises)

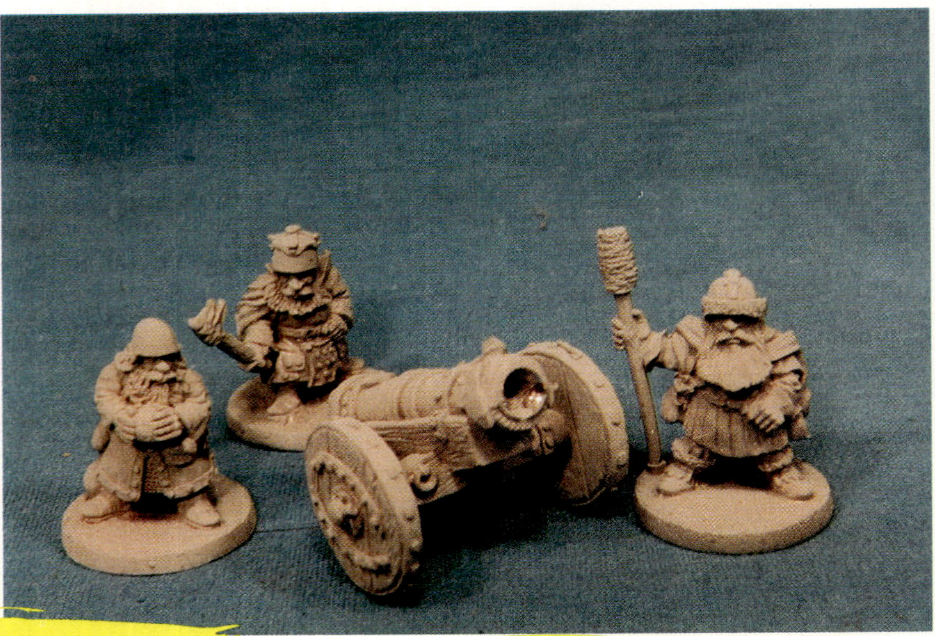

Dwarf Bombard (Ral Partha Enterprises)

body and a cross timber with plate and axles bolted on both ends. The actual barrel fits in a notched section of the timber and is held down by iron straps and large bolts, while the cannon barrel has reinforcement bands. This barrel also has a Mr. Yuk-type goblin face in bas-relief on the upper side of the cannon muzzle.

The leader wears a heavy leather coat over chain mail. The coat has long sleeves and a studded hem on the bottom. The figure clutches a cannonball in both hands, with another at his feet. A pouch, water bottle, and short sword hang from a wide belt supported by a shoulder strap. The helmet protects a face that is not as detailed as it could be, though it has a long beard and a moustache. The helmet even has an extension to keep burning cinders from reaching his skin.

The swabber holds his swab in his right gauntleted hand while he waits his turn. His feet are protected by fur-topped boots, and his upper body is covered by a joined strip leather suit cinched by a simple belt and buckle. No sword is visible, but there is a pouch. A cape falls to his knees. His head is covered by a fringed helmet. A long beard falls and curls at the stomach line, as a look of concentration fills his face. There was little flash or mold line problems except on the base and feet.

The gun captain holds a flaming brand in his right hand while his left is tucked in his belt. The figure wears full-length armor with studs on the lower half and a long-sleeve undershirt. His back is also covered by an oddly cut fringed cape with hood. His facial expression is pure acid and glare, and his beard bristles slightly. The high helmet is topped by crossed straps.

With the rising number of powder-based miniatures, this is almost a must. With the detail, it is almost worth the $6.95 price tag. Don't surround it with troops, in case the gun explodes.

54-471 Sword & Bucklermen   *****½

This six-figure set is composed of three different types of 25-mm lead figures. All have slightly oval, nontextured bases, all wear burgonet-type helmets, and all have neatly trimmed if slightly varying beards. Little or no flash is present, but there are some mold lines that require work.

Each figure in casting set #1 is of a man wearing a mid-thigh-length chain-mail shirt overlaid with padded leather. He wears boots, but the left one is slightly armored and comes to mid-thigh, while the right folds over beneath the knee. Gauntlets guard both hands; a sword is in his right hand while a notched shield with wrist straps and wide forearm straps is on his left arm. The shield has a huge bas-relief of a bar that would be about 6" thick in real life. The sword blade is triangular, and the dwarf's face is set but lacking fine detail. His beard is almost a van Dyke in style.

neatly trimmed to pointed beards and moustaches. The faces are well detailed and determined. Each is armed as before with sword and bolt.

The last castings are identical in positioning to figure style #2 but have full beards, true burgonet helmets, and heads set more to the left. Both groups #2 and #3 share the angular leg problem of #1, but to a lesser degree.

These figures would make an excellent addition to the sets of those who play in the Maztica setting for the AD&D® game,

enjoy gaming in the early colonial period of history, or are looking for excellent town guards or medium troops. The set is well recommended at $5.75 per pack.

02-161 Dwarf Bombard   *****

This set is made of lead and consists of six parts scaled to 25 mm. The wheels for the cannon are banded planks, joined with rivets and reinforced by metal strips. The hub has a pin/spike retainer that is easily seen, with well-done wood grain. The gun consists of a huge timber main

Each man in casting set #2 has knee-high boots that end with puffed-out edges. He wears pantaloons with tight behind and a puffy-shoulder, long-sleeve shirt. He is protected in the front and back by plate to the waist and in front by overlapping plate to the thigh. A long sword is in his right hand, and a dagger is in his left (his left also holds a round shield by its straps). The shield has a spoke design engraved on the front. This figure's face has slightly more detail and expression than type #1's, and the beard is groomed to a point. The posing is good, and there are no angular surfaces that shouldn't be present except for a spot on one leg.

The figures in the last pair have shoes, pantaloon pants, and tights from mid-thigh down. Each man's upper body has ornately done studded plate with buckle and leather connecting straps, with a separation from waist down for easy movement. The back is protected by plate, while buttocks and upper arms are protected by overlapping leather strips. A round wheel-embossed shield is on his left arm, while in his right hand he holds a long sword. The face is well detailed, and the expression is stern.

These figures are good not only for the AD&D Maztica setting but also as outstanding town militia and police. They well worth their $5.75 price tag.

Grenadier Models

P.O. Box 305
Springfield PA 19064

Grenadier Models UK Ltd.

25 Babage Rd.
Deeside, Clwyd, Wales
UNITED KINGDOM CH5 2QB

3112 Armored Centaurs   *****

Centaur cavalry gives you the best of two worlds, speed and power, as well as the intelligence to use them. These centaurs from Grenadier give you a start on a medium or heavy "cavalry" unit. The figures are scaled for 25 mm and are currently made of lead, but that will change shortly as Grenadier adopts a new metal for its miniatures. Both figures are mounted on slightly textured oval bases with a hint of a mold line that is easily removed. Both centaurs measure 35 mm to the top of the head and are 26 mm long, the size of a small or medium horse (I imagine the heavy cavalry figure should have been bigger).

The medium unit would be equivalent to a man-at-arms in regular fighting units. His body is covered by a hemmed blanket on which rests a chain-mail suit. The suit stretches from chin to just short of the flanks, including shoulders and arms, and is secured by a strap and buckle. His chest is covered by a breastplate with angular shaping and back straps and buckles, and

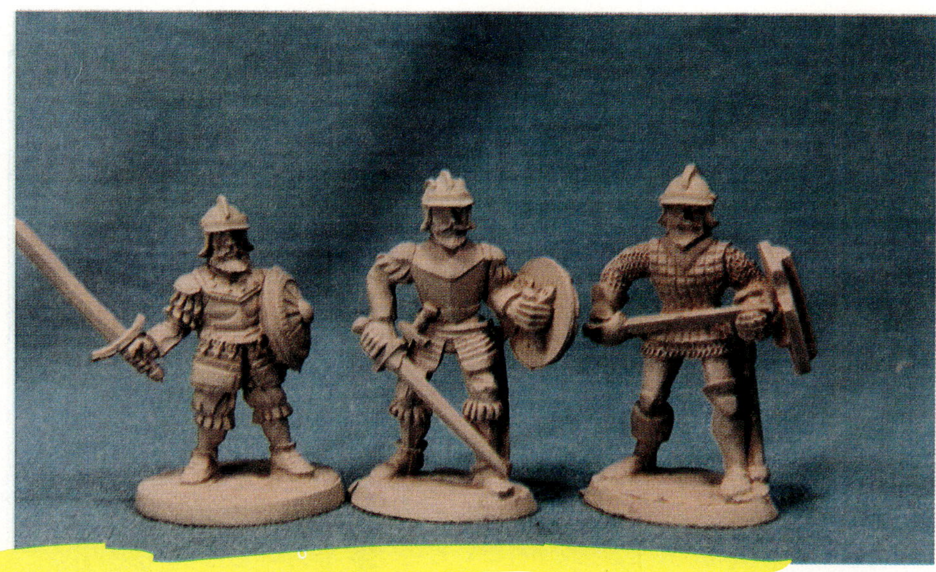

Sword & Bucklermen (Ral Partha Enterprises)

his back is covered by an additional padded piece with quilt embroidering. The horse-body detail is very good, with smooth muscle groups and a nicely done tail. Remember to clip the extra lead sprue from the front left hoof. The human part has good features, with long hair falling to shoulder length. The figure has a sheathed sword on his belt. His gloved hands hold a spear in the throwing position and an embossed round shield with a dragon. There is a small nick in the shield, but otherwise it is an excellent figure.

The heavy knight has overlapping plates

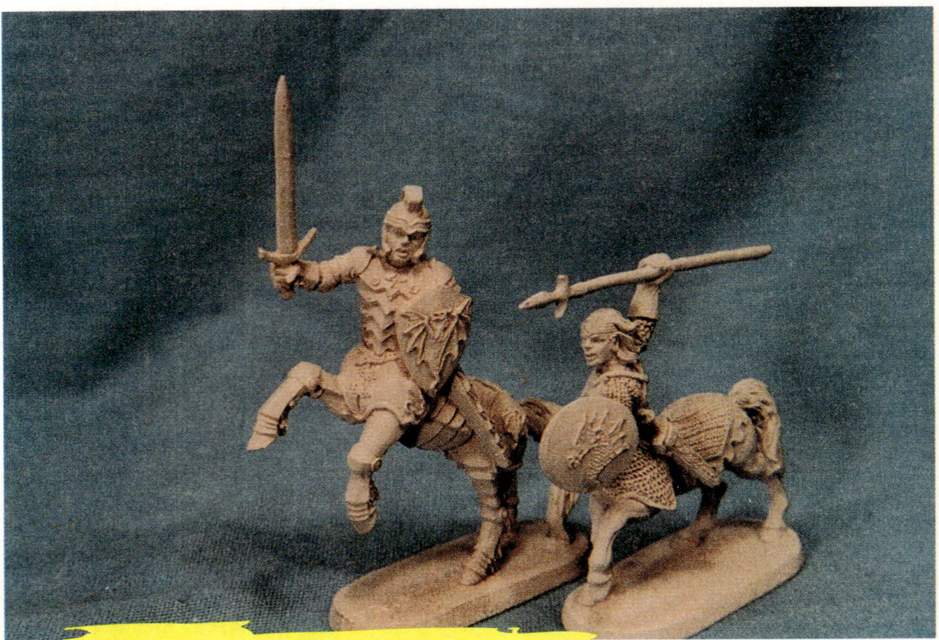

Armored Centaurs (Grenadier Models)

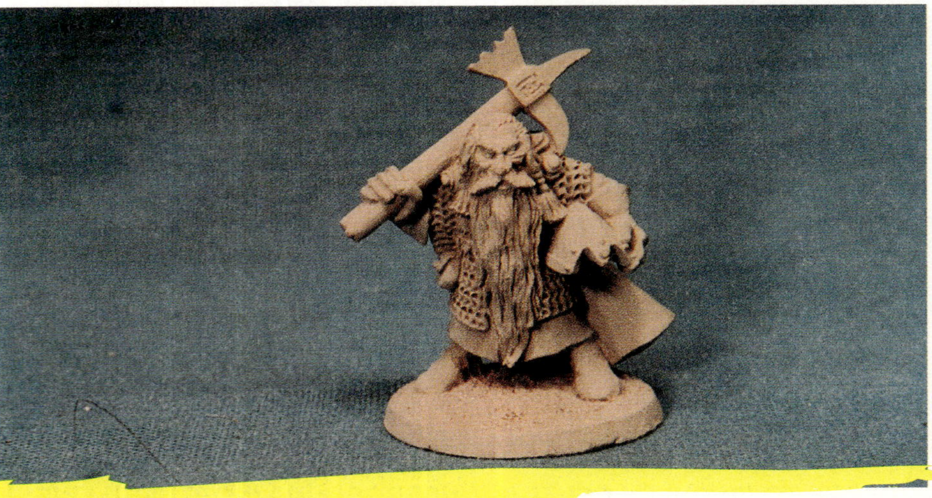

Dwarf Warchief (Grenadier Models)

his ankles, and bushy eyebrows frame a heavy brow and eyes. A look of intense concentration is on his face.

This figure has now become an officer in charge of my heavy support units. It is highly recommended at $1.75, but any single figure will be pricey at the new $2.25 level that will appear when Grenadier starts using its new metal soon.

3403 Cyberpunk Rockers ***½

This package contains three different music-related figures all scaled for 25 mm. The lead figures all come mounted on undetailed oval bases with minimal mold lines visible. All three figures are of young people of different heights.

Figure #1 is of a young lady posed as if singing in concert. At 27 mm she is taller than her companions. She is dressed in high, high-heel boots with fold-over tops, a miniskirt, and an open blouse with a halter and puffy sleeves. Her left hand is out, and the right holds a wireless mike. Her hair is well done and short, and the facial detail including teeth is very good. As a final touch, large hoop earrings dangle from her ears. There was no flash and only one troublesome mold line.

Figure #2 is a guitar accompanist who wears high cowboy boots and probably blue jeans. His upper torso is covered by a V-necked undershirt and an open shirt with the sleeves rolled up. Good facial features portray a certain seriousness on a face framed by shoulder-length hair. His left hand firmly grasps the neck of an electric guitar with three knobs; the right hand is ready to strike a chord. There was flash between the body and the guitar, but it could almost be removed by a pencil.

The last figure is a male dressed in high boots, a smooth shirt, and a great coat edged with embroidery. Standing 26 mm, he is posed in the classic nonmilitary shooter's pose with an automatic pistol in his left hand. A very well done guitar with crisper detail than the other figure's is strapped to his back, neck up. Facial features are set in a serious manner as he lines up his shot, and his hair is styled and wavy.

Only one of these figures (the armed one) has potential value as a player character for a cyberpunk-style near-future game, while the other two are good diorama or background pieces. The figures are nice even at $5.95 per pack.

5622 Fightingman Marksman ****½

This 28-mm lead figure with an oval base could easily be used as one of Robin Hood's men. Long boots and tights clothe his legs, and a jerkin covers a long-sleeve shirt. He has just released an arrow from the bow in his left hand. On his back is a quiver of arrows; a long sword and a pouch hang from his belt. Facial features are smooth and not highly detailed, and only a small beard breaks the symmetry.

covering his entire body from shoulders to the top of his hooves. Large formed plates with embossed dragons cover the rear flanks, front legs, horse's chest, and upper part of the human chest. These plates are secured to other plates by detailed belts, straps, and buckles. Both arms are covered in overlapping plates that end in gloves. The major joints also have rivets. The left arm has a kite shield with a dragon, while his right hand holds the sword he drew from the sheath and thrusts into the air. The human face has a look almost of surprise and is framed by a Corinthian-type helmet. Even the stomach is covered. Rearing up, the figure projects a feeling of power. Even the tail is large.

I'm going to be broke shortly, as I need at least eight of this figure set. It's highly recommended at $6.99 per pack.

5620 Dwarf Warchief *****

This lead figure is scaled to the larger 28-mm lines, although with its height of 20 mm it could be used with 25-mm figures. The figure has a slightly off-round base textured to resemble short grass. His base garment is an ankle-length robe covered by a long sleeveless chain coat. Heavy gauntlets protect his hands; he holds his helmet in his left hand and a bearded war axe in his right. His helmet could be deeper but is nice in its simplicity. His head is bare. Long hair, including braided sections, falls to mid-back. A full mustache complements a beard that drops to

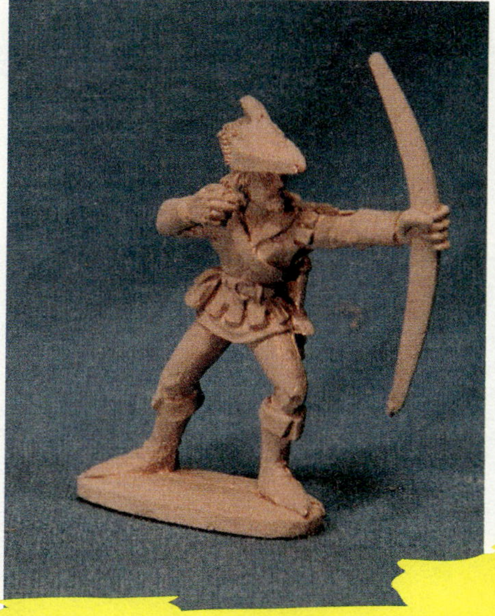
Fightingman Marksman (Grenadier Models)

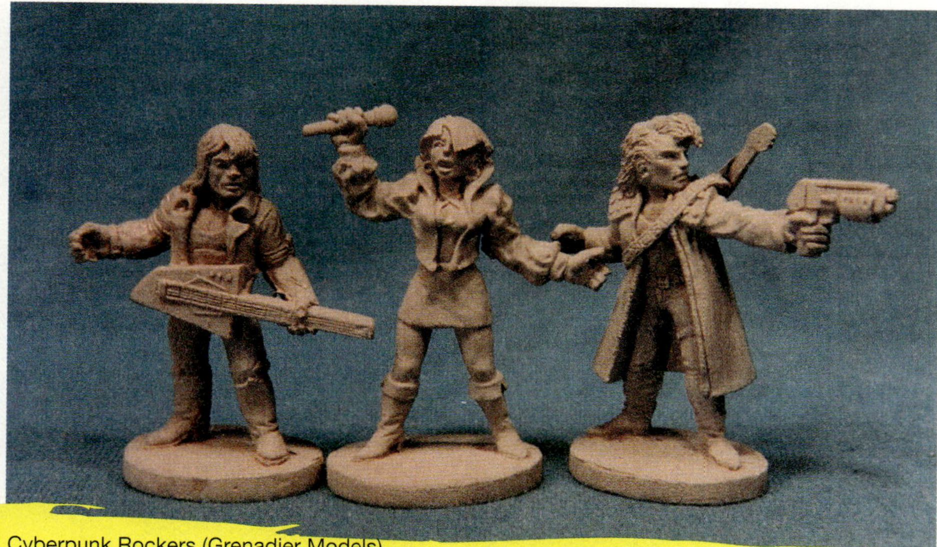
Cyberpunk Rockers (Grenadier Models)

The hat has a feather in it.

This figure looks really nice with a little work. Remember to carefully cut away the sprue connecting the bottom of the bow to the base, as twisting it off may break the bow. This figure is recommended at $1.75 each.

If you wish to reach me, I would prefer to have you call me unless you have information for the gaming opponents' list. My number is (708) 336-0790, and I am available MWThF from 2-10 P.M. If you want to write, the address is: Robert Bigelow, c/o Friends' Hobby Shop, 1411 Washington St., Waukegan IL 60085.   Ω

* indicates a product produced by a company other than TSR, Inc. Most product names are trademrks owned by the companies publishing those products. The use of the name of any product without mention of its trademark status should not be construed as a challenge to such status.

RAL PARTHA

NEW RELEASES

Advanced Dungeons & Dragons® 2nd Edition
MINIATURES

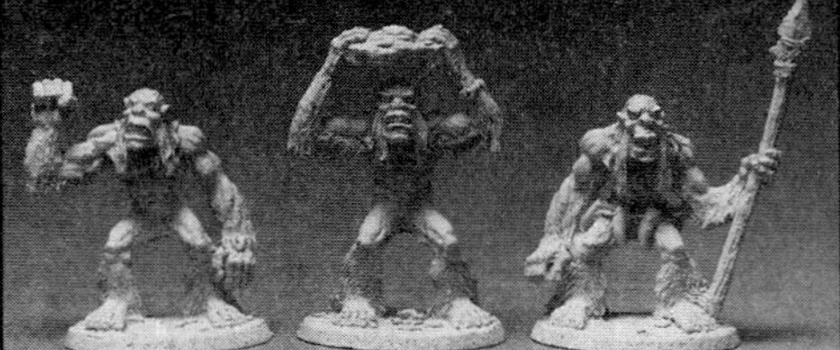

11-468 Taers

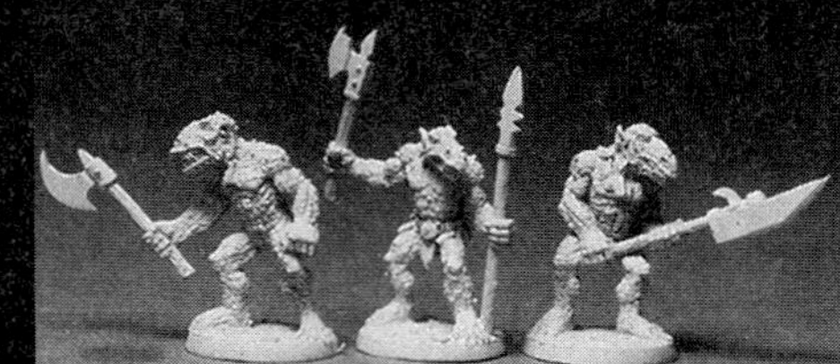

11-469 Sligs

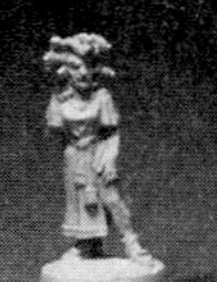

11-470 Medusa

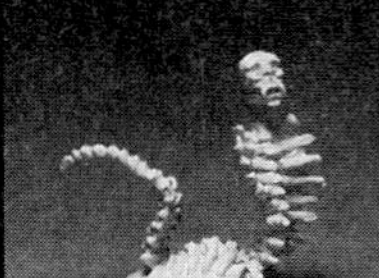

11-471 Necrophidius

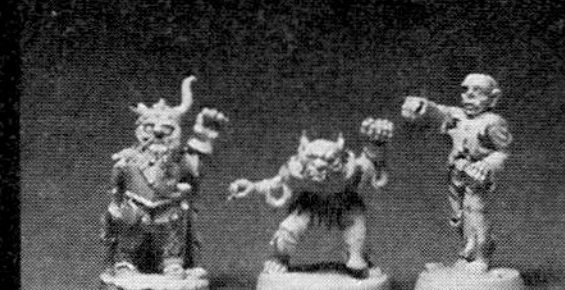

11-472 Zombies

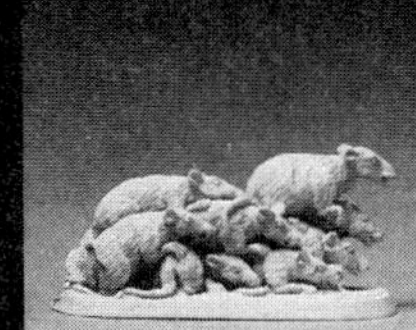

11-473 Giant Rat Stand

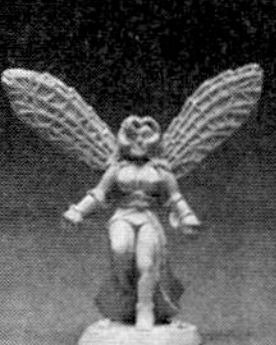

11-474 Sylph

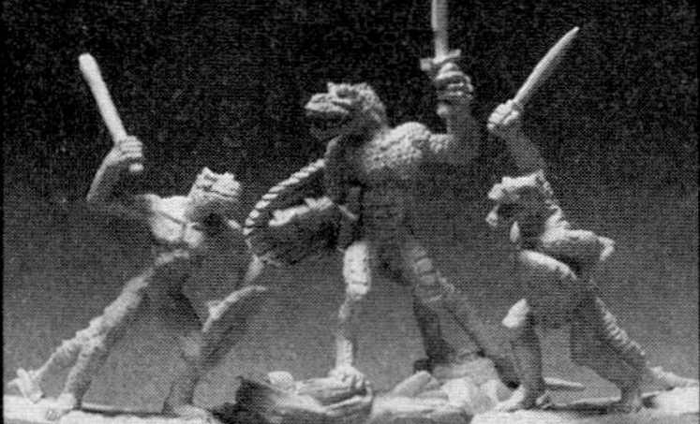

11-475 Lizardmen

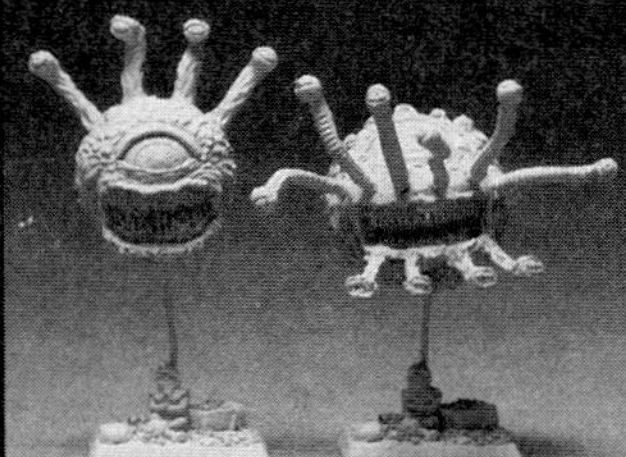

11-476 Beholder Kin

Code	Item	Price	Code	Item	Price	Code	Item	Price
11-442	Giant Toad	4.25	11-454	Efreet & Jann	8.50	11-466	Blink Dogs (2)	4.25
11-443	Sahuagin (4)	6.50	11-455	Gorgon	5.50	11-467	Minotaur	4.25
11-444	Troglodytes (3)	6.50	11-456	Mimics (3)	6.50	11-468	Taers (3)	6.50
11-445	Griffon	5.95	11-457	Orgs (3)	7.50	11-469	Sligs (3)	6.50
11-446	Hobgoblins (3)	6.50	11-458	Dragonne	5.95	11-470	Medusa	2.15
11-447	Fire Minion	4.25	11-459	Skrag (Sea Troll)	4.75	11-471	Necrophidius	2.15
11-448	Gnomes (5)	6.50	11-460	Mites (6)	6.95	11-472	Zombies (Orc, Human, and Dwarf)	5.50
11-449	Wyvern	9.75	11-461	Lamasu	5.95	11-473	Giant Rat Stand (2)	5.25
11-450	Beastmen (4)	6.50	11-462	Lamia	2.95	11-474	Sylph	2.15
11-451	Satyr	2.15	11-463	Ketch (3)	6.50	11-475	Lizardmen (3)	6.50
11-452	Giant Scorpion	5.50	11-464	Naga	2.15	11-476	Beholder Kin(2)	7.50
11-453	Cyclops-Kin (3)	6.50	11-465	Bonesnapper	4.25			

CONTAINS RALIDIUM™
RALIDIUM IS RAL PARTHA'S NEW LEAD FREE ALLOY.
CAUTION: FOR AGES 5 & UP. NOT SUITABLE FOR CHILDREN WHO STILL PUT OBJECTS IN THEIR MOUTH. CONTAINS SMALL PARTS.

RAL PARTHA MINIATURES ARE ALSO AVAILABLE FROM.

UNITED KINGDOM: MINIFIGS-- 1/5 GRAHAM ROAD, SOUTHAMPTON, ENGLAND. SO2 OAX

CANADA: RAFM-- 20 PARK HILL ROAD EAST. CAMBRIDGE, ONTARIO, CANADA N1R1P2

FRANCE: JEAUX DESCARTES-- 1, RUE DU COLONEL PIERRE AVIA, PARIS CEDEX 15, 75503 FRANCE

TO ORDER OUR COMPLETE CATALOG, CALL TOLL FREE, MONDAY THRU FRIDAY, 8:30 TO 5:00 EST, at 1(800) 543-0272 OR SEND $4.00 TO:

RAL PARTHA ENTERPRISES, INC.
5938 CARTHAGE COURT, CINCINNATI, OH 45212-1197

PHONE: (513) 631-7335

FAX: (513) 631-0028

VISA, MASTERCARD AND DISCOVER ACCEPTED